A CLINICAL GUIDE FOR CONTRACEPTION

FOURTH EDITION

A CLINICAL GUIDE FOR CONTRACEPTION

FOURTH EDITION

Leon Speroff, M.D.
Professor of Obstetrics and Gynecology
Oregon Health & Science University
Portland, Oregon

Philip D. Darney, M.D., M.Sc.
Professor and Chief
Obstetrics, Gynecology and Reproductive Sciences
San Francisco General Hospital
University of California, San Francisco
San Francisco, California

Illustration by Becky Slemmons and Daniyel Hicks
Page Design by Daniyel Hicks
Portland, Oregon

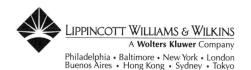

LIPPINCOTT WILLIAMS & WILKINS
A **Wolters Kluwer** Company
Philadelphia • Baltimore • New York • London
Buenos Aires • Hong Kong • Sydney • Tokyo

Acquisition Editor: Anne M. Sydor
Managing Editor: Nicole Dernoski
Production Manager: Fran Gunning
Manufacturing Manager: Ben Rivera
Marketing Manager: Kathy Neely
Design Coordinator: Holly McLaughlin
Production Services: Nesbitt Graphics, Inc.
Printer: R.R. Donnelley, Crawfordsville

© 2005 by LIPPINCOTT WILLIAMS & WILKINS
530 Walnut Street
Philadelphia, PA 19106 USA
LWW.com

Printed in the USA

Library of Congress Cataloging-in-Publication Data
Speroff, Leon, 1935–
   A clinical guide for contraception / Leon Speroff, Philip D. Darney ;
illustration by Becky Slemmons and Daniyel Hicks.—4th ed.
      p. ; cm.
   Includes bibliographical references and index.
   ISBN 0-7817-6488-2
   1. Contraception. I. Darney, Philip D. II. Title. [DNLM: 1.
Contraception—methods. WP 630 S749c 2006]
RG136.S63 2006
613.9'4—dc22

                                        2005045188

Care has been taken to confirm the accuracy of the information presented and to describe generally accepted practices. However, the authors, editors, and publisher are not responsible for errors or omissions or for any consequences from application of the information in this book and make no warranty, expressed or implied, with respect to the currency, completeness, or accuracy of the contents of the publication. Application of this information in a particular situation remains the professional responsibility of the practitioner.

The authors, editors, and publisher have exerted every effort to ensure that drug selection and dosage set forth in this text are in accordance with current recommen-dations and practice at the time of publication. However, in view of ongoing research, changes in government regulations, and the constant flow of information relating to drug therapy and drug reactions, the reader is urged to check the package insert for each drug for any change in indications and dosage and for added warnings and precautions. This is particularly important when the recommended agent is a new or infrequently employed drug.

Some drugs and medical devices presented in this publication have Food and Drug Administration (FDA) clearance for limited use in restricted research settings. It is the responsibility of the health care provider to ascertain the FDA status of each drug or device planned for use in their clinical practice.

10 9 8 7 6 5 4 3 2 1

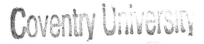

Dedication

This book is dedicated to our children, one son, seven daughters, and three grandchildren. As Sherlock Holmes said: "You know my methods, use them!"

Contents

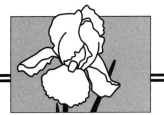

Preface

Contraception, socially recognized and accepted only in the last 30 years, is both an essential and a complicated part of modern life. Contraception has separated sex from procreation and has provided couples greater control and enjoyment of their lives. It is a critical element in limiting population, thus preserving our planet's resources and maintaining quality of life for ourselves and our children. Contraception is both a personal and a social responsibility.

The above accomplishments could not be achieved by the simple contraceptive methods employed before the late 20th century. Greater effectiveness and ease of use required more complicated methods, associated with greater consequences to our health. Intensive study of these issues has yielded an enormous wealth of information, making an informed choice possible but not easy.

In this book, we have distilled and formulated the information essential for the intelligent use of contraception. The current state of knowledge and variety of contraceptive options allow clinicians and patients to select methods best suited to an individual's personal, social, and medical characteristics and requirements. But even now science is still sometimes inadequate, and medical judgments must be made without the comfort of scientific support. In these situations we have expressed our opinion, reflecting our knowledge and our clinical experience.

In addition to our children and grandchildren, we dedicate this book to all health care professionals who have assumed the social responsibility of assisting couples to use safe, effective contraception. We hope our text will help you and your patients.

Leon Speroff, M.D.
Portland, Oregon

Philip D. Darney, M.D.
San Francisco, California

1

Contraception in the U.S.A.

Fertility decreases as societies become more affluent. This decrease is a response to the use of contraception and abortion. During her reproductive lifespan, the average !Kung woman, a member of an African tribe of hunter-gatherers, experiences 15 years of lactational amenorrhea, 4 years of pregnancy, and only 48 menstrual cycles.[1] In contrast, a modern urban woman experiences 420 menstrual cycles. Contemporary women undergo earlier menarche and start having sexual intercourse earlier in their lives than in the past. Even though breastfeeding has increased in recent years, its duration is relatively brief, and its contribution to contraception in the developed world is trivial. Therefore, it is more difficult today to limit the size of a family unless some method of contraception is utilized.

More young women (under age 25) in the United States become pregnant than do their contemporaries in other Western countries.[2-4] The teenage pregnancy rates in 5 northern European countries and Canada range from 13 to 53% of the U.S. rate. The differences disappear almost completely after age 25. This is largely because American men and women after age 25 utilize surgical sterilization at a great rate.

It is not true that young American women want to have these higher pregnancy rates. About 78% of all pregnancies among American teenagers are unintended.[5] Nevertheless, increasing contraceptive use among young Americans is having an impact. Teenage pregnancy has reached the lowest rate since estimates began in 1976, a 21% decline from 1990 to 1997 for teenagers 15–17 years and a 13% decline for older teenagers.[6] Overall, there has been a 17% decline in teenage birth rates and a 12.8% decline in teenage induced abortions from 1990 through 1999. In 1997, 74% of pregnancies in married women ended as live births and 7% in abortion; 47% of pregnancies in unmarried women ended as live births and 41% in abortion.

American teenagers abort nearly half of their pregnancies, and this proportion is similar to that seen in other countries.[5] American women age 20–34 have the highest proportion of pregnancies aborted compared with other countries, indicating an unappreciated, but real, problem of unintended pregnancy existing beyond the teenage years. In fact, American women older than age 40 have a high ratio of abortions per live births, a ratio exceeded only by teenagers.[7]

A decrease in unintended pregnancies and the abortion rate in the United States in the 1990s is due to better use of contraception; however, the rates are still relatively high. About half of all pregnancies in the United States are estimated to be unplanned, and more than half of these are aborted.[5]

Delaying marriage prolongs the period in which women are exposed to the risk of unintended pregnancy. This, however, cannot be documented as a major reason for the large differential between young adults in Europe and the United States. The available evidence also indicates that a difference in sexual activity is not an important explanation. The major difference between American women and European women is that American women under age 25 are less likely to use any form of contraception. Significantly, the use of oral contraceptives (the main choice of younger women) is lower in the U.S. than in other countries.

Why are Americans different? The cultures in areas such as the United Kingdom and the Scandinavian countries are certainly very similar with similar rates of sexual experience. A major difference must be attributed to the availability of contraception. In the rest of the world, contraceptive services can be obtained from more accessible resources and relatively inexpensively. Major American problems are the enormous diversity of people and the unequal distribution of income in the United States These factors influence the ability of our society to effectively provide education regarding sex and contraception and to effectively make contraception services available.

In 1966, a report from NASA placed our technological achievements into historical perspective.[8] Eight hundred lifespans can bridge more than 50,000 years. But of those 800 people:

- 650 spent their lives in caves,
- only the last 70 had a truly effective means of communication.
- only the last 6 saw the printed word,
- only the last 4 could measure time with precision,
- only the last 2 used an electric motor,
- and the majority of items that make up our current world were developed within the lifespan of the 800th person.

The era of modern contraception dates from 1960 when oral contraception was first approved by the U.S. Food and Drug Administration, and intrauterine devices were re-introduced. For the first time, contraception for many couples did not have to be a part of the act of coitus. However, national family planning services and research were not funded by the U.S. Congress until 1970, and the last U.S. law prohibiting contraception was not reversed until 1973.

Contraception is not new, but its widespread development and application are new. It is in the latest tick of the Earth's time clock that safe control of fertility is now possible. This book is dedicated to that end. This chapter presents an overview of the efficacy of contraceptive methods, a summary of contraceptive use in the United States and the world, and a brief look at the future.

Efficacy of Contraception

A clinician's anecdotal experience with contraceptive methods is truly insufficient to provide the accurate information necessary for patient counseling. The clinician must be aware of the definitions and measurements used in assessing contraceptive efficacy and must draw on the talents of appropriate experts in this area to summarize the accurate and comparative failure rates for the various methods of contraception. The publications by Trussell et al., summarized below, accomplish these purposes and are highly recommended.[9–13]

Definition and Measurement

Contraceptive efficacy is generally assessed by measuring the number of unplanned pregnancies that occur during a specified period of exposure and use of a contraceptive method. The two methods that have been used to measure contraceptive efficacy are the Pearl index and life-table analysis.

4

The Pearl Index

The Pearl index is defined as the number of failures per 100 woman-years of exposure. The denominator is the total months or cycles of exposure from the onset of a method until completion of the study, an unintended pregnancy, or discontinuation of the method. The quotient is multiplied by 1200 if the denominator consists of months or by 1300 if the denominator consists of cycles.

With most methods of contraception, failure rates decline with duration of use. The Pearl index is usually based on a specific exposure (usually one year) and, therefore, fails to accurately compare methods at various durations of exposure. This limitation is overcome by using the method of life-table analysis.

Life-Table Analysis

Life-table analysis calculates a failure rate for each month of use. A cumulative failure rate can then compare methods for any specific length of exposure. Women who leave a study for any reason other than unintended pregnancy are removed from the analysis, contributing their exposure until the time of the exit.

Contraceptive failures do occur and for many reasons. Thus, "method effectiveness" and "use effectiveness" have been used to designate efficacy with correct and incorrect use of a method. It is less confusing to simply compare the very best performance (the lowest expected failure rate) with the usual experience (typical failure rates) as noted in the table of failure rates during the first year of use. The lowest expected failure rates are determined in clinical trials, in which the combination of highly motivated subjects and frequent support from the study personnel yields the best results. It should be noted that slightly more than half of the unintended pregnancies in the United States are due to contraceptive failures.[5] Contraceptive failure rates have been estimated using the data from the 1995 National Survey of Family Growth, correcting for the underreporting of induced abortion.

Failure Rates During the First Year of Use, United States[12-14]

Method	Percent of Women with Pregnancy	
	Lowest Expected	Typical
No method	85.0%	85.0%
Combination pill	0.1	7.6
Progestin-only	0.5	3.0
IUDs		
Levonorgestrel IUD	0.1	0.1
Copper T 380A	0.6	0.8
Implant	0.2	0.2
Injectable	0.3	0.3
Female sterilization	0.2	0.4
Male sterilization	0.1	0.15
Spermicides	6.0	25.7
Periodic abstinence		20.5
Calendar	9.0	
Ovulation method	3.0	
Symptothermal	2.0	
Post-ovulation	1.0	
Withdrawal	4.0	23.6
Cervical cap		
Parous women	20.0	40.0
Nulliparous women	9.0	20.0
Sponge		
Parous women	20.0	40.0
Nulliparous women	9.0	20.0
Diaphragm and spermicides	6.0	12.1
Condom		
Male	3.0	13.9
Female	5.0	21.0

6

Contraceptive Use in the United States

The National Survey of Family Growth is conducted by the National Center for Health Statistics of the Centers for Disease Control and Prevention Data are available from 1972, 1976, 1982, 1995, and 2002.[15–18, 51] The samples are very large; therefore, the estimates are very accurate.

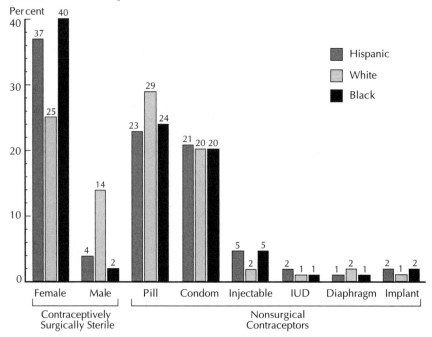

Contraceptive Methods in Women 15–44 in 1995 [17,18]

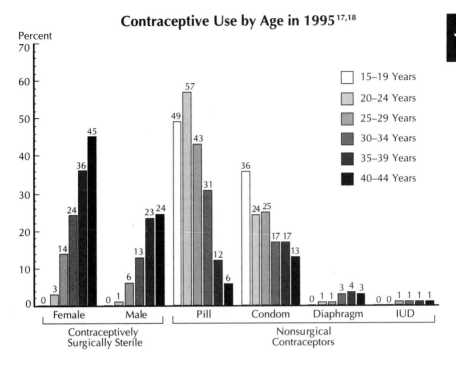

Contraceptive Use by Age in 1995[17,18]

Legend:
- 15–19 Years
- 20–24 Years
- 25–29 Years
- 30–34 Years
- 35–39 Years
- 40–44 Years

Contraceptively Surgically Sterile: Female, Male

Nonsurgical Contraceptors: Pill, Condom, Diaphragm, IUD

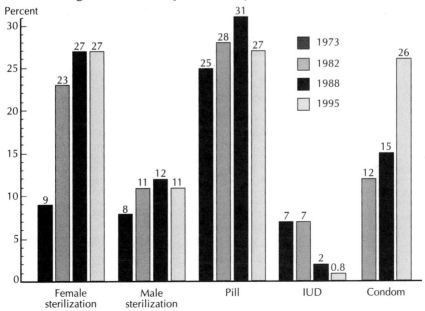

Changes in Contraceptive Use by U.S. Women 15–44[15–18]

Legend:
- 1973
- 1982
- 1988
- 1995

Categories: Female sterilization, Male sterilization, Pill, IUD, Condom

8

Pregnancy rates in the 1990s declined for women younger than age 30 years and increased in older women.[6] From 1990 to 1997, the decrease in women in their early twenties was 8%, and the increase in women in their early thirties was 3%. The percent of married couples using sterilization as a method of contraception more than doubled from 1972 to 1988 and has remained stable since then. The use of oral contraception reached a high in 1992 and then decreased in 1995, especially among Hispanic and black Americans. Approximately 10.7 million American women used oral contraceptives in 1988, 10.4 million in 1995, and 11.6 million in 2002. Among never married women, oral contraception has been the leading method of birth control, but from 1988 to 1995, oral contraceptive use decreased in women younger than 25 and rose among women aged 30–44. A part of the decrease in oral contraceptive use is due to the new availability and use of implant (about 0.5 million women in 1995) and injectable methods (about 1.0 million women in 1995). However, the greater impact is due to an increase in condom use, especially by never married and formerly married women, women younger than 25, black women, and Hispanic women; indeed, the recent increase in overall contraceptive use is due to the increase in condom use, which rose from 5.1 million women aged 15–44 in 1988 (15%) to 7.9 million in 1995 (20%). This increase occurred in all racial and ethnic groups. These changes reflect the concern regarding sexually transmitted infections, including human immunodeficiency virus (HIV). About one-third of condom users in 1995 were using more than one method, especially younger and never married women!

In 1982, 56% of U.S. women, 15–44 years of age, were using contraception, and this increased in 1995 to 64% (about 39 million women). In 1995, contraceptive sterilization (male and female) was utilized by 38% (15 million) of these women (the next leading method was oral contraception, 27%). The number of reproductive-aged women using the intrauterine device (IUD) decreased by two-thirds from 1982 to 1988 and further decreased in 1995, from 7.1% to 2% to 0.8%, respectively. IUD use is concentrated in the U.S. in married women older than age 35. In 1982 more than 2 million women used the IUD and a similar number used the diaphragm, but in 1995 only 0.3 million women used the IUD and 0.7 million women (1.9%) used the diaphragm. The decrease in IUD use since 1982 has been especially marked in Hispanic and black women.

The oral contraceptive and condoms are the most popular methods among teenagers. However, studies have repeatedly documented that the use of the implant and injectable methods is associated with lower discontinuation rates and a lower rate of repeat pregnancies following delivery.[19, 20] This warrants a renewed effort to extend the use of these methods.

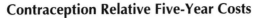

Contraception Relative Five-Year Costs

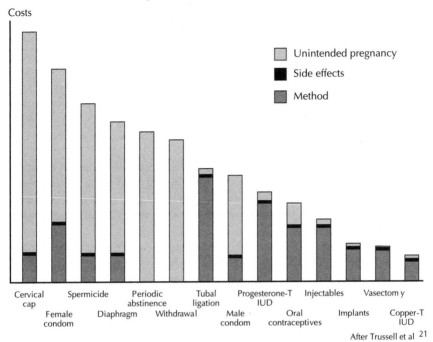

Costs

Legend:
- Unintended pregnancy
- Side effects
- Method

Categories (left to right): Cervical cap, Female condom, Spermicide, Diaphragm, Periodic abstinence, Withdrawal, Tubal ligation, Male condom, Progesterone-T IUD, Oral contraceptives, Injectables, Implants, Vasectomy, Copper-T IUD

After Trussell et al [21]

In 1995, 95% of those who were at risk of getting pregnant were using some method of contraception, whereas 36% of women of reproductive age were not using a method of contraception for the following reasons:

10.9% — No sexual experience.
8.6% — Pregnant or trying to get pregnant.
6.2% — Not sexually active.
4.3% — Sterilized for medical reasons.
0.6% — Male sterility.
5.2% — At risk for an unintended pregnancy
       (this percent steadily decreased since 1990
       until it increased in 2002 to 7.4%).

U.S. couples have made up for the lack of contraceptive choices by greater reliance on voluntary sterilization. Between 1973 and 1982, oral contraception and sterilization changed places as the most popular contraceptive method among women over the age of 30. Approximately one-half of American couples choose sterilization within 15 to 20 years of their last wanted birth. During the years of maximal fertility, oral contraceptives are the most common method peaking at age 20–24. The use of condoms is the second most widely used method of reversible contraception, rising from about 9% in the mid-1980s to approximately 20% of couples in 1995.[18]

The pattern of contraceptive use in Canada in 1995 was similar to that of the United States, with a slightly higher percentage of oral contraceptive use (38.2% of women 15–44 years of age) and a slightly lower use of sterilization (32.5%).[22] Canada, too, has seen an increase in condom use and a decrease in use of the IUD. In England, the primary method of contraceptive service in the National Health Service is oral contraception (43%) followed by condoms (34%), injectable methods (8%), and the IUD (7%); only about 11% of the reproductive-aged women have been sterilized.[23] In France, 36.3% of reproductive-aged women used oral contraceptives (in 1994), and although IUD use has slightly decreased (only among younger women), French women use the IUD at a rate that is more than 16-fold greater compared with North American women.[24] Most French women use oral contraceptives when young and then turn to the IUD in their older years (only 4.1% of French women relied on sterilization—male sterilization is virtually nonexistent).

Induced Abortion in the United States

The number of abortions performed in the United States has been decreasing since a peak was reached in 1990, totaling 1.33 million in 1993 and 1.18 million in 1997, with the greatest decline among teenagers.[7, 25, 26] This is partly because the number of pregnancies in the United States has been decreasing and the proportion of reproductive-aged women younger than age 30 is also decreasing.[27] Accounting for underreporting, a more accurate estimate indicated about 1.36 million induced abortions in 1996 and 1.31 million in 2000, the lowest number since 1976.[28, 29] The proportion of abortions performed in hospitals has steadily declined, reaching 5% in 2000. The proportion handled by specialized abortion clinics has increased, while the percentage of abortions performed by physicians in their own offices has remained low, about 2% of all abortions. More than 50% of abortions are obtained by women younger than 25 (about 20% under the age of 20), with the rate peaking at ages 18–19, and about 80% are unmarried.[25, 26, 30]

U.S. Characteristics

American women have fewer birth control choices than women in most other industrialized nations, and contraception is more expensive. These are the reasons that American women have higher rates of unintended childbirth and induced abortion compared to women in other industrialized nations. Another contrast is oral contraceptive use among older married women. In the Netherlands, for example, it is nearly twice as high in 20–29-year-old women as among comparable U.S. women, and among women over 35, the level in the Netherlands is nearly 10 times that in the United States. Conversely, the total induced abortion rate in the United States is almost 3 times that of Dutch women. Most American IUD users are concentrated between ages 35 and 50, and even here there are differences: 4 times as many French women over 40 use IUDs compared to American women. Among American 30–44-year-olds, sterilization is the most utilized method of family planning. The rate of sterilization among American women over 35 is about the same compared with Great Britain and the Netherlands, but under the age of 30 it is 50% higher in American women. In young women, the frequency of sexual intercourse is associated with the choice of contraceptive.[31] Young people who are very active sexually prefer oral contraception because it is perceived as very effective and allows sex to be worry free. As concern with AIDS grew, a more favorable attitude towards the condom emerged.

In the United States, there are no major differences in expected family size among the various religious groups, an exception being the higher level of family size desired by Mormons. Religion does influence choice of contraceptive method; Protestant levels of female sterilization are higher than that of Catholics and Catholic utilization of oral contraception and condoms is higher than that of Protestants.[32]

A major problem in the U.S. is the prevalence of misconceptions. More than half of women, even well-educated women, are not accurately aware of the efficacy or the benefits and side effects associated with contraception.[33-35] Unfortunately, a significant percentage of women still do not know that there are many health benefits with the use of estrogen-progestin contraception. Misconceptions regarding contraception have, in many instances, achieved the stature of myths. Myths are an obstacle to poor utilization and can only be dispelled by accurate and effective educational efforts.

The Impact of the Worldwide Use of Contraception

The world population is expected to stabilize at between 11 and 12 billion around 2150, with a fertility rate of 2.1 children per woman.[36-39] Approximately 96% of the population growth now occurs in developing countries, so that by 2100, 13% of the population will live in developed countries, a decrease from the current 25%. Some time after 2020, all of the growth in global population will occur in developing countries. An estimated 120 million married women in developing countries are not receiving needed contraception.[38] Today, the fertility rate is less than 2.1 children per women in China, Eastern and Western Europe, North America, Japan, Australia, and New Zealand. In 2001, the fertility rate in the U.S. reached a low of 2.03.[39]

A more serious and prolonged impact of the HIV epidemic has produced a lower estimate for population growth, and it may take longer for the world population to stabilize than previously projected.[40]

World Population

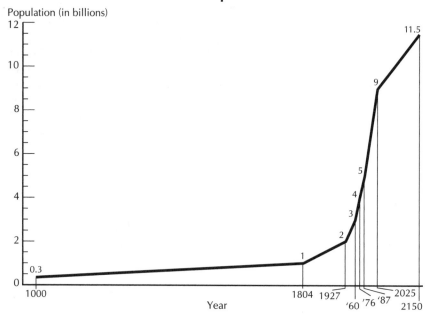

Population (in billions)

Year

Throughout the world, 45% of married women of reproductive age practice contraception. However, there is significant variation from area to area; e.g., more than 70% in the United States and China but only 6% in Nigeria.[38] Female sterilization and the IUD are most popular in developing countries, whereas oral contraceptives and condoms are most popular in developed countries. Less than 15% of women of reproductive age in the world are using oral contraceptives, and more than half live in the United States, Brazil, France, and Germany.

The 76% of the world's population living in developing countries account for:

- 85% of all births,
- 95% of all infant and childhood deaths,
- 99% of all maternal deaths.

The problem in the developing world is self-evident. The ability to regulate fertility has a significant impact on infant, child, and maternal mortality and morbidity. A pregnant woman has a 200 times greater chance of dying if she lives in a developing country rather than in a developed country.[41] The health risks associated with pregnancy and childbirth in the developing world are far, far greater than risks secondary to the use of modern contraception.[42] To meet the projected growth in the world's population, the number of women using family planning will need to increase substantially from 1998 to 2025; for example, 40 million more women in India will need to use some method of contraception![38]

In recent years, there has been an appropriate shift from a narrow focus on contraception to a broader view that encompasses the impact of poverty, emphasizes overall well-being and the rights of individuals, endorses gender equality, and examines the interactions among these issues.[43] It is not enough to simply limit fertility; contraception is only one component of reproductive health.

The Impact of Use and Non-use

Inadequate access to contraception is associated with a high induced abortion rate. Effective contraceptive use largely, although not totally, replaces the resort to abortion.[44] The combination of restrictive abortion laws and the lack of safe abortion services continues to make unsafe abortion a major cause of morbidity and mortality throughout the world. Both safe and unsafe abortions can be minimized by maximizing contraceptive services. However, the need for safe abortion services persists. Contraceptive failures account for about half of the 1.3 million annual induced abortions in the United States.

In the United States, money spent on public funding for family planning saves money spent on medical, welfare, and nutritional services.[45] States with higher family planning expenditures have fewer induced abortions, low-birth-weight newborns, and premature births.[46] The investment in family planning leads to short-term reductions in expenditures on maternal and child health services and, after 5 years, a reduction in costs for education budgets. Cutting back on publicly funded family planning services largely affects poor women, increasing the number of unintended births and abortions.

STIs and Contraception

The interaction between clinician and patient for the purpose of contraception provides an opportunity to control sexually transmitted infections (STIs). The modification of unsafe sexual practices reduces the risk of unplanned pregnancy and the risk of infections of the reproductive tract. A patient visit for contraception is an excellent time for STI screening; if an infection is symptomatic, it should be diagnosed and treated during the same visit in which contraception is requested. A positive history for STIs should trigger both screening for asymptomatic infections and counseling for safer sexual practices. Attention should be given to the contraceptive methods that have the greatest influence on the risk of STIs.

Contraception and Litigation

Clinicians are concerned about the prospect of bad outcomes associated with contraceptive use leading to litigation. Multimillion dollar verdicts and settlements in favor of plaintiffs who have used products as innocent as spermicides capture national attention. Actually, these events are very unusual compared with the widespread use of contraception.

The best way to avoid litigation is good patient communication. Patients who sue usually claim there were contraindications or risks that were not conveyed by the clinician. The best way to influence litigation is to keep good records. Good clinician's records are the most formidable weapon for the defense. Documentation is vital, but it is useless without thorough history taking. Good records and good history taking put the responsibility on the patient's honesty in response to the clinician.

Document that the risks and benefits of all methods were discussed.
Document a plan for follow-up.
Document all interactions with the patient, including phone calls.

The Future

From 1970 to 1986, the number of births in women older than 30 quadrupled; since 1990, the fertility rate among women older than 30 has remained relatively stable.[6, 47] As couples deferred pregnancy until later in life, the use of sterilization under age 35 declined, and the need for reversible contraception increased. Between 1988 and 1995, oral contraceptive use decreased in women younger than 25 and increased in women aged 30–44.[18] These numbers changed because clinicians and patients came to understand and accept that low-dose estrogen-progestin contraception is safe for healthy, nonsmoking, older women.

The highest number of births in the United States occurred between 1947 and 1965—the post–World War II baby boom (a demographic phenomenon shared by all parts of the developed world). The entire cohort of women born in this period will not reach its 45th birthday until around 2010. For approximately a 20-year period, therefore, there will be an unprecedented number of women in the later childbearing years. This group of women is not only increasing in number but changing its fertility pattern.

The deferment of marriage is a significant change in our society. However, only a small percentage of the decline in the total fertility rate is accounted for by the increase in the average age at first marriage. Most of the decline in total fertility rate is accounted for by changes in marital fertility rates. In other words, postponement of pregnancy in marriage is the more significant change. This combination of increasing numbers, deferment of marriage, and postponement of pregnancy in marriage is responsible for the fact that we will be seeing more and more older women who will need reversible contraception. In short, there will continue to be longer duration of use in younger women and greater use in older women, a pattern that began in 1990.

U.S. Change in Female Demographics 1985–2000 [48]

Age	1985	1990	1995	2000	% Change 1985–2000
15–24	19.5 mill.	17.4 mill.	16.7 mill.	17.7 mill.	−9.2%
25–29	10.9	10.6	9.3	8.6	−21.1
30–34	10.0	11.0	10.8	9.4	− 6.0
35–44	16.2	19.1	21.1	21.9	+35.2
Total 15–44	56.6	58.1	57.9	57.6	+1.8

There are many obstacles to the development of new contraceptive methods, including the attitudes of the American public (in addition to America's traditionally conservative, religion-oriented views toward sex and family, polarization is produced by responses evoked by specific issues such as sterilization and induced abortion), the funding available for research, the time and cost required to meet federal regulations, and the problems of product liability. However, experts in the field remain optimistic, citing the many needs and opportunities for improvements and new developments.[49]

Fortunately, clinicians and patients have recognized that low-dose estrogen-progestin contraception is very safe for healthy, nonsmoking, older women. Between 1988 and 1995, the use of oral contraceptives doubled among women aged 35–39, and increased 6-fold in women older than age 40.[18] However, as the previously mentioned statistics indicate, its use is still not sufficient to meet the need. In addition to fulfilling a need, this population of women has a series of benefits to be derived from estrogen-progestin contraception that tilt the risk/benefit ratio to the positive side (Chapter 2).

The growing need for reversible contraception would also be served by increased use of the IUD. The decline in IUD use in the U.S. is in direct contrast to the experience in the rest of the world, a complicated response to publicity and litigation. An increased risk of pelvic infection with contemporary IUDs in use is limited to the act of insertion and the transportation of pathogens to the upper genital tract. This risk is effectively minimized by careful screening with preinsertion cultures and the use of good technique. A return to IUD use by American couples is both warranted and desirable.

Contraceptive advice is a component of good preventive health care. The clinician's approach is a key. This is an era of informed choice by the patient. Patients deserve to know the facts and need help in dealing with the state of the art and the uncertainty. But there is no doubt that patients, especially young patients, are influenced in their choice by their clinicians' advice and attitude. Although the role of a clinician is to provide the education necessary for the patient to make proper choices, one should not lose sight of the powerful influence exerted by the clinician in the choices ultimately made. In the 1970s, we approached the patient with great emphasis on risk. In the new century, the approach should be different, highlighting the benefits and the greater safety of appropriate contraception. If one attempts to sum the impact of the benefits of contraception on public health, as some have done with models focusing on hospital admissions, there is no doubt that the benefits outweigh the risks. The impact can be measured in terms of both morbidity and mortality. However, the impact on public health is of little concern during the clinician–patient interchange in the medical office. Here personal risk is paramount, and compliance with effective contraception requires accurate information presented in a positive, effective fashion.

The challenge for the next 20 years is to do as Sherlock Holmes said: "You know my methods, use them."[50] A stable global population of about 8–10 billion is possible. Without better contraceptive education and services, global population could reach 15 billion before stabilization.[12–14]

Useful Web Sites

Planned Parenthood:
   http://plannedparenthood.org

The Alan Guttmacher Institute:
   http://www.agi-usa.org/

The World Health Organization:
   http://who.int/en/

References

1. **Djerassi C,** The Politics of Contraception, Vol. I. The Present, Stanford Alumni Association, Stanford, California, 1979.

2. **Westoff CF,** Unintended pregnancy in America and abroad, Fam Plann Persp 20:254, 1988.

3. **Spitz AM, Velebil P, Koonin LM, Strauss LT, Goodman KA, Wingo P, Wilson JB, Morris L, Marks JS,** Pregnancy, abortion, and birth rates among US adolescents—1980, 1985, and 1990, JAMA 275:989, 1996.

4. **The Alan Guttmacher Institute,** Facts in Brief: Teenagers' Sexual and Reproductive Health, The Alan Guttmacher Institute, New York, 2002.

5. **Henshaw SK,** Unintended pregnancy in the United States, Fam Plann Perspect 30:24, 1998.

6. **Ventura SJ, Hamilton BE, Sutton PD,** Revised birth and fertility rates for the United States, 2000 and 2001, Natl Vital Stat Rep 51:1, 2003.

7. **Centers for Disease Control and Prevention,** Abortion Surveillance—United States, 1999, MMWR 52(No. SS09):1, 2002.

8. **Lesher RL, Howick GJ,** (NASA), Assessing technology transfer, Report No. SP-50671, 1966.

9. **Trussell J, Hatcher RA, Cates Jr W, Stewart FH, Kost K,** A guide to interpreting contraceptive efficacy studies, Obstet Gynecol 76:558, 1990.

10. **Trussell J, Hatcher RA, Cates Jr W, Stewart FH, Kost K,** Contraceptive failure in the United States: an update, Stud Fam Plann 21:51, 1990.

11. **Trussell J,** Contraceptive efficacy of the Reality® female condom, Contraception 58:147, 1998.

12. **Trussell J, Vaughan B,** Contraceptive failure, method-related discontinuation and resumption of use: results from the 1995 National Survey of Family Growth, Fam Plann Perspect 31:64, 1999.

13. **Trussell J,** Contraceptive failure in the United States, Contraception 70:89, 2004.

14. **Fu H, Darroch JE, Haas T, Ranjit N,** Contraceptive failure rates: new estimates from the 1995 National Survey of Family Growth, Fam Plann Perspect 31:58, 1999.

15. **Mosher WD, Pratt WF,** Contraceptive use in the United States, 1973–88, Advance data from vital and health statistics, Report No. 182, National Center for Health Statistics, Washington, D.C., 1990.

16. **Mosher WD,** Use of family planning services in the United States: 1982 and 1988, Advance data from vital and health statistics, Report No. 184, National Center for Health Statistics, Washington, D.C., 1990.

17. **Abma JC, Chandra A, Mosher WD, Peterson L, Piccinino L,** Fertility, family planning, and women's health: new data from the 1995 National Survey of Family Growth, Report No. 19, Series 23, Centers for Disease Control and Prevention, National Center For Heath Statistics, Washington, D.C., 1997.

18. **Piccinino LJ, Mosher WD,** Trends in contraceptive use in the United States: 1982–1995, Fam Plann Perspect 30:4, 1998.

19. **Polaneczky M, Slap G, Forke C, Rappaport A, Sondheimer S,** The use of levonorgestrel implants (Norplant) for contraception in adolescent mothers, New Engl J Med 331:1201, 1994.

20. **Polaneczky M, Guarnaccia M, Alon J, Wiley J,** Early experience with the contraceptive use of depo-medroxyprogesterone acetate in an inner-city population, Fam Plann Perspect 28:174, 1996.

21. **Trussell J, Leveque JA, Koenig JD, London R, Borden S, Henneberry J, LaGuardia KD, Stewart F, Wilson TG, Wysocki S, Strauss M,** The economic value of contraception: a comparison of 15 methods, Am J Public Health 85:494, 1995.

22. **Boroditsky R, Fisher W, Sand M,** The 1995 Canadian Contraception Study, J Soc Obstet Gynaecol Can 18:1, 1996.

23. **Government Statistical Service, NHS** Contraceptive Services, England: 2001–02, Department of Health, Government Statistical Service, England, 2002.

24. **Toulemon L, Leridon H,** Contraceptives practices and trends in France, Fam Plann Perspect 30:114, 1998.

25. **Henshaw SK, Van Vort J,** Abortion services in the United States, 1991 and 1992, Fam Plann Perspect 26:100, 1994.

26. **Jones RK, Darroch JE, Henshaw SK,** Patterns in the socioeconomic characteristics of women obtaining abortions in 2000–2001, Persp Sexual Reprod Health 34:226, 2002.

27. **Deardorff KE, Montgomery P, Hollmann FW,** U.S. population estimates by age, sex, race, and Hispanic origin: 1990 to 1995, U.S. Department of Commerce, Economics and Statistics Administration, Bureau of the Census, Washington, D.C., 1996.

18

28. **Henshaw SK,** Abortion incidence and services in the United States, 1995–1996, Fam Plann Perspect 30:263, 1998.

29. **Finer LB, Henshaw SK,** Abortion incidence and services in the United States in 2000, Persp Sexual Reprod Health 35:6, 2003.

30. **Henshaw SK,** Induced abortions: a world review, 1990, Fam Plann Perspect 22:76, 1990.

31. **Glor JE, Severy LJ,** Frequency of intercourse and contraceptive choice, J Biosoc Sci 22:231, 1990.

32. **Goldscheider C, Mosher WD,** Patterns of contraceptive use in the United States: the importance of religious factors, Studies Fam Plann 22:102, 1991.

33. **Peipert JF, Gutmann J,** Oral contraceptive risk assessment: a survey of 247 educated women, Obstet Gynecol 82:112, 1993.

34. **Murphy P, Kirkman A, Hale RW,** A national survey of women's attitudes toward oral contraception and other forms of birth control, Womens Health Issues 5:94, 1995.

35. **Tessler SL, Peipert JF,** Perceptions of contraceptive effectiveness and health effects of oral contraception, Women's Health Issues 7:400, 1997.

36. **United Nations,** World Population Prospects: The 1996 Revision, New York, 1998.

37. **Raleigh VS,** Trends in world population: how will the millennium compare with the past? Hum Reprod Update 5:500, 1999.

38. **McDevitt TM,** Report WP/98, World Population Profile: 1998, U.S. Bureau of the Census, U.S. Government Printing Office, Washington, D.C., 1999.

39. **Haub C,** 2003 World population data sheet, Population Reference Bureau http://www.prb.org, 2003.

40. **United Nations Population Division,** World Population Prospects. The 2002 Revision, www.un.org/esa/population/unpop.htm, 2003.

41. **Diczfalusy E,** The worldwide use of steroidal contraception, Int J Fertil 34(Suppl):56, 1989.

42. **DaVanzo J, Parnell AM, Foege WH,** Health consequences of contraceptive use and reproductive patterns: summary of a report from the US National Research Council, JAMA 265:2692, 1991.

43. **Garcia-Moreno C, Türmen T,** International perspectives on women's reproductive health, Science 269:790, 1995.

44. **Potts M, Rosenfield A,** The fifth freedom revisited: I. Background and existing programs, Lancet 336:1227, 1990.

45. **Forrest JD, Singh S,** Public-sector savings resulting from expenditures for contraceptive services, Fam Plann Perspect 22:6, 1990.

46. **Meier KJ, McFarlane DR,** State family planning and abortion expenditures: their effect on public health, Am J Public Health 84:1468, 1994.

47. **Ventura SJ,** Advance report of final natality statistics, 1992, Mon Vital Stat Rep, Vol. 43, 1994.

48. **Day JC,** Bureau of the Census, Current population reports. Population projections of the United States, by age, sex, race, and Hispanic origin: 1993 to 2050, U.S. Government Printing Office, Washington, D.C., 1993.

49. **Harrison PF, Rosenfield A,** eds, Contraceptive Research and Development: Looking to the Future, National Academy Press, Washington, D.C., 1996.

50. **Doyle AC,** The Sign of Four.

51. **Mosher WD, Martinez GM, Chandra A, Abma JC, Willson SJ,** Use of contrception and use of family planning services in the United States: 1982–2002, Advance Data from Vital and Health Statistics, No. 350, December 10, 2004.

2

Oral Contraception

Contraception is commonly viewed as a modern event, a recent development in human history. On the contrary, efforts to limit reproduction predate our ability to write about it. It is only contraception with synthetic sex steroids that is recent.

History[1-4]

It wasn't until the early 1900s that inhibition of ovulation was observed to be linked to pregnancy and the corpus luteum. Ludwig Haberlandt, professor of physiology at the University of Innsbruck, Austria, was the first to demonstrate that ovarian extracts given orally could prevent fertility (in mice). In the 1920s, Haberlandt and a Viennese gynecologist, Otfried Otto Fellner, were administering steroid extracts to a variety of animals and reporting the inhibition of fertility. By 1931, Haberlandt was proposing the administration of hormones for birth control. An extract was produced, named Infecundin, ready to be used, but Haberlandt's early death in 1932, at age 47, brought an end to this effort. Fellner disappeared after the annexation of Austria to Hitler's Germany.

The concept was annunciated by Haberlandt, but steroid chemistry wasn't ready. The extraction and isolation of a few milligrams of the sex steroids required starting points measured in gallons of urine or thousands of pounds of organs. Edward Doisy processed 80,000 sow ovaries to produce 12 mg of estradiol.

Russell Marker

The supply problem was solved by an eccentric chemist, Russell E. Marker, who completed his thesis, but not his course work, for his Ph.D. Marker, born in 1902 near Hagerstown, Maryland, received his bachelor's degree in organic chemistry and his master's degree in colloidal chemistry from the University of Maryland. After leaving the University of Maryland, Marker worked with the Ethyl Gasoline Corporation and in 1926 developed the process of octane rating, based on the discovery that knocking in gasoline was due to hydrocarbons with an uneven number of carbons.

From 1927 to 1935, Marker worked at the Rockefeller Institute, publishing a total of 32 papers on configuration and optical rotation as a method of identifying compounds. He became interested in solving the problem of producing abundant and cheap amounts of progesterone, but he was told to continue with his work in optical technology. In 1935, he moved to Pennsylvania State University at a reduced salary but with the freedom to pursue any field of research. At that time, the ovaries from 2,500 pregnant pigs were required to produce 1 mg of progesterone. In 1939, Marker devised the method (called the Marker degradation) to convert a sapogenin molecule into a progestin. Marker became convinced that the solution to the problem of obtaining large quantities of steroid hormones was to find plants (in the family that includes the lily, the agave, and the yam) that contained sufficient amounts of diosgenin, a plant steroid (a sapogenin) that could be used as a starting point for steroid hormone production. This conviction was strengthened with his discovery that a species of *Trillium,* known locally as Beth's root, was collected in North Carolina and used in the preparation of Lydia Pinkham's Compound, popular at the time to relieve menstrual troubles. A principal ingredient in Beth's root was diosgenin, but the rhizome was too small to provide sufficient amounts for commercial production. Marker's search for an appropriate plant took him to California, Arizona, and Texas.

On a visit to Texas A & M University, Marker found a picture of a large dioscorea *(Dioscorea mexicana)* in a book that he just happened to pick up and browse through while spending the night at the home of a retired botanist. After returning to Pennsylvania, he decided to go to Veracruz, Mexico (it took 3 days by train), to search for this dioscorea. He made several attempts in 1941 and early 1942 but was frustrated first by the lack of a plant-collecting permit from the Mexician government and then by his failure to find the plant. He remembered that the book with the picture reported that this dioscorea was known locally as "cabeza de negro," black tubers that grew near Orizaba and Cordoba. Marker took a bus to Cordoba, and near Orizaba, an Indian who owned a small store brought him two plants. Each tuber was 9–12 inches high and consisted of white material like a turnip, used by local Mexicans as a poison to catch fish.

Marker managed to get one bag of tubers back to Pennsylvania State University and isolated diosgenin. Unable to obtain support from the pharmaceutical industry, Marker used his life savings, and in 1942, he returned to Veracruz, collected the roots of the Mexican yam, and prepared a syrup from the roots. Marker paid Mexican medical students to collect the yams. The students were arrested when farmers reported that their yams were being stolen, but not before Marker had enough to prepare a syrup. Back in Pennsylvania with his 5-gallon cans of syrup, Marker worked out the degradation of diosgenin to progesterone. One 5-gallon can yielded 3 kg of progesterone. United States pharmaceutical companies still refused to back Marker, and even the University refused, despite Marker's urging, to patent the process.

In 1943, Marker resigned from Pennsylvania State University and went to Mexico where he collected the roots of *Dioscorea mexicana,* 10 tons worth! Looking through the yellow pages in a Mexico City telephone directory, Marker found a company called Laboratorios Hormona, owned by a lawyer, Emeric Somlo, and a physician, Frederick Lehman. Marker arranged a meeting, and the three agreed to form a Mexican company to produce hormones. In an old pottery shed in Mexico City (the laboratories of Laboratorios Hormona), in 2 months he prepared several pounds of progesterone (worth $300,000) with the help of four young women who had little education and spoke no English (Marker did not speak Spanish). The two partners and Marker formed a company in 1944 that they called Syntex (from synthesis and Mexico). In 1944, Marker produced over 30 kg of progesterone. The price of progesterone fell from $200 to $50 a gram.

During this time, Marker received expenses, but he was not given his share of the profits or the 40% share of stock due to him. Failing to reach a settlement, Marker left Syntex after only 1 year and started a new company in Texcoco, called Botanica-Mex. He changed to *Dioscorea barbasco,* which gave a greater yield of diosgenin, and the price of progesterone dropped to $10 a gram, and later to $5. This company was allegedly harassed (legally and physically) by Syntex, and in 1946 was sold, eventually coming under the ownership of Organon of Holland, which still uses it.

In 1949, Marker retired to Pennsylvania to devote the rest of his life to making replicas of antique works in silver, a successful business that allowed him, in the 1980s, to endow scientific lectureships at both Pennsylvania State University and the University of Maryland. However, he took his know-how with him. Fortunately for Syntex, he had published a scientific description of his process, and there still was no patent on his discoveries. Syntex recruited George Rosenkranz, a Hungarian immigrant living in Cuba, to reinstitute the commercial manufacture of progesterone (and testosterone) from Mexican yams, a task that took him (with the help of the women left behind by Marker) 2 years.

In 1970, the Mexican government honored Marker and awarded him the Order of the Aztec Eagle; he declined. In 1984, Pennsylvania State University established the annual Marker Lectures in Science and, in 1987, the Russell and Mildred Marker Professorship of Natural Product Chemistry. In 1987, Marker was granted an honorary doctorate in science from the University of Maryland, the degree he failed to receive in 1926. At the age of 92, Russell Earl Marker died in Wernersville, Pennsylvania, in 1995, from complications after a broken hip.

Carl Djerassi[5]

The Djerassi family lived in Bulgaria for hundreds of years after escaping Spain during the Inquisition. Carl Djerassi, the son of a Bulgarian physician, was born in Vienna (as was his physician mother). Djerassi, at the age of 16, and his mother emigrated to the United States in 1939. A Jewish refugee aid organization placed Djerassi with a family in Newark, New Jersey. With a scholarship to Tarkio College in Tarkio, Missouri, he was exposed to middle America, where he earned his way giving talks to church groups about Bulgaria and Europe. His education was further supported by another scholarship from Kenyon College in Ohio, where he pursued chemistry. After a year working for CIBA, Djerassi received his graduate degree from the University of Wisconsin. Returning to CIBA and being somewhat unhappy, he responded to an invitation to visit Syntex. Rosenkranz proposed that Djerassi head a research group to concentrate on the synthesis of cortisone.

In 1949, it was discovered that cortisone relieved arthritis, and the race was on to develop an easy and cheap method to synthesize cortisone. Carl Djerassi, at age 26, joined Syntex to work on this synthesis using the Mexican yam plant steroid diosgenin as the starting point. This was quickly achieved (in 1951), but soon after, an even better method of cortisone production using microbiologic fermentation was discovered at Upjohn. This latter method used progesterone as the starting point, and, therefore, Syntex found itself as the key supplier to other companies for this important process, at the rate of 10 tons of progesterone per year and a price of 48 cents per gram.

Djerassi and other Syntex chemists then turned their attention to the sex steroids. They discovered that the removal of the 19-carbon from yam-derived progesterone increased the progestational activity of the molecule. Ethisterone had been available for a dozen years, and the Syntex chemists reasoned that removal of the 19-carbon would increase the progestational potency of this orally active compound. In 1951, norethindrone was synthesized; the patent for this drug is the first patent for a drug listed in the National Inventor's Hall of Fame in Akron, Ohio. A closely related compound, norethynodrel, was actually the first orally active progestational agent to receive a patent, assigned to Frank Colton, a chemist at G.D. Searle & Company.

Djerassi eventually left Syntex to become a professor at Stanford University, and is now a playwright and novelist, living in San Francisco.

Gregory Pincus

Gregory Goodwin (Goody) Pincus was born in 1903 in New Jersey, the son of Russian Jewish immigrants who lived on a farm colony founded by a German-Jewish philanthropic organization. Pincus was the oldest of 6 children and grew up in a home of intellectual curiosity and energy, but even his family regarded him as a genius.

Pincus graduated from Cornell and went to Harvard to study genetics, joining Hudson Hoagland and B. F. Skinner as graduate students of W. J. Crozier in physiology, receiving degrees in 1927. Crozier's hero was Jacques Loeb who discovered artificial parthenogenesis working with sea urchin eggs. Most importantly, Loeb was a strong believer in applying science to improve human life. Thus, Crozier, influenced by Loeb, taught Pincus, Hoagland, and Skinner (respectively, in reproductive biology, neurophysiology, and psychology) to apply science to human problems. This was to be the cornerstone of Pincus's own philosophy.

Hoagland, after a short stay at Harvard, spent a year in Cambridge, England, and then moved to Clark University in Worcester, Massachusetts, to be the chair of biology at the age of 31. Pincus went to England and Germany, and returned to Harvard as an assistant professor of physiology.

Pincus performed pioneering studies of meiotic maturation in mammalian oocytes, in both rabbit and human oocytes. In 1934, Pincus reported the achievement of in vitro fertilization of rabbit eggs, earning him a headline in the *New York Times* that alluded to Haldane and Huxley. An article in *Colliers* depicted him as an evil scientist. By 1936, Harvard had cited Pincus's work as one of the university's outstanding scientific achievements of all time, but Harvard denied him tenure in 1937.

At Clark University, Hudson Hoagland was in constant conflict with the president of the university, Wallace W. Atwood, the senior author of a widely used textbook on geography. In 1931, the Department of Biology consisted of one faculty member and his graduate student, and their chair, Hudson Hoagland. Hoagland, upset and angry over Harvard's refusal to grant tenure to his friend (suspecting that this was because of anti-Semitism), invited Pincus to join him. Hoagland secured funds for Pincus from philanthropists in New York City, enough for a laboratory and an assistant. This success impressed the two men, especially Hoagland, planting the idea that it would be possible to support research with private money.

Min-Chueh Chang received his Ph.D. from Harvard on an infamous day, December 7, 1941, and thus he was forced to remain in this country. He was drawn to Pincus because of Pincus's book, *The Eggs of Mammals,* published in 1936, a book that had a major impact on biologists at that time. The successful recruitment of M-C Chang by Hoagland and Pincus was to pay great dividends.

Soon Hoagland had put together a group of outstanding scientists, but because of his on-going antagonism with President Atwood, the group was denied faculty status. Working in a converted barn, they were totally supported by private funds. By 1943, 12 of Clark's 60 faculty were in the Department of Biology.

Frustrated by the politics of academia, Hoagland and Pincus (who both enjoyed stepping outside of convention) had a vision of a private research center devoted to their philosophy of applied science. Indeed, the establishment of the Worcester Foundation for Experimental Biology, in 1944, can be attributed directly to Hoagland and Pincus, their friendship for each other, and their confidence, enthusiasm, ambition, and drive. It was their spirit that turned many members of Worcester society into financial supporters of biologic science. Hoagland and Pincus accomplished what they set out to do. They created and sustained a vibrant, productive scientific institution in which it was a pleasure to work.

Although named the Worcester Foundation for Experimental Biology, the Foundation was located in the summer of 1945 across Lake Quinsigamond in a house on an estate in Shrewsbury. The board of trustees was chaired by Harlow Shapley, a distinguished astronomer, vice-chaired by Rabbi Levi Olan, and included three Nobel laureates and a group of Worcester businessmen.

From 1945 to the death of Pincus in 1967, the staff grew from 12 to 350 (scientists and support people), 36 of whom were independently funded and 45 were postdoctoral fellows. The annual budget grew from $100,000 to $4.5 million. One hundred acres of adjoining land were acquired, and the campus grew to 11 buildings. In its first 25 years, approximately 3,000 scientific papers were published.

But in those early years, Pincus was the animal keeper, Mrs. Hoagland the bookkeeper, M-C. Chang was the night watchman, and Hoagland mowed the lawn. During the years of World War II, Pincus and Hoagland combined their interests in hormones and neurophysiology to focus on stress and fatigue in industry and the military.

The initial discoveries that led to an oral contraceptive can be attributed to M-C. Chang (also the first to describe the capacitation process of sperm). In 1951, he confirmed the work of Makepeace (in 1937) demonstrating that progesterone could inhibit ovulation in rabbits. When norethindrone and norethynodrel became available, Chang found them to be virtually 100% effective in inhibiting ovulation when administered orally to rabbits.

Katherine Dexter McCormick (1875–1967) was a very rich woman; in 1904, she married Stanley McCormick, the son of Cyrus McCormick, the founder of International Harvester. She was also intelligent, the second woman to graduate from the Massachusetts Institute of Technology, socially conscious, and a generous contributor to family planning efforts. McCormick's husband suffered from schizophrenia, and she established the Neuroendocrine Research Foundation at Harvard to study schizophrenia. This brought her together with Hoagland, who told her of the work being done by Chang and Pincus.

Pincus attributed his interest in contraception to his growing appreciation for the world's population problem and to a 1951 visit with Margaret Sanger, at that time president of the Planned Parenthood Federation of America. At that visit, Sanger expressed hope that a method of contraception could be derived from the laboratory work being done by Pincus and Chang.

In 1952, Margaret Sanger brought Pincus and Katherine McCormick together. During this meeting, Pincus formulated his thoughts derived from his mammalian research. He envisioned a progestational agent in pill form as a contraceptive, acting like progesterone in pregnancy. Sanger and McCormick provided a research grant for further animal research. By the time of her death, McCormick had contributed more than $2 million to the Worcester Foundation, and left another $1 million in her will. In his book, *The Control of Fertility,* published in 1965, Pincus wrote: "This book is dedicated to Mrs. Stanley McCormick because of her steadfast faith in scientific inquiry and her unswerving encouragement of human dignity."[6]

It was Pincus who made the decision to involve a physician because he knew human experiments would be necessary. John Rock, chief of gynecology and obstetrics at Harvard, met Pincus at a scientific conference and discovered their mutual interest in reproductive physiology. Rock and his colleagues pursued Pincus's work. Using oocytes from oophorectomies, they reported in vitro fertilization in 1944, the first demonstration of fertilization of human oocytes in vitro. Rock was interested in the work with progestational agents, not for contraception, however, but because he hoped the female sex steroids could be used to overcome infertility.

Sanger and McCormick needed some convincing that Rock's Catholicism would not be a handicap, but they were eventually won over because of his stature. Rock was a physician who literally transformed his personal values in response to his recognition of the problems secondary to uncontrolled reproduction. With the help of Luigi Mastroianni, the first administration of synthetic progestins to women was to Rock's patients in 1954. Of the first 50 patients to receive 10–40 mg of synthetic progestin (a dose extrapolated from the animal data) for 20 days each month, all failed to ovulate during treatment (causing Pincus to begin referring to the medication as "the pill"), and 7 of the 50 became pregnant after discontinuing the medication (pleasing Rock, who all along was motivated to treat infertility).

Pincus and Chang decided to announce their findings at the International Planned Parenthood meeting in Tokyo, in the fall of 1955. Rock refused to join in this effort, believing that Pincus and Chang were moving too fast. Despite this disagreement (which apparently was spirited and strong), it was done, and the Tokyo presentation generated worldwide publicity.

In 1956, with Celso-Ramon Garcia and Edris Rice-Wray, working in Puerto Rico, the first human trial was performed. The initial progestin products were contaminated with about 1% mestranol. In the amounts being used, this added up to 50–500 μg of mestranol, a sufficient amount of estrogen to inhibit ovulation by itself. When efforts to provide a more pure progestin lowered the estrogen content and yielded breakthrough bleeding, it was decided to retain the estrogen for cycle control, thus establishing the principle of the combined estrogen-progestin oral contraceptive. Early clinical trials were conducted by J. W. Goldzieher in San Antonio and E. T. Tyler in Los Angeles.

Pincus, a longtime consultant to Searle, picked the Searle compound for extended use, and with great effort, convinced Searle that the commercial potential of an oral contraceptive warranted the risk of possible negative public reaction. Pincus also convinced Rock, and together they pushed the U.S. Food and Drug Administration for acceptance of oral contraception. In 1957, Enovid was approved for the treatment of miscarriages and menstrual disorders and, in 1960, for contraception. Neither Pincus nor the Worcester Foundation got rich on the pill; alas, there was no royalty agreement.

The pill did bring Pincus fame and travel. There is no doubt that he was very much aware of the accomplishment and its implications. As he traveled and lectured in 1957, he said: "How a few precious facts obscurely come to in the laboratory may resonate into the lives of men everywhere, bring order to disorder, hope to the hopeless, life to the dying. That this is the magic and mystery of our time is sometimes grasped and often missed, but to expound it is inevitable."[6]

Pincus was the perfect person to bring oral contraception into the public world, at a time when contraception was a private, suppressed subject. Difficult projects require people like Pincus. A scientific entrepreneur, he could plow through distractions. He could be hard and aggressive with his staff. He could remain focused. He hated to lose, even in meaningless games with his children. Yet he combined a gracious, charming manner with his competitive hardness. He was filled with the kind of self-confidence that permits an individual to forge ahead, to translate vision into reality. Pincus died in 1967 (as did Katherine McCormick at the age of 92) of aplastic anemia that some have argued was caused by his long-term exposure to solvents and chemicals. Rock died in 1984 at the age of 94. Chang died in 1991 at the age of 82 and was buried in Shrewsbury, near his laboratory and close to the grave of Pincus.

Pincus wrote his book, *The Control of Fertility*, in 1964–65, only because "a break came in the apparent dam to publication on reproductive physiology and particularly its subdivisions concerned with reproductive behavior, conception, and contraception."[6]

> "We have conferred and lectured in many countries of the world, seen at first hand the research needs and possibilities in almost every European, Asiatic, Central, and South American country. We have faced the hard fact of overpopulation in country after country, learned of the bleak demographic future, assessed the prospects for the practice of efficient fertility control. This has been a saddening and a heartening experience; saddening because of the sight of continuing poverty and misery, heartening because of the dedicated colleagues and workers seeking to overcome the handicap of excess fertility and to promote healthy reproductive function. Among these we have made many friends, found devoted students."[6]

Syntex, a wholesale drug supplier, was without marketing experience or organization. By the time Syntex had secured arrangements with Ortho for a sales outlet, Searle marketed Enovid in 1960 (150 μg mestranol and 9.85 mg norethynodrel). Ortho-Novum, using norethindrone from Syntex, appeared in 1962. Wyeth Laboratories introduced norgestrel in 1968, the same year in which the first reliable prospective studies were initiated. It was not until the late 1970s that a dose-response relationship between problems and the amount of steroids in the pill was appreciated. As a result, health care providers and patients, over the years, have been confronted by a bewildering array of different products and formulations. The solution to this clinical dilemma is relatively straightforward, the theme of this chapter: use the lowest doses that provide effective contraception.

Pharmacology of Steroid Contraception

The Estrogen Component of Combination Oral Contraceptives

Estradiol is the most potent natural estrogen and is the major estrogen secreted by the ovaries. The major obstacle to the use of sex steroids for contraception was inactivity of the compounds when given orally. A major breakthrough occurred in 1938 when it was discovered that the addition of an ethinyl group at the 17 position made estradiol orally active. Ethinyl estradiol is a very potent oral estrogen and is one of the two forms of estrogen used in every oral contraceptive. The other estrogen is the 3-methyl ether of ethinyl estradiol, mestranol.

Ethinyl estradiol   Mestranol

Mestranol and ethinyl estradiol are different from natural estradiol and must be regarded as pharmacologic drugs. Animal studies have suggested that mestranol is weaker than ethinyl estradiol, because mestranol must first be converted to ethinyl estradiol in the body. Indeed, mestranol does not bind to the cellular estrogen receptor. Therefore, unconjugated ethinyl estradiol is the active estrogen in the blood for both mestranol and ethinyl estradiol. In the human body, differences in potency between ethinyl estradiol and mestranol do not appear to be significant, certainly not as great as indicated by assays in rodents. This is now a minor point because all of the low-dose oral contraceptives contain ethinyl estradiol.

The metabolism of ethinyl estradiol (particularly as reflected in blood levels) varies significantly from individual to individual and from one population to another.[7] There is even a range of variability at different sampling times within the same individual. Therefore, it is not surprising that the same dose can cause side effects in one individual and not in another.

The estrogen content (dosage) of the pill is of major clinical importance. Thrombosis is one of the most serious side effects of the pill, playing a key role in the increased risk of death (in the past with high doses) from a variety of circulatory problems. This side effect is related to estrogen, and it is dose related; therefore, the dose of estrogen is a critical issue in selecting an oral contraceptive.

The Progestin Component of Combination Oral Contraceptives

The discovery of ethinyl substitution and oral potency led (at the end of the 1930s) to the preparation of ethisterone, an orally active derivative of testosterone. In 1951, it was demonstrated that removal of the 19-carbon from ethisterone to form norethindrone did not destroy the oral activity, and most importantly, it changed the major hormonal effect from that of an androgen to that of a progestational agent. Accordingly, the progestational derivatives of testosterone were designated as 19-nortestosterones (denoting the missing 19-carbon). The androgenic properties of these compounds, however, were not totally eliminated, and minimal anabolic and androgenic potential remains within the structure.

Testosterone   Ethisterone

Ethisterone   Norethindrone

The "impurity" of 19-nortestosterone, i.e., androgenic as well as progestational effects, was further complicated in the past by a belief that they were metabolized within the body to estrogenic compounds. This question was restudied, and it was argued that the previous evidence for metabolism to estrogenic compounds was due to an artifact in the laboratory analysis. More recent studies indicate that norethindrone can be converted to ethinyl estradiol; however, the rate of this conversion is so low that insignificant amounts of ethinyl estradiol can be found in the circulation or urine following the administration of the commonly used doses of norethindrone.[8] Any estrogenic activity, therefore, would have to be due to a direct effect. In animal and human studies, however, only norethindrone, norethynodrel, and ethynodiol diacetate have estrogen activity, and it is very slight due to weak binding to the estrogen receptor.[9] Clinically, androgenic and estrogenic activities of the progestin component, therefore, are insignificant due to the low dosage in the current oral contraceptives. As with the estrogen component, serious side effects have been related to the high doses of progestins used in old formulations, not the particular progestin, and routine use of oral contraceptives should now be limited to the low-dose products.

The norethindrone family contains the following 19-nortestosterone prog-estins: norethindrone, norethynodrel, norethindrone acetate, ethynodiol diacetate, lynestrenol, norgestrel, norgestimate, desogestrel, and gestodene.

Most of the progestins closely related to norethindrone are converted to the parent compound. Thus the activity of norethynodrel, norethindrone acetate, ethynodiol diacetate, and lynestrenol is due to rapid conversion to norethindrone.

Norgestrel is a racemic equal mixture of the dextrorotatory enantiomer and the levorotatory enantiomer. These enantiomers are mirror images of each other and rotate the plane of polarized light in opposite directions. The dextrorotatory form is known as d-norgestrel, and the levorotatory form is l-norgestrel (known as levonorgestrel). Levonorgestrel is the active isomer of norgestrel.

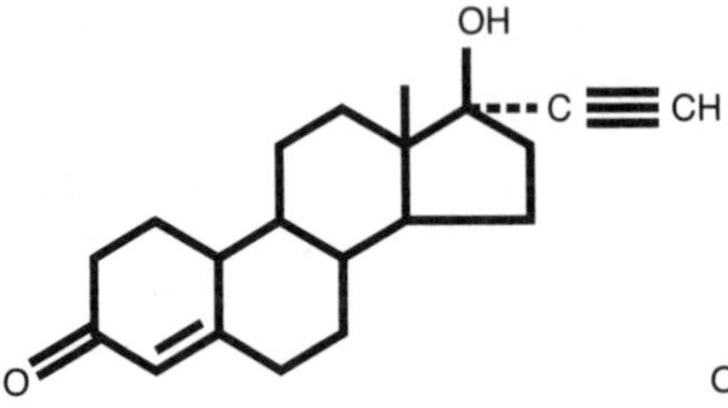

Norethindrone

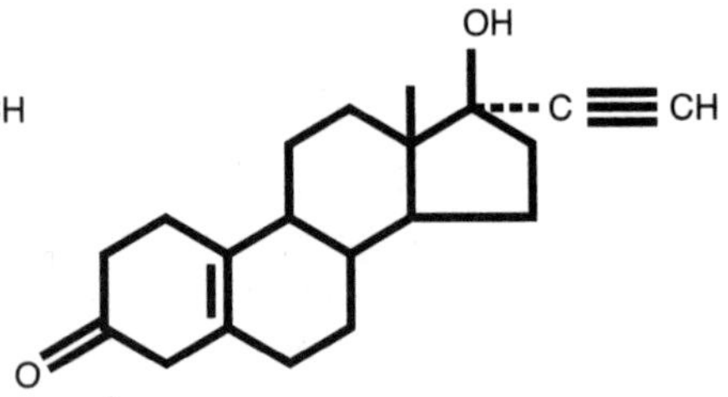

Norethynodrel

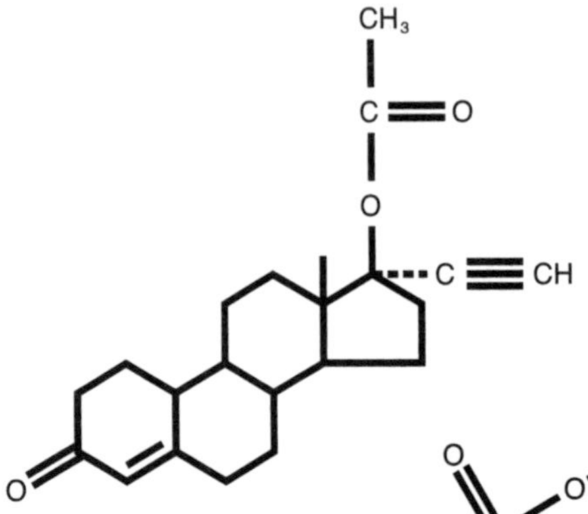

Norethindrone
acetate

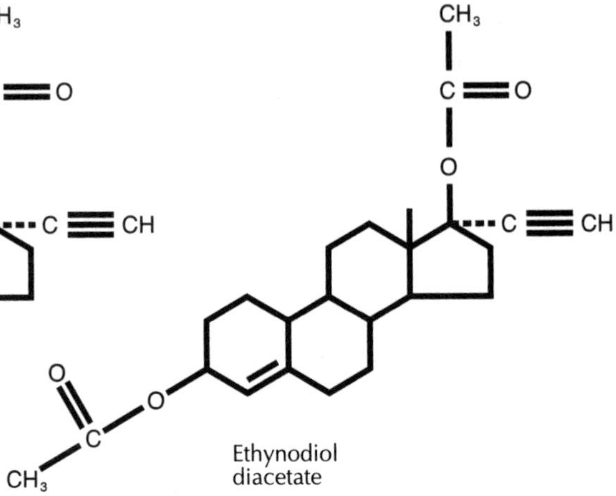

Ethynodiol
diacetate

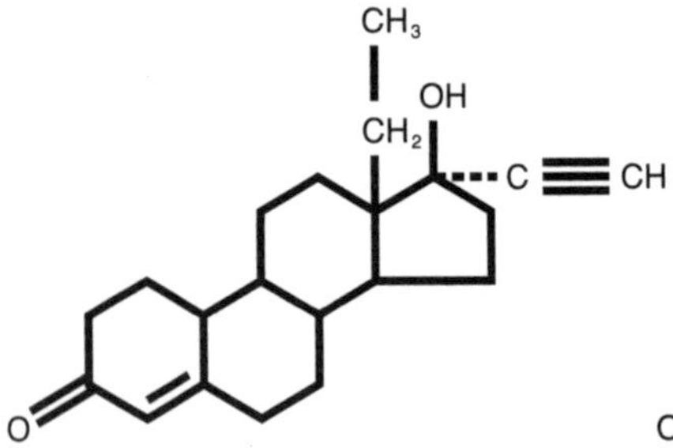

Levonorgestrel

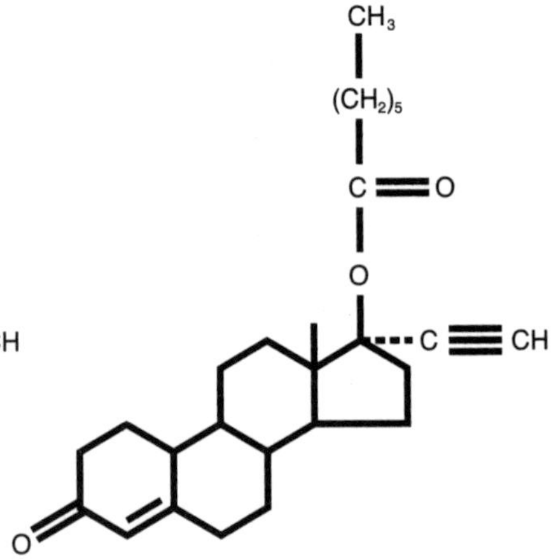

Norethindrone
enanthate

Desogestrel undergoes two metabolic steps before the progestational activity is expressed in its active metabolite, 3-keto-desogestrel, now known as etonogestrel. This metabolite differs from levonorgestrel only by a methylene group in the 11 position. Gestodene differs from levonorgestrel by the presence of a double bond between carbons 15 and 16; thus, it is Δ-15 gestodene. It is metabolized into many derivatives with progestational activity, but not levonorgestrel. Several metabolites have the potential to contribute to the activity of norgestimate. Although norgestimate is a "new" progestin, epidemiologists included it in the oral contraceptive second-generation family because its activity was believed to be largely due to levonorgestrel and levonorgestrel metabolites.[10, 11] Almost all of the biologic effects are now attributed to the 17-deacetylated metabolite, now known as norelgestromin; the levonorgestrel metabolite is tightly bound to sex hormone-binding globulin (unlike norelgestromin) severely limiting its biologic activity.[12]

DEFINITIONS USED IN EPIDEMIOLOGIC STUDIES

Low-Dose Oral Contraceptives
Products containing less than 50 μg ethinyl estradiol
First-Generation Oral Contraceptives
Products containing 50 μg or more of ethinyl estradiol
Second-Generation Oral Contraceptives
Products containing levonorgestrel, norgestimate, and other members of the norethindrone family and 20, 30, or 35 μg ethinyl estradiol
Third-Generation Oral Contraceptives
Products containing desogestrel or gestodene with 20, 25, or 30 μg ethinyl estradiol

A second group of progestins became available for use when it was discovered that acetylation of the 17-hydroxy group of 17-hydroxyprogesterone produced an orally active but weak progestin. An addition at the 6 position is necessary to give sufficient progestational strength for human use, probably by inhibiting metabolism. Derivatives of progesterone with substituents at the 17 and 6 positions include the widely used medroxyprogesterone acetate.

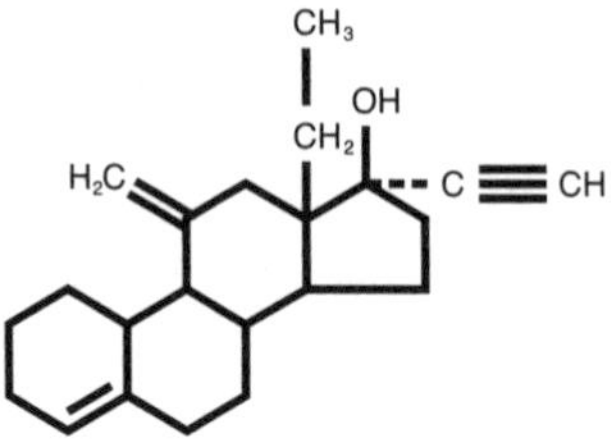

Desogestrel

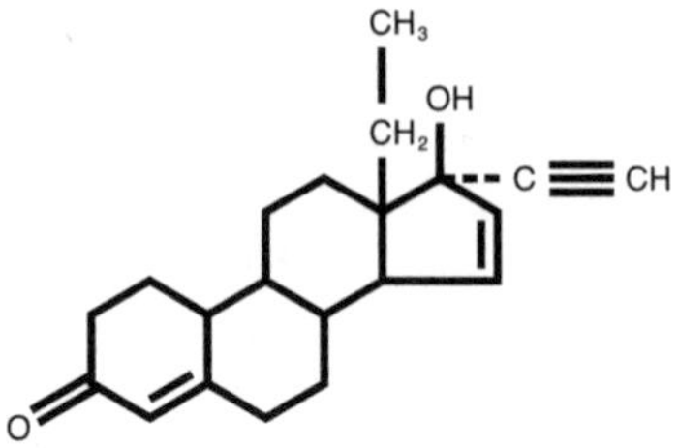

Gestodene

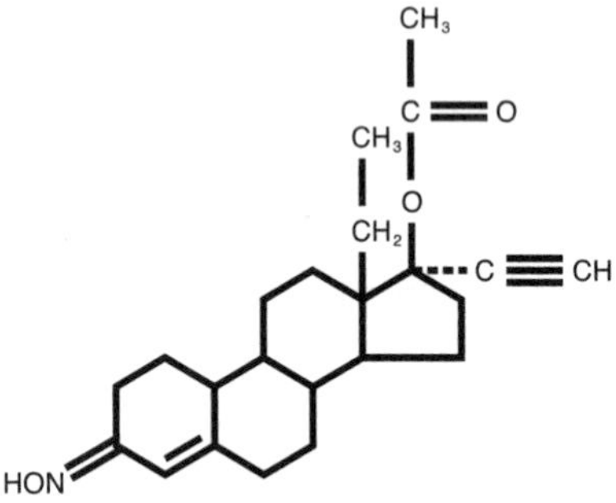

Norgestimate

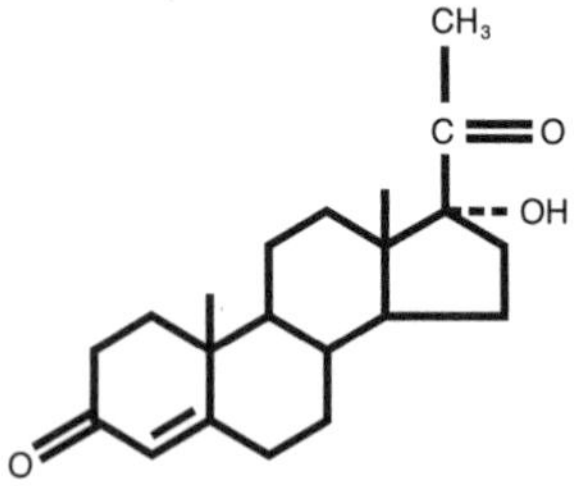

17α-Hydroxyprogesterone

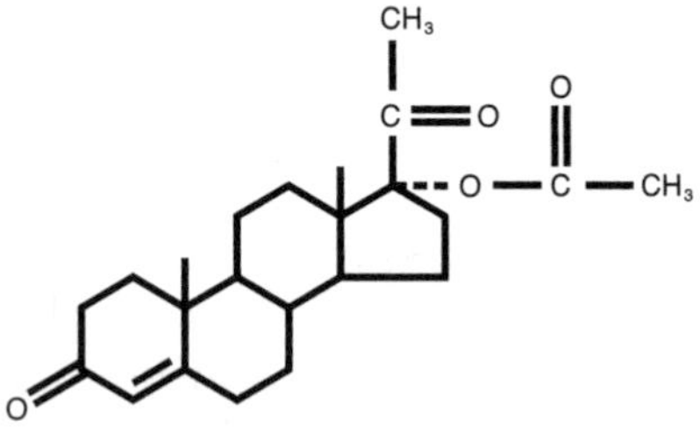

17-Acetoxy progesterone

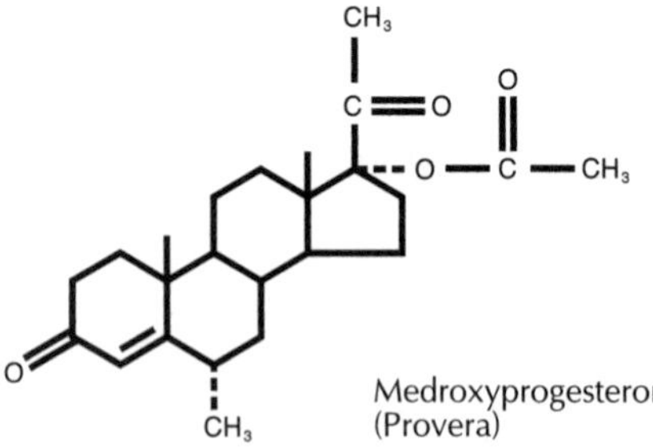

Medroxyprogesterone acetate
(Provera)

Dienogest is a 19-nortestosterone that has a cyanomethyl group instead of an ethinyl group in the 17 position, combining the properties of both the 19-nortestosterone family and the derivatives of progesterone.[13] It exerts antiandrogenic activity and is used in a 2-mg dose combined with ethinyl estradiol as an oral contraceptive.

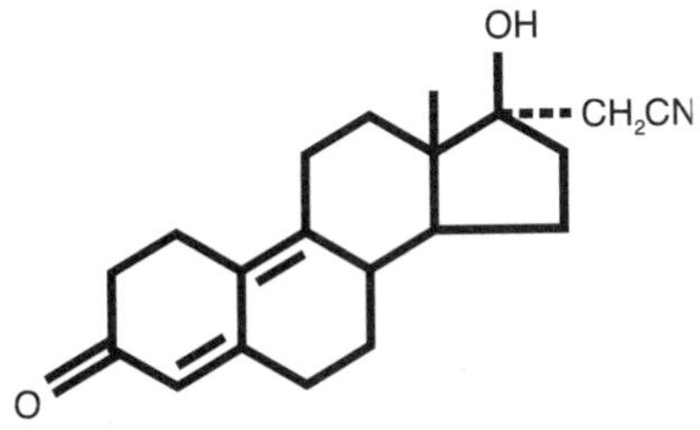

Dienogest

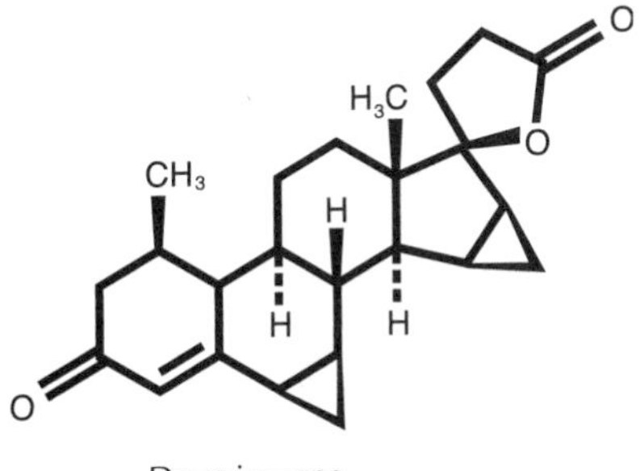

Drospirenone

New Progestins

Probably the greatest influence on the effort that yielded the new progestins was the belief throughout the 1980s that androgenic metabolic effects were important, especially in terms of cardiovascular disease. Cardiovascular side effects are now known to be due to a dose-related stimulation of thrombosis by estrogen. In the search to find compounds that minimize androgenic effects, however, the pharmaceutical companies succeeded.

The new progestins include desogestrel, gestodene, and norgestimate, and even newer progestins are in development.[14] In regard to cycle control (breakthrough bleeding and amenorrhea), the new formulations are comparable with previous low-dose products. All progestins derived from 19-nortestosterone have the potential to decrease glucose tolerance and increase insulin resistance. The impact on carbohydrate metabolism of the previous low-dose formulations was very minimal, and the impact of the new progestins is negligible. Most changes are not statistically significant, and when they are, they are so subtle as to be of no clinical significance. The decreased androgenicity of the progestins in the new products is reflected in increased sex hormone–binding globulin and decreased free testosterone concentrations to a greater degree than the older oral contraceptives. This difference could be of greater clinical value in the treatment of acne and hirsutism, but comparative clinical studies have indicated similar effects for all oral contraceptives.[15]

The new progestins, because of their reduced androgenicity, predictably do not adversely affect the cholesterol-lipoprotein profile. Indeed, the estrogen-progestin balance of combined oral contraceptives containing one of the new progestins even promotes favorable lipid changes. Thus, the new formulations have the potential to offer protection against cardiovascular disease, an important consideration as we enter an era of women using oral contraceptives for longer durations and later in life. But one must be cautious regarding the clinical significance of subtle changes, and it will be difficult to accumulate data with these rare events.

Drospirenone is a progestin that is an analogue of spironolactone. Its biochemical profile is very similar to progesterone, including a high affinity for the mineralocorticoid receptor that produces an antimineralocorticoid effect.[16, 17] Contraceptive efficacy equal to that of other formulations is achieved in the combination of 3.0 mg drospirenone and 30 μg ethinyl estradiol (Yasmin). Because drospirenone is spironolactone-like with antiandrogenic and antimineralocorticoid activity, caution is recommended in regard to serum potassium levels, avoiding its use in women with abnormal renal, adrenal, or hepatic function. It has been suggested that the oral contraceptive that contains drospirenone is effective for treating premenstrual syndrome/premenstrual dysphoric disorder (PMDD).

In an open-label, 1-year study of 326 women, Yasmin was associated with a significant reduction in scores assessing negative affect, water retention, and increased appetite during the premenstrual and menstrual phases of their cycles.[18] A similar effect was observed in new users and in those who switched from oral contraceptives. We have learned over the last decade that treatments for premenstrual syndrome must be studied in comparison with a placebo because of the powerful placebo response associated with this disorder. In the only double-blind, placebo-controlled randomized trial, 82 women with established diagnoses of PMDD were assessed using the Calendar of Premenstrual Experiences scale.[19] A statistically significant reduction associated with the oral contraceptive treatment was achieved in only one category, that measuring acne, appetite, and food cravings. The authors interpreted their results as indicating a general and consistent trend in all symptom groups, suggesting a beneficial effect of the oral contraceptive for the treatment of PMDD. However, a close look at the results easily reveals very wide standard deviations around each point, and by no means, can this study be considered conclusive or definitive.

In a multicenter 2-year study in Europe of 900 women, Yasmin was compared to Marvelon (the same dose of ethinyl estradiol and 150 μg desogestrel).[20] Marvelon was associated with a small increase in body weight after the fifth cycle; the average body weight associated with Yasmin remained throughout the 2 years below the baseline level at the beginning of the study but increased to a level above the baseline at the end of the study. The early weight loss amounted to only 1% of body weight and may reflect diuretic action. This study also showed a small reduction in premenstrual symptoms with Yasmin. There is evidence, therefore, to indicate favorable effects that could be expected to have a beneficial impact on PMDD. However, the strength of this activity in the only double-blind, placebo-controlled trial was minimal. Whether these effects are sufficient to have a meaningful clinical impact requires further study with appropriate numbers and placebo controls.

New Formulations

The multiphasic preparation alters the dosage of both the estrogen and progestin components periodically throughout the pill-taking schedule. The aim of these new formulations is to alter steroid levels in an effort to achieve lesser metabolic effects and minimize the occurrence of breakthrough bleeding and amenorrhea, while maintaining efficacy. We are probably at or very near the lowest dose levels that can be achieved without sacrificing efficacy. Metabolic studies with the multiphasic preparations indicate no differences or slight improvements over the metabolic effects of low-dose monophasic products. Low-dose oral contraceptives now include products with ethinyl estradiol daily doses of 20, 25, 30, and 35 μg.

An estrophasic approach (Estrostep) combines a continuous low dose of a progestin with a low, but gradually increasing dose of estrogen.[21] This approach minimizes estrogen exposure at the beginning of the cycle, yielding a low rate of side effects such as nausea. The increasing estrogen results in a marked increase in sex hormone–binding globulin that produces a very low androgenic state by reducing the bioavailability of circulating free androgens, and this formulation is very effective for treating acne.[22, 23]

Reduction of the pill-free interval is a strategy aimed at the concern that pill omission with low-dose oral contraceptives might more readily result in "escape" ovulation. Utilizing a 4-day pill-free interval (rather than the usual 7 days) is associated with greater ovarian suppression.[24] Another approach adds estrogen for 5 of the usual 7 pill-free days.[25] However, these approaches have failure rates and breakthrough bleeding rates that are comparable to the standard regimens, and no clear-cut advantage for these alterations can be established.

Generic Products

Generic products are therapeutically equivalent drugs, containing the same amount of active ingredients in the same concentration and dosage form. These products are less expensive, marketed by pharmaceutical companies after patent expiration of the original drug. Generic oral contraceptives need only meet the test of bioequivalence; studies to demonstrate efficacy, side effects, and safety are not required. Meeting the test of bioequivalence requires demonstration in a small number of subjects that absorption, concentrations, and time curves are comparable to the reference drug. The generic product is approved if the bioequivalence testing ranges from 80% to 120% of the values for the reference drug (differences no greater than 20%). Approved, patented products must not vary more than ±10%; therefore, a generic oral contraceptive could contain only 72% of the standard dose. In the lowest-dose oral contraceptives, this could impair efficacy. We should hasten to point out that there has been no evidence or even anecdotal suggestions that generic oral contraceptives have reduced efficacy or caused more side effects such as breakthrough bleeding.

Potency

For many years, clinicians, scientists, medical writers, and even the pharmaceutical industry have attempted to assign potency values to the various progestational components of oral contraceptives. An accurate assessment, however, has been difficult to achieve for many reasons. Progestins act on numerous target organs (e.g., the uterus, the mammary glands, and the liver), and potency varies depending on the target organ and end point being studied. In the past, animal assays, such as the Clauberg test (endometrial change in the rabbit) and the rat ventral prostate assay, were used to determine progestin potency. Although these were considered acceptable methods at the time, a better understanding of steroid hormone action and metabolism and a recognition that animal and human responses differ have led to greater reliance on data collected from human studies.

Historically, this has been a confusing issue because publications and experts used potency ranking to provide clinical advice. There is absolutely no need for confusion. Oral contraceptive progestin potency is no longer a consideration when it comes to prescribing oral contraception, because the potency of the various progestins has been accounted for by appropriate adjustments of dose. In other words, the biologic effect (in this case the clinical effect) of the various progestational components in current low-dose oral contraceptives is approximately the same. The potency of a drug does not determine its efficacy or safety, only the amount of a drug required to achieve an effect.

Clinical advice based on potency ranking is an artificial exercise that has not stood the test of time. There is no clinical evidence that a particular progestin is better or worse in terms of particular side effects or clinical responses. Thus oral contraceptives should be judged by their clinical characteristics: efficacy, side effects, risks, and benefits. Our progress in lowering the doses of the steroids contained in oral contraceptives has yielded products with little serious differences.

Mechanism of Action

The combination pill, consisting of estrogen and progestin components, is given daily for 3 of every 4 weeks. The combination pill prevents ovulation by inhibiting gonadotropin secretion via an effect on both pituitary and hypothalamic centers. The progestational agent in the pill primarily suppresses luteinizing hormone (LH) secretion (and thus prevents ovulation), while the estrogenic agent suppresses follicle-stimulating hormone (FSH) secretion (and thus prevents the emergence of a dominant follicle). Therefore, the estrogenic component significantly contributes to the contraceptive efficacy. However, even if follicular growth and development were not sufficiently inhibited, the progestational component would prevent the surge-like release of LH necessary for ovulation.

The estrogen in the pill serves two other purposes. It provides stability to the endometrium so that irregular shedding and unwanted breakthrough bleeding can be minimized, and the presence of estrogen is required to potentiate the action of the progestational agents. The latter function of estrogen has allowed reduction of the progestational dose in the pill. The mechanism for this action is probably estrogen's effect in increasing the concentration of intracellular progestational receptors. Therefore, a minimal pharmacologic level of estrogen is necessary to maintain the efficacy of the combination pill.

Because the effect of a progestational agent always takes precedence over estrogen (unless the dose of estrogen is increased many, many fold), the endometrium, cervical mucus, and perhaps tubal function reflect progestational stimulation. The progestin in the combination pill produces an endometrium that is not receptive to ovum implantation, a decidualized bed with exhausted and atrophied glands. The cervical mucus becomes thick and impervious to sperm transport. It is possible that progestational influences on secretion and peristalsis within the fallopian tubes provide additional contraceptive effects. Even if there is some ovarian follicular activity (especially with the lowest dose products), these actions serve to ensure good contraceptive efficacy.[26]

Efficacy

A clinician's anecdotal experience with contraceptive methods is truly insufficient to provide the accurate information necessary for patient counseling. The clinician must be aware of the definitions and measurements used in assessing contraceptive efficacy and must draw on the talents of appropriate experts in this area to summarize the accurate and comparative failure rates for the various methods of contraception. The publications by Trussell et al., summarized below, accomplish these purposes and are highly recommended.[27–29]

Contraceptive failures do occur and for many reasons. Thus, "method effectiveness" and "use effectiveness" have been used to designate efficacy with correct and incorrect use of a method. It is less confusing to simply compare the very best performance (the lowest expected failure rate) with the usual experience (typical failure rates) as noted in the table of failure rates during the first year of use. The lowest expected failure rates are determined in clinical trials, where the combination of highly motivated subjects and frequent support from the study personnel yields the best results. It should be noted that slightly more than half of the unintended pregnancies in the United States are due to contraceptive failures.

In view of the multiple actions of oral contraceptives, it is hard to understand how the omission of a pill or two can result in a pregnancy. Indeed, careful review of failures suggests that pregnancies usually occur because initiation of the next cycle is delayed allowing escape from ovarian suppression. Strict adherence to 7 pill-free days is critical to obtain reliable, effective contraception. For this reason, the 28-day pill package, incorporating 7 pills that do not contain steroids, is a very useful aid to ensure adherence to the necessary schedule. The most prevalent problems that can be identified associated with apparent oral contraceptive failures are vomiting and diarrhea.[30, 31] *Even if no pills have been missed, patients should be instructed to use a backup method for at least 7 days after an episode of gastroenteritis. An alternative is to place the pill in the vagina during the illness (discussed later).*

The contraceptive effectiveness of the new progestin oral contraceptives, multiphasic formulations, and lowest estrogen dose products are unequivocally comparable with older low-dose (less than 50 μg estrogen) and higher dose monophasic combination birth control pills.[26] While carefully monitored studies with motivated subjects achieve an annual failure rate of 0.1%, typical usage is associated with a 7.6% failure rate during the first year of use.[29] Contraceptive failure rates have been estimated using the data from the 1995 National Survey of Family Growth and correcting for the underreporting of induced abortion.[29, 32, 33]

Failure Rates During the First Year of Use, United States[29,32,33]

Method	Percent of Women with Pregnancy Lowest Expected	Typical
No method	85.0%	85.0%
Combination pill	0.1	7.6
Progestin-only	0.5	3.0
IUDs		
Levonorgestrel IUD	0.1	0.1
Copper T 380A	0.6	0.8
Implant	0.2	0.2
Injectable	0.3	0.3
Female sterilization	0.2	0.4
Male sterilization	0.1	0.15
Spermicides	6.0	25.7
Periodic abstinence		20.5
Calendar	9.0	
Ovulation method	3.0	
Symptothermal	2.0	
Post-ovulation	1.0	
Withdrawal	4.0	23.6
Cervical cap		
Parous women	20.0	40.0
Nulliparous women	9.0	20.0
Sponge		
Parous women	20.0	40.0
Nulliparous women	9.0	20.0
Diaphragm and spermicides	6.0	12.1
Condom		
Male	3.0	13.9
Female	5.0	21.0

Metabolic Effects of Oral Contraception

Cardiovascular Disease

In October 1995, the United Kingdom Committee on Safety of Medicines sent a letter to all U.K. physicians and pharmacists stating that women taking oral contraceptives containing desogestrel or gestodene should be urged to complete their current cycle and to continue a formulation with these progestins only if prepared to accept an increased risk of venous thromboembolism. The Committee on Safety of Medicines took this action because of observational studies that indicated a 2-fold increase in the risk of venous thromboembolism when desogestrel- and gestodene-containing contraceptives were compared with products with other progestins (mostly levonorgestrel). This action and the studies on which it was based immediately became controversial. The controversy went beyond the validity of the epidemiologic data. The publicity surrounding these events reverberated throughout Europe, leading to an immediate overall decrease in oral contraceptive use, an increase in unwanted pregnancies, and an increase in induced abortions.[34, 35]

The controversy involving new progestin oral contraceptives that began in late 1995, continued through 1996, and began to reach resolution in 1997. The fundamental question is whether oral contraceptives containing desogestrel and gestodene have a different risk of thrombosis compared with oral contraceptives containing older progestins. Thrombosis can be divided into two major categories, venous thromboembolism and arterial thrombosis. Venous thromboembolism includes both deep vein thrombosis and pulmonary embolism. Arterial thrombosis includes acute myocardial infarction and stroke.

The Coagulation System

The goal of the clotting mechanism is to produce thrombin, which converts fibrinogen to a fibrin clot. Thrombin is generated from prothrombin by factor Xa in the presence of factor V, calcium, and phospholipids. The vitamin K–dependent factors include factors VII, IX, and X, as well as prothrombin. Antithrombin III is one of the body's natural anticoagulants, an irreversible inhibitor of thrombin and factors IXa, Xa, and XIa. Protein C and protein S are two other major inhibitors of coagulation and are also vitamin K–dependent. Protein C, and its helper, protein S, inhibit clotting at the level of factors V and VIII. Tissue plasminogen activator (t-PA) is produced by endothelial cells and released when a clot forms. Both t-PA and plasminogen bind to the fibrin clot. The t-PA converts the plasminogen to plasmin, which lyses the clot by degrading the fibrin. Deficiencies of antithrombin III, protein C, and protein S are inherited in an autosomal dominant pattern, accounting for 10–15% of familial thrombosis. The most common inherited causes of venous thromboembolism are the factor V Leiden mutation, followed distantly by a mutation in the prothrombin gene.[36]

46

Coagulation Factors:
   Factors that favor clotting when increased
      Fibrinogen
      Factors VII, VIII, X
   Factors that favor clotting when decreased
      Antithrombin III
      Protein C
      Protein S

Fibrinolysis Factors:
   Factors that favor clotting when increased
      Plasminogen
      Plasminogen activator inhibitor-1 (PAI-1)
   Factor that favors clotting when decreased
      Antiplasmin

An inherited resistance to activated protein C has been identified as the basis for about 50% of cases of familial venous thrombosis, due in almost all cases to a gene alteration recognized as the factor V Leiden mutation.[37, 38] The factor V Leiden mutation is found in approximately 30% of individuals who develop venous thromboembolism.[39] Activated protein C inhibits coagulation by degrading factors V and VIII. One of the three cleavage sites in factor V is the precise site of a mutation (known as the factor V Leiden mutation) that substitutes glutamine instead of arginine at this site (adenine for guanine at nucleotide 1691 in the gene).[39] This mutation makes factor V resistant to degradation (and activation in fibrinolysis). The entire clotting cascade is then resistant to the actions of the protein C system.

Heterozygotes for the factor V Leiden mutation have an 5–8-fold increased risk of venous thrombosis, and homozygotes have an 80-fold increased risk, and this risk is further enhanced by oral contraceptive use.[40–42] The highest prevalence (3–4% of the general population) of factor V Leiden is found in Europeans, and its occurrence in populations not of European descent is very rare, perhaps explaining the low frequency of thromboembolic disease in Africa, Asia, and in Native Americans.[43] The mutation is believed to have arisen in a single ancestor approximately 21,000 to 34,000 years ago.[44] It has been suggested that this was a useful adaptation in heterozygotes in response to life-threatening bleeding, such as with childbirth.

The next most common inherited disorder after the factor V Leiden mutation is a mutation, a guanine to adenine change, in the gene encoding prothrombin.[36, 45] The prevalence of this abnormality in the white population is estimated to range from 0.7% to 4%.[46] Oral contraceptive use has been reported to markedly increase the risk of venous thrombosis in carriers of the prothrombin mutation.[47] Perhaps other unidentified disorders make a contribution because an increased risk of venous thrombosis with oral contraceptives has been reported in women with elevated prothrombin levels despite an absence of the prothrombin gene mutation.[48]

The administration of pharmacologic amounts of estrogen as in high-dose oral contraceptives causes an increase in the production of clotting factors such as factor V, factor VIII, factor X, and fibrinogen.[49] The progestin component also influences the clotting factor responses.[50] Some studies of the blood coagulation system have concluded that both monophasic and multiphasic low-dose oral contraceptives have no significant clinical impact on the coagulation system. Slight increases in thrombin formation are offset by increased fibrinolytic activity.[51, 52] Other studies of formulations containing 30 and 35 μg of ethinyl estradiol indicate an increase in clotting factors associated with an increase in platelet activity.[53] However, these changes are essentially all within normal ranges and their clinical significance is unknown.[50]

Smoking produces a shift to hypercoagulability.[54] A 20 μg estrogen formulation has been reported to have no effect on clotting parameters, even in smokers.[54, 55] One study comparing a 20 μg product with a 30 μg product found similar mild procoagulant and fibrinolytic activity, although there was a trend toward increased fibrinolytic activity with the lower dose.[56] These mixed reports make it essential to base clinical decisions on the epidemiologic studies of clinical events.

There is no evidence of an increase in risk of cardiovascular disease among past users of oral contraception.[57–59] In the Nurses' Health Study, the Royal College of General Practitioners' Study, and the Oxford Family Planning Association Study, long-term past use of oral contraceptives was not associated with an increase in overall mortality.[60–62] Part of the concern for a possible lingering effect of oral contraceptive use was based on a presumed adverse impact on the atherosclerotic process, which would then be added to the effect of aging and, thus, would be manifested later in life. Instead, the findings have been consistent with the contention that cardiovascular disease due to oral contraception is secondary to acute effects, specifically estrogen-induced thrombosis, a dose-related event.

Venous Thromboembolism — The Conventional Wisdom

Older epidemiologic evaluations of oral contraceptives and vascular disease indicated that venous thrombosis was an effect of estrogen, limited to current users, with a disappearance of the risk by 3 months after discontinuation.[63, 64] Thromboembolic disease was believed to be a consequence of the pharmacologic administration of estrogen, and the level of risk was believed to be related to the estrogen dose.[65-67] Smoking was documented to produce an additive increase in the risk of arterial thrombosis [68-70] but had no effect on the risk of venous thromboembolism.[71, 72]

Is there still a risk of venous thromboembolism with the current low-dose (less than 50 μg ethinyl estradiol) formulations of oral contraceptives? In the first years of oral contraception, the available products, containing 80 and 100 μg ethinyl estradiol (an extremely high dose), were associated with a 6-fold increased risk of venous thrombosis.[73] Because of the increased risks for venous thrombosis, myocardial infarction, and stroke, lower dose formulations (less than 50 μg estrogen) came to dominate the market, and clinicians became more careful in their screening of patients and prescribing of oral contraception. Two forces, therefore, were at work simultaneously to bring greater safety to women utilizing oral contraception: (1) the use of lower dose formulations, and (2) the avoidance of oral contraception by high-risk patients. Because of these two forces, the Puget Sound study in the United States documented a reduction in venous thrombosis risk to 2-fold.[74] The new studies also reflect the importance of these two forces, but they still indicate an increased risk.

Venous Thromboembolism — The Controversial Studies

The World Health Organization (WHO) Collaborative Study of Cardiovascular Disease and Steroid Hormone Contraception was a hospital-based, case-control study with subjects collected from 21 centers in 17 countries in Africa, Asia, Europe, and Latin America.[75] As part of this study, the risk of idiopathic venous thromboembolism associated with a formulation containing 30 μg ethinyl estradiol and levonorgestrel (doses ranging from 125 to 250 μg) was compared with the risk with preparations containing 20 or 30 μg ethinyl estradiol and either desogestrel or gestodene (data from 10 centers in 9 countries).[76] There were only 9 cases and 3 controls using combined oral contraceptives with other progestins, precluding precise analysis. The users of the levonorgestrel formulations had an increased odds ratio (an estimation of relative risk used in case-control studies) of 3.5 compared with nonusers. Current users of a desogestrel product had an increased risk of 9.1 compared with nonusers, and with gestodene, the odds ratio was also 9.1. Thus, the increased risk for desogestrel and gestodene was 2.6 times that of levonorgestrel, when adjusted for body weight and height. Also of note, the increased risk for the desogestrel formulation containing 20 μg ethinyl estradiol was 38.2, a number that is obviously not reliable because it was based upon only 8 cases and 1 control; the confidence interval (CI) of 4.5–325 reflected this imprecision. Overall, these increased risks were lower than those estimated by earlier case-control studies of higher dose oral contraceptives.

The Transnational Study on Oral Contraceptives and the Health of Young Women analyzed 471 cases of deep vein thrombosis and/or venous thromboembolism from the United Kingdom and Germany.[77] Second-generation oral contraceptives were defined as products containing 35 μg or less of ethinyl estradiol and a progestin other than desogestrel or gestodene. Comparing users of second-generation products to nonusers, the odds ratio was 3.2 (CI = 2.3–4.3). Comparing users of desogestrel and gestodene products to users of second-generation oral contraceptives, the risk of venous thromboembolism was 1.5-fold greater.

A third major study was from Boston University, but the data were derived from **the General Practice Research Database,** a computerized system involving the general practitioners in the United Kingdom.[78] Using this cohort, the authors calculated the death rate from pulmonary embolism, stroke, and acute myocardial infarction in the users of levonorgestrel, desogestrel, and gestodene low-dose oral contraceptives. Over a 3-year period, they collected a total of 15 unexpected idiopathic cardiovascular deaths in users of these products, a nonsignificant change, and no difference in the risk comparing desogestrel and gestodene with levonorgestrel. The risk estimates for venous thromboembolism (adjusted for smoking and body size) were about 2 times greater for desogestrel and for gestodene, compared with levonorgestrel uses. There were only 4 cases and 9 controls using the 20 μg ethinyl estradiol and desogestrel product, and although the risk was similar to that associated with the 30 μg ethinyl estradiol and desogestrel product, this is too small a number for analysis. In an updated analysis from this same group and database, the findings were unchanged, except that smoking was found to be a risk factor for venous thromboembolism.[79]

Similar results were reported when women with deep vein thrombosis in the **Leiden Thrombophilia Study** in the Netherlands were reanalyzed for their use of oral contraceptives.[80] As expected, the risk of deep vein thrombosis was markedly higher in women who were carriers of the factor V Leiden mutation and in women with a family history of thrombosis.

Venous Thromboembolism — Subsequent Studies

The reports in late 1995 and early 1996 were followed by a flood of letters to editors, as well as reviews and editorials, highlighting confounding and bias problems in these studies.[81–83] Some prominent figures were convinced the reports of increased risks with desogestrel and gestodene were real;[84, 85] others were skeptical, pointing out possible confounding biases. Subsequently, reanalysis and new studies did reveal confounders and biases in the initial studies.

In Denmark, Lidegaard and colleagues performed a hospital-based, case-control study of women with confirmed diagnoses of venous thromboembolism in 1994 and 1995 (in Denmark, all women with this diagnosis are hospitalized, and, therefore, very few, if any, cases were missed).[86] A 2-fold increased risk of venous thromboembolism was found in current users of oral contraceptives, regardless of estrogen doses ranging from 20 to 50 μg. The increased risk was concentrated in the first year of use. **Because there were more short-term users of the new progestins and more long-term users of the older progestins, adjustment for duration of use resulted in no significant differences between the different types of progestins.** Those factors associated with an increased risk of thromboembolism included coagulation disorders, treated hypertension during pregnancy, family history of venous thromboembolism, and an increasing body mass index. Notably, conditions not associated with an increased risk of venous thromboembolism included smoking, migraine, diabetes, hyperlipidemia, parity, or age at first birth. There was still insufficient strength in this study to establish the absence or presence of a dose-response relationship comparing the 20 μg estrogen dose to higher doses; however, a 5-year update reported the following useful information:[87]

- The risk of venous thrombosis associated with current use of oral contraceptives declined with increasing duration of use.
- The risk was slightly greater with desogestrel or gestodene.
- Smoking more than 10 cigarettes per day increased the risk.
- Oral contraceptives with 20 μg estrogen had a lower risk than products with 30–40 μg.
- Progestin-only contraceptive products did not increase the risk.

Case-control studies using cases of venous thromboembolism derived from the computer records of general practices in the U.K. concluded that the increased risk associated with oral contraceptives was the same for all types, and that the pattern of risk with specific oral contraceptives suggested confounding because of "preferential prescribing" (defined later).[88, 89] *In these studies, matching cases and controls by year of birth eliminated differences between different types of oral contraceptives.* A similar analysis based on 42 cases from a German database again found no difference between new progestin and older progestin oral contraceptives.[90] Thus, in these two studies, more precise adjustments for age eliminated a confounding bias. An assessment of the incidence of venous thromboembolism in the United Kingdom before and after the decline in third-generation progestin use could detect no impact on the statistics (neither an increase nor a decrease).[91]

A reanalysis of the Transnational Case-Control Study considered the duration and patterns of oral contraceptive use.[92, 93] This reanalysis focused on first-time users of second- and third-generation oral contraceptives. *Statistical analysis with adjustment for duration of use in 105 cases who were first-time users could find no differences between second- and third-generation products.* Similarly, a reanalysis of the U.K. General Practice Database could demonstrate no difference between different oral contraceptive formulations.[94]

A case-control study in Germany assessed the outcome when the cases were restricted to hospitalized patients compared to results when all cases, both in-hospital and out-of-hospital, were considered.[95] The conclusion indicated that hospital-based studies overestimated the risk of venous thromboembolism, and that there was no difference comparing progestins when all cases were included.

Evaluation of the Studies

An immediate problem with the initial studies was how to reconcile the results with the conventional wisdom that thrombosis is an estrogen dose-related complication. Progestational agents, and desogestrel and gestodene in particular, have no significant impact on clotting parameters.[14] Therefore, there was inherent biologic implausibility surrounding the new studies. The initial reports resurrected the claim by Kuhl in 1988 and 1989 that gestodene could cause more thrombosis because it affected ethinyl estradiol metabolism, resulting in higher estrogen levels.[96, 97] Other laboratories, however, could not replicate Kuhl's findings.[98, 99]

Former users discontinue oral contraceptives for a variety of reasons, and often are switched to what clinicians perceive to be "safer" products ("preferential prescribing").[100–102] Individuals who do well with a product tend to remain with that product. Thus, at any one point in time, individuals on an older product are relatively healthy and free of side effects ("healthy user effect"). This is also called attrition of susceptibles because higher risk individuals with problems are gradually eliminated from the group.[82] *Comparing users of older and newer products, therefore, can involve disparate cohorts of individuals.*

Because desogestrel- and gestodene-containing products were marketed as less androgenic and therefore "better" (a marketing claim not substantiated by epidemiologic studies), clinicians chose to provide these products to higher risk patients and older women.[100, 101] In addition, clinicians switched patients perceived to be at greater risk for thrombosis from older oral contraceptives to the newer formulations with desogestrel and gestodene. Furthermore, these products were prescribed more often to young women who were starting oral contraception for the first time (these young women will not have experienced the test of pregnancy or previous oral contraceptive use to help identify those who have a congenital predisposition to venous thrombosis). These changing practice patterns exert different effects over the lifetime of a product, and analytical adjustments are extremely difficult. The Transnational Group believed it accomplished an appropriate adjustment by focusing on first-time users and duration of use.[92] It is also unlikely that the "healthy user effect" is dominant in first-time users. And, of course, this analysis found no differences between second- and third-generation oral contraceptives.

The challenge for a clinician is to make a decision: is an observational study with statistically significant results clinically (biologically) real? This controversy illustrates how difficult this can be. When faced with results from observational studies, clinicians want to see uniformity, consistency, agreement—all arguing in favor of a real clinical effect; an example is the protective effect of oral contraceptives on the risk of ovarian cancer. The initial studies were impressive in their agreement. All indicated increased relative risks associated with desogestrel and gestodene compared with levonorgestrel. Nevertheless, all of the early studies, somewhat similar in design, were influenced by the same unrecognized biases. *Persistent errors produce consistent conclusions.*

Forty cases of venous thrombosis in drospirenone (Yasmin) users (two of which were fatal) were reported in Europe in 2002.[103] The Dutch College of General Practitioners issued a statement encouraging clinicians not to prescribe Yasmin. However, this is the similar story we experienced with "third-generation" progestins, only to learn that preferential prescribing and the healthy user effect probably biased the early case-control studies. In postmarketing surveillance, only one case of venous thrombosis occurred in a million cycles of Yasmin compared with 5 among users of other oral contraceptives.[103]

The risk of venous thrombosis associated with modern oral contraceptives is increased but manifested primarily in the first years of use. The risk is influenced in a major way by the estrogen dose, and the difference between second-generation and third-generation progestin products is small, either real and not meaningful clinically or a reflection of biases and confounders. The impact of smoking on the risk of venous thrombosis is less than that on the risk of arterial thrombosis.

Venous Thromboembolism and the Factor V Leiden Mutation

A risk of idiopathic venous thrombosis persists with low-dose oral contraceptives, at a level of approximately 3–4-fold greater than the normal, general incidence.[76-78, 80, 104] However, an inherited resistance to activated protein C, the factor V Leiden mutation, may account for a significant portion of the patients who experience venous thrombosis while taking oral contraceptives.

Relative Risk and Actual Incidence of
Venous Thromboembolism[40–42, 105, 109]

Population	Relative Risk	Incidence
Young women-general population	1	4–5 per 100,000 per year
Pregnant women	12	48–60
High-dose oral contraceptives	6–10	24–50
Low-dose oral contraceptives	3–4	12–20
Leiden mutation carrier	6–8	24–40
Leiden carrier and oral contraceptives	10–15	40–75
Leiden mutation - homozygous	80	320–400

An inherited resistance to activated protein C, the factor V Leiden mutation, is the most common inherited coagulation problem, transmitted in an autosomal-dominant fashion.[37, 106] Heterozygotes have a 5- to 8-fold increased risk of venous thromboembolism, and homozygotes an 80-fold increased risk. Oral contraceptive users who have this mutation have been reported to have a 30-fold increased risk of venous thrombosis.[107, 108] Some have argued, however, that this increase has been overestimated, and it may be closer to 10–15-fold.[41, 109] The risk of developing venous thrombosis is greatest in the initial months of use, and it has been suggested that venous thrombosis occurring in the first month of exposure should make the clinician suspect the presence of a clotting disorder.[110]

An American case-control study confirmed the approximately 3–4-fold increased risk of venous thrombosis with the current use of low-dose oral contraceptives.[42] The risk for women with Factor V Leiden mutations increased 11-fold (comparable to the risk in a pooled analysis of case-control studies[41]). Almost half of the cases in current users occurred in women with a BMI greater than 30.

Should screening for the factor V Leiden mutation (or for other inherited clotting disorders) be routine prior to prescribing contraceptives? The carrier frequencies of the Leiden mutation in the American population (the percentages are similar in men and women) are as follows:[105]

Caucasian Americans	—	5.27%
Hispanic Americans	—	2.21%
Native Americans	—	1.25%
Black Americans	—	1.23%
Asian Americans	—	0.45%

These estimates are consistent with the European assessments, indicating that this is a trait carried in people of European origin. In the United States, of the approximately 10 million women currently using oral contraceptives, about 450,000 are likely to carry the factor V Leiden mutation. However, because the incidence rate of venous thromboembolism is so low (4–5 per 100,000 young women per year),[40, 105] the number of women required to be screened to prevent one death is prohibitively large. The prevalence of all deficiencies is only about 0.5% in the asymptomatic population, and only one-third of patients at risk are detected by the present tests.[111]

Furthermore, because only a small number of women even with the Leiden mutation (less than 1 in 1,000) have a clinical event (99.85% of the individuals who test positively will NOT have a clinical event!), the finding of a positive screening test, especially considering the high rate of false-positive tests, would be a barrier to the use of oral contraceptives, and a subsequent increase in unwanted pregnancies (which has an even greater risk of venous thromboembolism) would likely follow. *Most experts believe that screening for inherited disorders should be pursued only in women with a previous episode of venous thromboembolism or a close positive family history (parent or sibling) of venous thrombosis.*

Arterial Thrombosis

Because the incidence of cerebral thrombotic attacks (thrombotic strokes and transient ischemic attacks) among young women is higher than venous thromboembolism and myocardial infarction, and death and disability are more likely, cerebral arterial thrombosis is the most important possible side effect. A very low incidence of stroke in young women carries with it little increase in absolute risk. However, because the incidence of cerebral thrombotic attacks is higher in women over age 40, we should do our best, as the following discussion indicates, to make sure oral contraceptive users over age 40 are in good health and without significant risk factors for cardiovascular disease (especially hypertension, migraine with aura, and smoking).

It has been difficult to establish arterial thrombosis dose-response relationships with estrogen because these events are so rare. Nevertheless, the estrogen dose is important for the risk of myocardial infarction and thrombotic strokes.[112, 113] Thus, a rationale for advocating low-dose estrogen oral contraceptives continues to be valid.

Arterial Thrombosis — Myocardial Infarction

A population-based, case-control study analyzed 187 cases of myocardial infarction in users of low-dose oral contraceptives in the Kaiser Permanente Medical Care Program.[114] *There was no statistically significant increase in the odds ratio for myocardial infarction in current oral contraceptive users compared with past or never users.*

In the Transnational case-control study of myocardial infarctions collected from 16 centers in Austria, France, Germany, Switzerland, and the United Kingdom, the results were as follows:[115, 116]

	Cases	Controls	Odds Ratio	Confidence Interval
Any OC use	57	156	2.35	1.42–3.89
50 μg estrogen OCs	14	22	4.32	1.59–11.74
Old progestin OCs	28	71	2.96	1.54–5.66
New progestin OCs	7	49	0.82	0.29–2.31

These data were interpreted as indicating no increased risk of myocardial infarction associated with oral contraceptives containing desogestrel or gestodene. However, the reduced risk with the new progestin oral contraceptives was also emphasized (the comparison of third-generation products to second-generation products yielded a reduced risk that was statistically significant), suggesting a possible saving of deaths from myocardial infarction with desogestrel and gestodene. The problem is that the small actual incidence makes it difficult to acquire sufficient numbers. The conclusion was based on only 7 cases and 49 controls using third-generation oral contraceptives and 28 cases and 71 controls using second-generation products, and, in our view, the power is too limited to make any conclusion regarding the new progestin oral contraceptives. A similar limitation was apparent in a case-control study from the Netherlands and another from the United Kingdom[117, 118] This is a good example of a conclusion that may be statistically significant but clinically not real. A meta-analysis of recent studies on the risk of myocardial infarction concluded that the third-generation progestins were not associated with an increase in risk, but again the numbers were inadequate to support a beneficial impact.[119] The rare occurrence of a myocardial infarction in young women, especially young women free of cardiovascular risk factors, makes it unlikely that epidemiologic studies will detect meaningful differences comparing different formulations of oral contraceptives.

The Transnational study found that cigarette smoking carried a higher risk for myocardial infarction than oral contraceptives, and that nonsmoking users of oral contraceptives had no evidence of an increased risk.[115] In addition, there was an indication that patient screening is important in minimizing the impact of hypertension on the risk of myocardial infarction. Similar results were reported in a case-control study based on subjects in England, Scotland, and Wales and another in America.[117, 120]

In the WHO multicenter study, there were 368 cases of acute myocardial infarction.[121] Factors associated with an increased risk of myocardial infarction included smoking, a history of hypertension (including hypertension in pregnancy), diabetes, rheumatic heart disease, abnormal blood lipids, and a family history of stroke or myocardial infarction. Duration of use and past use of oral contraceptives did not affect risk. Although there was about a 5-fold overall increased odds ratio of myocardial infarction in current users of oral contraceptives, essentially all cases occurred in women with cardiovascular risk factors. There was no apparent effect of increasing age on risk; however, there were only 12 cases among oral contraceptives users less than 35 years old. There was no apparent relationship with estrogen dose, and there was no apparent influence of type or dose of progestin, but the rare occurrence of this condition produced such small numbers that there was insufficient statistical power to accurately assess the effects of progestin type, and estrogen and progestin doses. *The conclusion of this study was that the risk of myocardial infarction in women who use oral contraceptives is increased only in smokers.*

In a Danish case-control study of acute myocardial infarction in young women, a statistically significant increase in risk was noted only in current users of 50 µg ethinyl estradiol.[113] There was a progressive increase in risk with the number of cigarettes smoked, (accounting for 80% of the acute myocardial infarctions in young women), increasing body mass index, treated hypertension, treated hypertension in pregnancy, diabetes mellitus, hyperlipidemia, frequent migraine, and family history of myocardial infarction. However, only family history of myocardial infarction and smoking affected the risk associated with oral contraceptives; no influence on oral contraceptive risk was apparent with diabetes, hypertension, and heart disease. No differences could be demonstrated according to type of progestin.

A case-control study from the Netherlands found that the risk of myocardial infarction was highest among users of oral contraceptives who smoked, had diabetes mellitus, or who were hypercholesterolemic.[118] The risk of myocardial infarction was not affected by the presence of the factor V Leiden mutation or the prothrombin gene mutation.

Incidence of Myocardial Infarction in Reproductive Age Women [121]

Overall incidence [105]	5 per 100,000 per year
Women less than age 35	
Nonsmokers	4
Nonsmokers & OCs	4
Smokers	8
Smokers & OCs	43
Women 35 years old and older	
Nonsmokers	10
Nonsmokers & OCs	40
Smokers	88
Smokers & OCs	485

NOTE: The above incidences are estimates based on oral contraceptive use paired with cardiovascular risk factors prevalent in the general population. Effective screening would produce smaller numbers. The increased risks in the smokers and OC groups reflect the impact of undetected cardiovascular risk factors, especially hypertension.

Arterial Thrombosis — Stroke

Older case-control and cohort studies indicated an increased risk of cerebral thrombosis among current users of high-dose oral contraceptives.[123–125] However, thrombotic stroke did not appear to be increased in healthy, nonsmoking women with the use of oral contraceptives containing less than 50 μg ethinyl estradiol.[124, 125] A case-control study of all 794 women in Denmark who suffered a cerebral thromboembolic attack during 1985–1989 concluded that there was an almost 2-fold increased relative risk associated with oral contraceptives containing 30–40 μg estrogen, and the risk was significantly influenced by both smoking and the dose of estrogen in additive (not synergistic) fashion.[70] A case-control analysis of data collected by the Royal College of General Practitioners' Oral Contraception Study concluded that current users were at increased risk of stroke (with a persisting effect in former users); however, this outcome was limited mainly to smokers and to formulations with 50 μg or more of estrogen.[125]

A population-based, case-control study of 408 strokes from the California Kaiser Permanente Medical Care Program found no increase in risk for either ischemic stroke or hemorrhagic stroke.[126] The identifiable risk factors for ischemic stroke were smoking, hypertension, diabetes, elevated body weight, and low socioeconomic status. The risk factors for hemorrhagic stroke were the same plus greater body mass and heavy use of alcohol. *Current users of low-dose oral contraceptives did not have an increased risk of ischemic or hemorrhagic stroke compared with former users and with never users.* There was no evidence for an adverse effect of increasing age or for smoking (for hemorrhagic stroke, there was a suggestion of a positive interaction between current oral contraceptive use and smoking, but the numbers were small, and the result was not statistically significant).

The Transnational study analyzed their data for ischemic stroke in a case-control study of 220 ischemic strokes in the United Kingdom, Germany, France, Switzerland, and Austria.[127] Overall, there was a 3-fold increase in the risk of ischemic stroke associated with the use of oral contraceptives, with higher risks observed in smokers (more than 10 cigarettes per day), in women with hypertension, and in users of higher dose estrogen products. No differences were observed comparing second- and third-generation progestins. A Dutch case-control study also found no differences comparing second- and third-generation progestins.[128] A case-control study from the state of Washington concluded that there is no increased risk of stroke in current users of low-dose oral contraceptives.[129] A pooled analysis of the data from California and Washington concluded that low-dose oral contraceptives are not associated with an increase in the risk of stroke.[130]

The World Health Organization data on stroke come from the same collaborative study that yielded the publications on venous thromboembolism. The results with stroke were published as two separate reports, one on ischemic stroke and the other on hemorrhagic stroke.[131, 132]

This hospital-based, case-control study from 21 centers in 17 countries accumulated 697 cases of ischemic stroke, 141 from Europe and 556 from developing countries.[131] The overall odds ratio for ischemic stroke indicated about a 3-fold increased risk. In Europe, however, the risk was statistically significant only for higher-dose products and **NOT** statistically significant for products with less than 50 μg ethinyl estradiol. In developing countries, there was no difference in risk with low-dose and higher dose oral contraceptives. This is believed to be due to the strong influence of hypertension. In Europe, it was uncommon for women with a history of hypertension to be using oral contraceptives; however, this was not the case in developing countries. Duration of use and type of progestin had no impact, and past users did not have an increased risk, but smoking 10 or more cigarettes daily exerted a synergistic effect with oral contraceptives, increasing the risk of ischemic stroke, approximating the effect of hypertension and oral contraceptives. The risk was greater in women 35 years and older; however, this, too, was believed to be due to an effect of hypertension. *Thus, the conclusion of this study was that the risk of ischemic stroke is extremely low, concentrated in those who use higher dose products, smoke, or have hypertension.*

In the WHO study on hemorrhagic stroke, there were 1,068 cases.[132] Current use of oral contraceptives was associated with a slightly increased risk of hemorrhagic stroke only in developing countries, not in Europe. This again probably reflects the presence of hypertension, because the greatest increased risk (about 10- to 15-fold) was identified in current users of oral contraceptives who had a history of hypertension. Current cigarette smoking also increased the risk in oral contraceptive users, but not as dramatically as hypertension. For hemorrhagic stroke, the dose of estrogen had no effect on risk, and neither did duration of use or type of progestin. *This study concluded that the risk of hemorrhagic stroke due to oral contraceptives is increased only slightly in older women, probably occurring only in women with risk factors such as hypertension.*

A second Danish case-control study included thrombotic strokes and transitory cerebral ischemic attacks analyzed together as cerebral thromboembolic attacks.[112] In this study, the 219 cases during 1994 and 1995 included 146 cases of cerebral infarction and 73 cases of transient ischemic attacks. There was a dose-response relationship with estrogen in the dose ranges of 20, 30–40, and 50 μg ethinyl estradiol, although the number of 20 μg users (5 cases, 22 controls) was not sufficient to establish a lower risk at this lower dose. This analysis claimed a reduced risk associated with desogestrel and gestodene; however, the odds ratio did not achieve statistical significance. An updated 5-year report of the Danish case-control study indicated that the odds ratio of cerebral thrombosis decreased from a high of 4.5 with 50 μg estrogen pills to 1.6 with 20–40 μg pills.[133] Hypertension increased the risk 5-fold, migraine 3.2 times, diabetes 5.6 times, and hyperlipidemia and coagulation disorders about 12-fold.

Incidence of Stroke in Reproductive Age Women[122, 126, 131, 132]

Incidence of ischemic stroke	5 per 100,000 per year
	1–3 per 100,000 per year in women under age 35
	10 per 100,000 per year in women over age 35
Incidence of hemorrhagic stroke	6 per 100,000 per year
Excess cases per year due to OCs, *including smokers and hypertensives*	2 per 100,000 per year in low-dose OC users
	1 per 100,000 per year in low-dose OC users under age 35
	8 per 100,000 per year in high-dose users

Arterial Thrombosis — Current Assessment

There has been no evidence with respectable statistical power that the new progestins have an appreciable difference in risk for arterial disease, an event that is already **NOT** increased with low-dose older-type progestin oral contraceptives. It is possible that as these studies continue and acquire greater statistical power, a difference will emerge, but even if this is the case, the difference will be minor and likely unmeasureable. Conclusions based on a limited number of cases are premature, and a critical attitude toward arterial thrombosis is appropriate just as such an approach finally revealed likely explanations for the initial findings with venous thrombosis.

Most importantly, the new studies fail to find any substantial risk of ischemic or hemorrhagic stroke with low-dose oral contraceptives in healthy, young women. The WHO study did find evidence for an adverse impact of smoking in women under age 35; the Kaiser study did not. This difference is explained by the confounding effect of hypertension, the major risk factor identified. In the WHO study, a history of hypertension was based on whether a patient reported ever having had high blood pressure (other than in pregnancy) and not validated by medical records. In the Kaiser study, women were classified as having hypertension if they reported using antihypertensive medication (less than 5% of oral contraceptive users had treated hypertension, and there were no users of higher dose products). In the WHO study, the effect of using oral contraceptives in the presence of a high-risk factor is apparent in the different odds ratios when European women who received good screening from clinicians were compared with women in developing countries who received little screening; therefore, more women with cardiovascular risk factors in developing countries were using oral contraceptives.

Over the years, there has been recurring discussion over whether to provide oral contraceptives over-the-counter on a nonprescription basis. The data in the WHO report make an impressive argument against such a move. The increased risk of myocardial infarction was most evident in developing countries where 70% of the cases received their oral contraceptives from a nonclinical source. Deprived of screening, women with risk factors in developing countries were exposed to greater risk.

Oral contraceptives containing less than 50 µg ethinyl estradiol do not increase the risk of myocardial infarction or stroke in healthy, nonsmoking women, regardless of age. The effect of smoking in women under age 35 is, as we have long recognized, not detectable in the absence of hypertension. After age 35, the subtle presence of hypertension makes analysis difficult, but the Kaiser study indicates that increasing age and smoking by themselves have little impact on the risk of stroke in low-dose oral contraceptive users. The screening of patients in the Kaiser program was excellent, resulting in few women with hypertension using oral contraceptives. *The new studies indicate that hypertension should be a major concern, especially in regards to the risk of stroke.*

Smoking

Smoking continues to be a difficult problem, not only for patient management but for analysis of data as well. In large U.S. surveys in 1982 and 1988, the decline in the prevalence of smoking was similar in users and nonusers of oral contraception; however, 24.3% of 35- to 45-year-old women who used oral contraceptives were smokers![134] In this group of smoking, oral contraceptive-using women, 85.3% smoked 15 or more cigarettes per day (heavy smoking). Despite the widespread teaching and publicity that smoking is a contraindication to oral contraceptive use over the age of 35, more older women who used oral contraceptives smoked and smoked heavily, compared with young women. This strongly implies that older smokers are less than honest with clinicians when requesting oral contraception, and this further raises serious concern over how well this confounding variable can be controlled in case-control and cohort studies. *A former smoker must have stopped smoking for at least 12 consecutive months to be regarded as a nonsmoker. Women who have nicotine in their bloodstream obtained from patches or gum should be regarded as smokers.*

Lipoproteins and Oral Contraception

The balance of estrogen and progestin potency in a given oral contraceptive formulation can potentially influence cardiovascular risk by its overall effect on lipoprotein levels. Oral contraceptives with relatively high doses of progestins (doses not used in today's low-dose formulations) do produce unfavorable lipoprotein changes.[135] The levonorgestrel triphasic exerts no significant changes on HDL-cholesterol, LDL-cholesterol, apoprotein B, and no change or an increase in apoprotein A. The monophasic desogestrel and desogestrel pills have a favorable effect on the lipoprotein profile, while the triphasic norgestimate and gestodene pills produce beneficial alterations in the LDL/HDL and apoprotein B/apoprotein A ratios.[136–139] Like the triphasic levonorgestrel pills, norethindrone multiphasic pills have no significant impact on the lipoprotein profile over 6–12 months.[140] *In summary, studies of low-dose formulations indicate that the adverse effects of progestins are limited to the fixed-dose combination with a dose of levonorgestrel that exceeds that in the multiphasic formulation or in the low-dose products.* The formulation that contains 100 μg levonorgestrel and 20 μg ethinyl estradiol produces short-term changes in the lipid profile that are similar to those seen with other low-dose oral contraceptives, and with long-term use, the levels revert to those observed at baseline before treatment.[141]

An important study in monkeys indicated a protective action of estrogen against atherosclerosis, but by a mechanism independent of the cholesterol-lipoprotein profile. Oral administration of a combination of estrogen and progestin to monkeys fed a high-cholesterol, atherogenic diet decreased the extent of coronary atherosclerosis despite a reduction in HDL-cholesterol levels.[142–144] In somewhat similar experiments, estrogen treatment markedly prevented arterial lesion development in rabbits.[145–147] In considering the impact of progestational agents, lowering of HDL is not necessarily atherogenic if accompanied by a significant estrogen impact. These animal studies help explain why older, higher dose combinations, which had an adverse impact on the lipoprotein profile did not increase subsequent cardiovascular disease.[57, 60] The estrogen component provided protection through a direct effect on vessel walls, especially favorably influencing vasomotor and platelet factors such as nitric oxide and prostacyclin.

This conclusion is reinforced by angiographic and autopsy studies. Young women with myocardial infarctions who have used oral contraceptives have less diffuse atherosclerosis than nonusers.[148, 149] Indeed, a case-control study indicated that the risk of myocardial infarction in patients taking older, high-dose levonorgestrel-containing formulations is the same as that experienced with pills containing other progestins.[57] An analysis of the database in the Women's Health Initiative revealed a reduced risk of cardiovascular disease in postmenopausal women who had been previous users of oral contraceptives; a finding that should be viewed with some caution because the clinical trial was not designed to address this issue.[150]

In the past two decades, we have been subjected to considerable marketing hype about the importance of the impact of oral contraceptives on the cholesterol-lipoprotein profile. If indeed certain oral contraceptives had a negative impact on the lipoprotein profile, one would expect to find evidence of atherosclerosis as a cause of an increase in subsequent cardio-vascular disease. There is no such evidence. Thus, the mechanism of the cardiovascular complications is undoubtedly a short-term acute mecha-nism—thrombosis (an estrogen-related effect).

Hypertension

Oral contraceptive-induced hypertension was observed in approximately 5% of users of higher dose pills. More recent evidence indicates that small increases in blood pressure can be observed even with 30 μg estrogen, monophasic pills, including those containing the new progestins. However, an increased incidence of clinically significant hypertension has not been reported.[151-154] The lack of clinical hypertension in most studies may be due to the rarity of its occurrence. The Nurses' Health Study observed an increased risk of clinical hypertension in current users of low-dose oral contraceptives, providing an incidence of 41.5 cases per 10,000 women per year.[155] Therefore, an annual assessment of blood pressure is still an important element of clinical surveillance, even when low-dose oral contraceptives are used. Postmenopausal women in the Rancho Bernardo Study who had previously used oral contraceptives (probably high-dose products) had slightly higher (2–4 mm Hg) diastolic blood pressures.[156] Because past users do not demonstrate differences in incidence or risk factors for cardiovascular disease, it is unlikely this blood pressure differ-ence has an important clinical effect.

Variables such as previous toxemia of pregnancy or previous renal disease do not predict whether a woman will develop hypertension on oral contraception.[157] Likewise, women who have developed hypertension on oral contraception are not more predisposed to develop toxemia of preg-nancy. Overall, there is no evidence that previous oral contraceptive users have an increased risk of hypertension during a subsequent pregnancy.[158,159] The exception is the Nurses' Health Study, which indicated that recent users for a long duration (8 or more years) have a 2-fold increased risk of preeclampsia, a finding that was based on a small number of cases.[160] These epidemiologic associations are hard to establish because of the role of underlying hypertension in pregnancy-induced hypertension and the difficulty in assessing the efficacy of hypertension screening in oral contraceptive users.

The mechanism for an effect on blood pressure is thought to involve the renin angiotensin system. The most consistent finding is a marked increase in plasma angiotensinogen, the renin substrate, up to 8 times normal values (on higher dose pills). In nearly all women, excessive vasoconstriction is prevented by a compensatory decrease in plasma renin concentration. If hypertension does develop, the renin-angiotensinogen changes take 3–6 months to disappear after stopping combined oral contraception.

One must also consider the effects of oral contraceptives in patients with preexisting hypertension or cardiac disease. Women on oral contraceptives and with uncontrolled hypertension have an increased risk of arterial thrombosis.[121, 131, 132] Women with treated hypertension using oral contraceptives have been reported to have poor control of blood pressure with higher diastolic pressures.[161] In our view, with medical control of the blood pressure and close follow-up (at least every 3 months), the clinician and the nonsmoking patient who is under age 35 and otherwise healthy may choose low-dose oral contraception. Close follow-up is also indicated in women with a history of preexisting renal disease or a strong family history of hypertension or cardiovascular disease. It seems prudent to suggest that patients with marginal cardiac reserve should utilize other means of contraception. Significant increases in cardiac output and plasma volume have been recorded with oral contraceptive use (higher dose pills), probably a result of fluid retention.

Cardiovascular Disease — Summary

The outpouring of epidemiologic data in the last few years allows the construction of a clinical formulation that is evidence-based. The following conclusions are consistent with the recent reports.

SUMMARY: Oral Contraceptives and Thrombosis

- **Pharmacologic estrogen increases the production of clotting factors.**

- **Progestins have no significant impact on clotting factors.**

- **Past users of oral contraceptives do not have an increased incidence of cardiovascular disease.**

- **All low-dose oral contraceptives, regardless of progestin type, have an increased risk of venous thromboembolism, concentrated in the first 1–2 years of use. The actual risk of venous thrombosis with low-dose oral contraceptives is lower in the new studies compared with previous reports. Some have argued that this is due to preferential prescribing and the healthy user effect. However, it is also logical** that the lower risk reflects better screening of patients and lower estrogen doses. The risk increases with increasing age and body weight.

•Smoking has a lesser effect on the risk of venous thrombosis compared with arterial thrombosis.

•Smoking and estrogen have an additive effect on the risk of arterial thrombosis. Why is there a difference between venous and arterial clotting? The venous system has low flow with a state of high fibrinogen and low platelets, in contrast to the high-flow state of the arterial system with low fibrinogen and high platelets. Thus, it is understandable why these two different systems can respond in different ways.

•Hypertension is a very important additive risk factor for stroke in oral contraceptive users.

•Low-dose oral contraceptives (less than 50 μg ethinyl estradiol) do not increase the risk of myocardial infarction or stroke in healthy, nonsmoking women, regardless of age.

•Almost all myocardial infarctions and strokes in oral contraceptive users occur in users of high-dose products, or users with cardiovascular risk factors over the age of 35. In the Oxford Family Planning Association cohort, cardiac deaths occurred only in women who smoked 15 or more cigarettes per day.[62]

•Arterial thrombosis (myocardial infarction and stroke) has a dose-response relationship with the dose of estrogen, but there are insufficient data to determine whether there is a difference in risk with products that contain 20, 30, or 35 μg ethinyl estradiol.

The recent studies reinforce the belief that the risks of arterial and venous thrombosis are a consequence of the estrogen component of combination oral contraceptives. Current evidence does not support an advantage or disadvantage for any particular formulation, except for the greater safety associated with any product containing less than 50 μg ethinyl estradiol. Although it is logical to expect the greatest safety with the lowest dose of estrogen, the rare occurrence of arterial and venous thrombosis in healthy women makes it unlikely that there will be any measurable differences in the attributable incidence of clinical events with all low-dose products.

The new studies emphasize the importance of good patient screening. The occurrence of arterial thrombosis is essentially limited to older women who smoke or have cardiovascular risk factors, especially hypertension. The impact of good screening is evident in the repeated failure to detect an increase in mortality due to myocardial infarction or stroke in healthy, nonsmoking women.[62, 78, 122] Although the risk of venous thromboembolism is slightly increased, the actual incidence is still relatively rare, and the mortality rate is about 1% (probably less with oral contraceptives, because most deaths from thromboembolism are associated with trauma, surgery, or a major illness). The minimal risk of venous thrombosis associated with oral contraceptive use does not justify the cost of routine screening for coagulation deficiencies. Nevertheless, the importance of this issue is illustrated by the increased risk of a very rare event, cerebral sinus thrombosis, in women who have an inherited predisposition for clotting and use oral contraceptives.[36, 162]

If a patient has a close family history (parent or sibling) or a previous episode of idiopathic thromboembolism, an evaluation to search for an underlying abnormality in the coagulation system is warranted. It has been reported that family history of venous thromboembolism has low predictive value.[163] Another study indicated that testing for thrombophilia did not allow for prediction of recurrent events, but risk factors such as family history did provide prediction.[164] The conservative recommendation for a woman considering exposure to exogenous estrogen stimulation is to rule out an underlying thrombophilia. The following measurements are recommended, and abnormal results require consultation with a hematologist regarding prognosis and prophylactic treatment. The list of laboratory tests is long, and because this is a dynamic and changing field, the best advice is to consult with a hematologist. If a diagnosis of a congenital deficiency is made, screening should be offered to other family members.

HYPERCOAGUABLE CONDITIONS	THROMBOPHILIA SCREENING
Antithrombin III deficiency	Antithrombin III
Protein C deficiency	Protein C
Protein S deficiency	Protein S
Factor V Leiden mutation	Activated protein C
Prothrombin gene mutation	resistance ratio
Antiphospholipid syndrome	Activated partial thrombo-
	plastin time
	Hexagonal activated partial
	thromboplastin time
	Anticardiolipin antibodies
	Lupus anticoagulant
	Fibrinogen
	Prothrombin G mutation
	(DNA test)
	Thrombin time
	Homocysteine level
	Complete blood count

Combination oral contraception is contraindicated in women who have a history of idiopathic venous thromboembolism and in women who have a close family history (parent or sibling) of idiopathic venous thromboembolism. These women will have a higher incidence of congenital deficiencies in important clotting measurements, especially antithrombin III, protein C, protein S, and resistance to activated protein C.[165] Such a patient who screens negatively for an inherited clotting deficiency might still consider the use of oral contraceptives, but this would be a difficult decision with unknown risks for both patient and clinician, and it is more prudent to consider other contraceptive options. Other risk factors for thromboembolism that should be considered by clinicians include an acquired predisposition such as the presence of lupus anticoagulant or malignancy and immobility or trauma. Varicose veins are not a risk factor unless they are very extensive.[73]

The conclusion once again is that low-dose oral contraceptives are very safe for healthy, young women. By effectively screening for the presence of smoking and cardiovascular risk factors, especially hypertension, in older women, we can limit, if not eliminate, any increased risk for arterial disease associated with low-dose oral contraceptives. And it is very important to emphasize that there is no increased risk of cardiovascular events associated with duration of use (long-term). In large cohort studies, the risk of overall mortality comparing users and nonusers of oral contraceptives is identical.[60-62]

Carbohydrate Metabolism

With the older high-dose oral contraceptives, an impaired glucose tolerance test was present in many women. In these women, plasma levels of insulin as well as the blood sugar were elevated. Generally, the effect of oral contraception is to produce an increase in peripheral resistance to insulin action. Most women can meet this challenge by increasing insulin secretion, and there is no change in the glucose tolerance test, although 1-hour values may be slightly elevated.

Insulin sensitivity is affected mainly by the progestin component of the pill.[166] The derangement of carbohydrate metabolism may also be affected by estrogen influences on lipid metabolism, hepatic enzymes, and elevation of unbound cortisol. The glucose intolerance is dose-related, and once again effects are less with the low-dose formulations. ***Insulin and glucose changes with low-dose monophasic and multiphasic oral contraceptives are so minimal that it is now believed they are of no clinical significance.***[154, 167–170] This includes long-term evaluation with hemoglobin A1c.

The observed changes in studies of oral contraception and carbohydrate metabolism are in the nondiabetic range. To measure differences, investigators have resorted to analysis by measuring the area under the curve for glucose and insulin responses during glucose tolerance tests. A highly regarded cross-sectional study utilizing this technique reported that even lower dose formulations have detectable effects on insulin resistance.[166] The reason this is important is that it is now recognized that hyperinsulinemia due to insulin resistance is a contributor to cardiovascular disease. However, there are several critical questions that remain unanswered. Can the results from a cross-sectional study be duplicated in a study of sufficient size with patients serving as their own controls? Is a statistically significant hyperinsulinemia, detected in a study, clinically meaningful?

Because long-term, follow-up studies of large populations have failed to detect any increase in the incidence of diabetes mellitus or impaired glucose tolerance (even in past and current users of high-dose pills),[156, 171, 172] the concern now appropriately focuses on the slight impairment as a potential risk for cardiovascular disease. If slight hyperinsulinemia were meaningful, wouldn't you expect to see evidence of an increase in cardiovascular disease in past users who took oral contraceptives when doses were higher? As we have emphasized before, there is no such evidence. The data strongly indicate that the changes in lipids and carbohydrate metabolism that have been measured are not clinically meaningful.

It can be stated definitively that oral contraceptive use does not produce an increase in diabetes mellitus.[171–174] The hyperglycemia associated with oral contraception is not deleterious and is completely reversible. Even women who have risk factors for diabetes in their history are not affected. In women with recent gestational diabetes, no significant impact on glucose tolerance could be demonstrated over 6–13 months comparing the use of low-dose monophasic and multiphasic oral contraceptives with a control group, and no increase in the risk of overt diabetes mellitus could be detected with long-term follow-up.[175, 176] A high percentage of women with previous gestational diabetes develop overt diabetes and associated vascular complications. Until overt diabetes develops, it is appropriate for these patients to use low-dose oral contraception.

In clinical practice, it may, at times, be necessary to prescribe oral contraception for the overt diabetic. No effect on insulin requirement is expected with low-dose pills.[177] According to the older epidemiologic data, the use of oral contraceptives increases the risk of thrombosis in women with insulin-dependent diabetes mellitus; therefore, women with diabetes have been encouraged to use other forms of contraception. However, this effect in women under age 35 who are otherwise healthy and nonsmokers is probably very minimal with low-dose oral contraception, and reliable protection against pregnancy is a benefit for these patients that outweighs the small risk. A case-control study could find no evidence that oral contraceptive use by young women with insulin-dependent diabetes mellitus increased the development of retinopathy or nephropathy.[178] In a 1-year study of women with insulin-dependent diabetes mellitus who were using a low-dose oral contraceptive, no deterioration could be documented in lipoprotein or hemostatic biochemical markers for cardiovascular risk.[179] And finally, no effect of oral contraceptives on cardiovascular mortality could be detected in a group of women with diabetes mellitus.[180]

The Liver

The liver is affected in more ways and with more regularity and intensity by the sex steroids than any other extragenital organ. Estrogen influences the synthesis of hepatic DNA and RNA, hepatic cell enzymes, serum enzymes formed in the liver, and plasma proteins. Estrogenic hormones also affect hepatic lipid and lipoprotein formation, the intermediary metabolism of carbohydrates, and intracellular enzyme activity. Nevertheless, an extensive analysis of the prospective cohorts of women in the Royal College of General Practitioners' Oral Contraception Study and the Oxford Family Planning Association Contraceptive Study could detect no evidence of an increased incidence or risk of serious liver disease among oral contraceptive users.[181]

The active transport of biliary components is impaired by estrogens as well as some progestins. The mechanism is unclear, but cholestatic jaundice and pruritus were occasional complications of higher dose oral contraception, and are similar to the recurrent jaundice of pregnancy, i.e., benign and reversible. The incidence with lower dose oral contraception is unknown, but it must be a very rare occurrence.

The only absolute hepatic contraindication to oral contraceptive use is acute or chronic cholestatic liver disease. Cirrhosis and previous hepatitis are not aggravated. Once recovered from the acute phase of liver disease, a woman can use oral contraception.

Data from the Royal College of General Practitioners' prospective study indicated that an increase in the incidence of gallstones occurred in the first years of oral contraceptive use, apparently due to an acceleration of gallbladder disease in women already susceptible.[182] In other words, the overall risk of gallbladder disease was not increased, but in the first years of use, disease was activated or accelerated in women who were vulnerable because of asymptomatic disease or a tendency toward gallbladder disease. The mechanism appears to be induced alterations in the composition of gallbladder bile, specifically a rise in cholesterol saturation that is presumably an estrogen effect.[183] The Nurses' Health Study reported no significant increase in the risk of symptomatic gallstones among ever-users, but slightly elevated risks among current and long-term users.[184] Although oral contraceptive use has been linked to an increased risk of gallbladder disease, the epidemiologic evidence has been inconsistent. Indeed an Italian case-control study and a report from the Oxford Family Planning Association cohort found no increase in the risk of gallbladder disease in association with oral contraceptive use and no interaction with increasing age or body weight.[185, 186] Keep in mind that even though some studies found a statistically significant modest increase in the relative risk of gallbladder disease, even if the effect were real, it is of little clinical importance because the actual incidence of this problem is very low.

Liver Adenomas

Hepatocellular adenomas can be produced by steroids of both the estrogen and androgen families. Actually, there are several different lesions, peliosis, focal nodular hyperplasia, and adenomas. Peliosis is characterized by dilated vascular spaces without endothelial lining, and may occur in the absence of adenomatous changes. The adenomas are not malignant; their significance lies in the potential for hemorrhage. The most common presentation is acute right upper quadrant or epigastric pain. The tumors may be asymptomatic, or they may present suddenly with hematoperitoneum. There is some evidence that the tumors and focal nodular hyperplasia regress when oral contraception is stopped.[187, 188] Epidemiologic data have not supported the contention that mestranol increased the risk more than ethinyl estradiol.

The risk appears to be related to duration of oral contraceptive use and to the steroid dose in the pills. This is reinforced by the rarity of the condition ever since low-dose oral contraception became available. The ongoing prospective studies have accumulated many woman-years of use and have not identified an increased incidence of such tumors.[181] In a collaborative study of 15 German liver centers, no increase in risk for liver adenomas in contemporary oral contraceptive users could be detected.[189] An Italian case-control study found an increase in risk for focal nodular hyperplasia associated with low-dose oral contraceptives, a risk that reached statistical significance only with 3 or more years of use (with a very wide confidence interval because of only 13 cases).[190] In our view it is not even worth mentioning during the informed consent (choice) process.

No reliable screening test or procedure is currently available. Routine liver function tests are normal. Computed tomography (CT) scanning or magnetic resonance imaging (MRI) is the best means of diagnosis; angiography and ultrasonography are not reliable. Palpation of the liver should be part of the periodic evaluation in oral contraceptive users. If an enlarged liver is found, oral contraception should be stopped, and regression should be evaluated and followed by imaging.

Other Metabolic Effects

Nausea and breast discomfort continue to be disturbing effects, but their incidence is significantly less with low-dose oral contraception. Fortunately, these effects are most intense in the first few months of use and, in most cases, gradually disappear. In placebo-controlled trials with low-dose oral contraceptives, the incidence of "minor" side effects such as headache, nausea, dysmenorrhea, and breast discomfort actually occurred at the same rate in the treated group and the placebo group![191–193]

Weight gain usually responds to dietary restriction, but for some patients, the weight gain is an anabolic response to the sex steroids, and discontinuation of oral contraception is the only way that weight loss can be achieved. This must be rare with low-dose oral contraception because data in published studies, especially in placebo-controlled trials, fail to indicate a difference in body weight between users and nonusers.[193–201]

There is no association between oral contraception and peptic ulcer disease or inflammatory bowel disease.[202, 203] Oral contraception is not recommended for patients with problems of gastrointestinal malabsorption because of the possibility of contraceptive failure.

Chloasma, a patchy increase in facial pigment, was, at one time, found to occur in approximately 5% of oral contraceptive users. It is now a rare problem due to the decrease in estrogen dose. Unfortunately, once chloasma appears, it fades only gradually following discontinuation of the pill and may never disappear completely. Skin-blanching medications may be useful.

Hematologic effects include an increased sedimentation rate, increased total iron-binding capacity due to the increase in globulins, and a decrease in prothrombin time. The use of oral contraceptives results in a decrease in iron deficiency anemia because of a reduction in menstrual bleeding.[204, 205] Indeed, in anemic women, an increase in hemoglobin and ferritin levels accompanies the use of oral contraceptives.[206]

The continuous, daily use of oral contraceptives may prevent the appearance of symptoms in porphyria precipitated by menses. Changes in vitamin metabolism have been noted: a small nonharmful increase in vitamin A and decreases in blood levels of pyridoxine (B6) and the other B vitamins, folic acid, and ascorbic acid. Despite these changes, routine vitamin supplements are not necessary for women eating adequate, normal diets.[207]

Mental depression is very rarely associated with oral contraceptives. In studies with higher dose oral contraceptives, the effect was due to estrogen interference with the synthesis of tryptophan that could be reversed with pyridoxine treatment. It seems wiser, however, to discontinue oral contraception if depression is encountered. Though infrequent, a reduction in libido is occasionally a problem and may be a cause for seeking an alternative method of contraception.

Adverse androgenic voice changes were occasionally encountered with the use of the first very high-dose oral contraceptives. Vocal virilization can be a serious and devastating problem for some women, especially when vocal performance is important. Careful study of women on low-dose oral contraceptives indicates that this is no longer a side effect of concern.[208]

The Risk of Cancer

Endometrial Cancer

The use of oral contraception protects against endometrial cancer. Use for at least 12 months reduces the risk of developing endometrial cancer by **50%,** with the greatest protective effect gained by use for more than 3 years.[209–214] This protection persists for 20 or more years after discontinuation (the actual length of duration of protection is unknown) and is greatest in women at highest risk: nulliparous and low parity women.[214, 215] This protection is equally protective for all 3 major histologic subtypes of endometrial cancer: adenocarcinoma, adenoacanthoma, and adenosquamous cancers. Finally, protection is seen with all monophasic formulations of oral contraceptives, including pills with less than 50 μg estrogen.[209, 211, 214, 216] There are no data as yet with multiphasic preparations or the new progestin formulations, but because these products are still dominated by their progestational component, there is every reason to believe that they will be protective.

Ovarian Cancer

Protection against ovarian cancer, the most lethal of female reproductive tract cancers, is one of the most important benefits of oral contraception. Because this cancer is detected late and prognosis is poor, the impact of this protection is very significant. Indeed, a decline in mortality from ovarian cancer has been observed in several countries since the early 1970s, perhaps an effect of oral contraceptive use.[217] Cohorts of women with increased exposure to oral contraceptives have demonstrated a marked decrease in the incidence of ovarian cancer.[218-220] The risk of developing epithelial ovarian cancer of all histologic subtypes in users of oral contraception is reduced by **40%** compared with that of nonusers.[211, 213, 221-226] This protective effect increases with duration of use and continues for 20 or more years after stopping the medication. This protection is seen in women who use oral contraception for as little as 3 to 6 months (although at least 3 years of use are required for a notable impact), reaching an 80% reduction in risk with more than 10 years of use, and is a benefit associated with all monophasic formulations, including the low-dose products.[225-227] The protective effect of oral contraceptives is especially observed in women at high risk of ovarian cancer (nulliparous women and women with a positive family history).[228, 229] Continuous use of oral contraception for 10 years by women with a positive family history for ovarian cancer can reduce the risk of epithelial ovarian cancer to a level equal to or less than that experienced by women with a negative family history.[228] Again, the multiphasic and new progestin products have not been in use long enough to yield any data on this issue, but because ovulation is effectively inhibited by these formulations, protection against ovarian cancer should be exerted. The same magnitude of protection has been observed in one case-control study of women with BRCA1 or BRCA2 mutations but not in another.[230, 231]

Case-control studies have indicated that a reduced risk of ovarian cancer is not only associated with oral contraception but also tubal sterilization, IUDs, and barrier methods (but only in multigravid women).[232] The mechanisms and biologic plausibility for this impact are certainly a puzzle.

Cancer of the Cervix

Studies have indicated that the risk for dysplasia and carcinoma in situ of the uterine cervix increases with the use of oral contraception for more than 1 year.[233-238] Invasive cervical cancer may be increased after 5 years of use, reaching a 2-fold increase after 10 years. It is well recognized, however, that the number of partners a woman has had and age at first coitus are the most important risk factors for cervical neoplasia. Other confounding factors include exposure to human papillomavirus, the use of barrier contraception (protective), and smoking. These are difficult factors to control, and, therefore, the conclusions regarding cervical cancer are not definitive. An excellent study from the Centers for Disease Control and Prevention (CDC) concluded there is no increased risk of invasive cervical cancer in users of oral contraception, and an apparent increased risk of carcinoma in situ is due to enhanced detection of disease (because oral contraceptive users have more frequent Pap smears).[236] In the World Health Organization Study of Neoplasia and Steroid Contraceptives, a Pap smear screening bias was identified, nevertheless the evidence still suggested an increased risk of cervical carcinoma in situ with long-term oral contraceptive use.[237]

A case-control study of patients in Panama, Costa Rica, Colombia, and Mexico concluded that there was a significantly increased risk for invasive adenocarcinoma.[239] Similar results were obtained in a case-control study in Los Angeles and in the World Health Organization Collaborative Study.[240, 241] In Los Angeles, the relative risk of adenocarcinoma of the cervix increased from 2.1 with ever use to 4.4 with 12 or more years of oral contraceptive use.[240] Because the incidence of adenocarcinoma of the cervix (10% of all cervical cancers) has increased in young women over the last 20 years, there is concern that this increase reflects the use of oral contraception.[242] Oral contraceptives increase cervical ectopia, but whether this increases the risk of cervical adenocarcinoma is unclear.

A large meta-analysis concluded that the relative risk of cervical cancer increased with increasing duration of use (for in situ and invasive cancer and both squamous cancer and adenocarcinoma); however, the risk was confined to the cases who tested positively for human papillomavirus (HPV).[243] A pooled analysis of case-control studies concluded that the risk of cervical cancer in women with HPV increases about 3-fold but not until after 5 years of use.[244] This obviously is an important reason for annual Pap smear surveillance. The liquid-based methods along with HPV DNA testing will provide even better identification of at-risk women. Fortunately, steroid contraception does not mask abnormal cervical changes, and the necessity for prescription renewals offers the opportunity for improved screening for cervical disease. It is reasonable to perform Pap smears every 6 months in women using oral contraception for 5 or more years who are also at higher risk because of their sexual behavior (multiple partners, history of sexually transmitted infections). Oral contraceptive use is appropriate for women with a history of cervical intraepithelial neoplasia (CIN), including those who have been surgically treated.

Liver Cancer

Oral contraception has been linked to the development of hepatocellular carcinoma.[245, 246] However, the very small number of cases, and, thus, the limited statistical power, requires great caution in interpretation. The largest study on this question, the WHO Collaborative Study of Neoplasia and Steroid Contraceptives, found no association between oral contraception and liver cancer.[247] Even case-control analysis of oral contraceptives containing cyproterone acetate (known to be toxic to the liver in high doses) could detect no evidence of an increased risk of liver cancer.[248] In the United States, Japan, Sweden, England, and Wales, the death rates from liver cancer did not change despite introduction and use of oral contraception.[249, 250] More recently, there has been an increase in liver cancer incidence and mortality in the United States, but this is believed to be due to infection with hepatitis C and hepatitis B.[251]

Breast Cancer

Because of breast cancer's prevalence and its long latent phase, concern over the relationship between oral contraception and breast cancer continues to be an issue in the minds of both patients and clinicians. Worth emphasizing is the protective effect of higher dose oral contraception on benign breast disease, an effect that became apparent after 2 years of use.[252–254] After 2 years there was a progressive reduction (about 40%) in the incidence of fibrocystic changes in the breast. Women who used oral contraception were one-fourth as likely to develop benign breast disease as nonusers, but this protection was limited to current and recent users. It is still uncertain whether this same protection is provided by the lower dose products. A French case-control study indicated a reduction of nonproliferative benign breast disease associated with low-dose oral contraceptives used before a first full-term pregnancy, but no effect on proliferative disease or with use after a pregnancy.[255] A Canadian cohort study that almost certainly reflected the use of modern low-dose oral contraceptives concluded that oral contraceptives do protect against proliferative benign disease, with an increasing reduction in risk with increasing duration of use.[256]

The Royal College of General Practitioners,[257] Oxford Family Planning Association,[258, 259] the Nurses' Health Study,[260] and Walnut Creek[261] cohort studies indicated no significant differences in breast cancer rates between users and nonusers. However, patients were enrolled in these studies at a time when oral contraception was used primarily by married couples spacing out their children. Beginning in the 1980s, oral contraception was primarily being used by women early in life, for longer durations, and to delay an initial pregnancy (remember, a full-term pregnancy early in life protects against breast cancer).

Case-control studies have focused on the use of oral contraception early in life, for long duration, and to delay a first, full-term pregnancy. Because the women who have used oral contraception in this fashion are just now beginning to reach the ages of postmenopausal breast cancer, many studies have had to focus on the risk of breast cancer diagnosed before age 45 (only 13% of all breast cancer). The results of these studies have not been clear-cut. Some studies have indicated an overall increased relative risk of early, premenopausal breast cancer,[262–270] whereas others indicated no increase in overall risk.[271–273] The most impressive finding indicates a link in most studies,[274–279] but not all,[280–284] of early breast cancer before age 40 with women who used oral contraception for long durations of time.

A collaborative group re-analyzed data from 54 studies in 26 countries, a total of 53,287 women with breast cancer and 100,239 without breast cancer, to assess the relationship between the risk of breast cancer and the use of oral contraceptives.[285, 286] Oral contraceptives were grouped into 3 categories: low, medium, and high dose (which correlated with less than 50 μg, 50 μg, and more than 50 μg of estrogen, respectively). At the time of diagnosis, 9% of the women with breast cancer were under age 35, 25% were 35–44, 33% were 45–54, and 33% were age 55 and older. A similar percentage of women with breast cancer (41%) and women without breast cancer (40%) had used combined oral contraceptives at some time in their lives. Overall, the relative risk (RR) of breast cancer in ever users of oral contraceptives was very slightly elevated and statistically significant: RR = 1.07; CI = 1.03–1.10.

The relative risk analyzed by duration of use was barely elevated and not statistically significant (even when long-term use, virtually continuous, was analyzed). Women who had begun use as teenagers had about a 20% statistically significant increased relative risk. In other words, recent users who began use before age 20 had a higher relative risk compared with recent users who began at later ages. The evidence was strong for a relationship with time since last use, an elevated risk being significant for current users and in women who had stopped use 1–4 years before (recent use). No influence on this risk was observed with the following: a family history of breast cancer, age of menarche, country of origin, ethnic groups, body weight, alcohol use, years of education, and the design of the study. There was no variation according to specific type of estrogen or progestin in the various products. Importantly, there was no statistically significant effect of low-, medium-, or high-dose preparations. Ten or more years after stopping use, there was no increased risk of breast cancer. Indeed, the risk of metastatic disease compared with localized tumors was reduced: RR = 0.88; CI = 0.81–0.95.

Oral Contraceptives and the Risk of Breast Cancer Re-analysis of the World's Data[252]

Current users	RR = 1.24, 95% CI = 1.15–1.33
1–4 years after stopping	RR = 1.16, 95% CI = 1.08–1.23
5–9 years after stopping	RR = 1.07, 95% CI = 1.02–1.13

Data were limited for progestin-only methods. The reanalysis indicated that the results were similar to those with combined oral contraceptives, but a close look at the numbers reveals that not one relative risk reached statistical significance.

Overall, this massive statistical exercise yielded good news. No major adverse impact of oral contraceptives emerged. *Even though the data indicated that young women who begin use before age 20 have higher relative risks of breast cancer during current use and in the 5 years after stopping, this is a time period when breast cancer is very rare; and, thus, there would be little impact on the actual number of breast cancers.* The difference between localized disease and metastatic disease was statistically greater and should be observable. Thus many years after stopping oral contraceptive use, the main effect may be protection against metastatic disease. Breast cancer is more common in older years, and 10 or more years after stopping, the risk was not increased.

What other explanation could account for an increased risk associated only with current or recent use, no increase with duration of use, and a return to normal 10 years after exposure? The slightly increased risk could be influenced by detection/surveillance bias (more interaction with the health care system by oral contraceptive users). It is also possible that this situation is analogous to that of pregnancy. Recent studies indicate that pregnancy transiently increases the risk of breast cancer (for a period of several years) after a woman's first childbirth, and this is followed by a lifetime reduction in risk.[287] And some have found that a concurrent or recent pregnancy adversely affects survival.[288, 289] It is argued that breast cells that have already begun malignant transformation are adversely affected by the hormones of pregnancy, while normal stem cells become more resistant because of a pregnancy. It is possible that early and recent use of oral contraceptives also affects the growth of a preexisting malignancy, explaining the limitation of the finding to current and recent use and the increase in localized disease. With the accumulation of greater numbers of older women previously exposed to oral contraceptives, a protective effect may become evident. In a case-control study of women in Toronto, Canada, age 40–69 years, those women who had used oral contraceptives for 5 or more years, 15 or more years previously, had a 50% reduced risk of breast cancer.[290] However, a case-control study from Sweden could detect neither a beneficial nor an adverse effect of previous use of oral contraceptives (mainly 50 μg estrogen products) on the risk of breast cancer in women age 50–74 years.[291]

The largest case-control study included 4,575 American women with breast cancer, and most importantly, the women were 35 to 64 years old.[292] The risk of breast cancer was not increased in current users or past users of oral contraception. There was no adverse effect of increasing duration of use or higher doses of estrogen, with no differences in current or recent users. Initiation at a younger age had no impact, and there was no increase in risk in women with a family history of breast cancer. This large American study had consistently negative results. An analysis of the large database in the Women's Health Initiative concluded that postmenopausal women who were past users of oral contraceptives did not have an increased risk of breast cancer.[293]

A cohort study from Minnesota concluded that women with a first-degree relative with breast cancer had an increased risk of breast cancer with oral contraception; however, this association was present only with oral contraceptives used prior to 1976 (high-dose formulations), and the confidence intervals were wide because of small numbers (13 ever users).[294] In a study of women with BRCA1 and BRCA2 mutations, an elevated risk of breast cancer associated with oral contraception was based on only a few cases and did not achieve statistical significance.[295] A larger case-control study concluded that BRCA1 mutation carriers had small increases in the risk of breast cancer in users for at least 5 years (OR = 1.33, CI = 1.11–1.60), in users before age 30 (OR = 1.29, CI = 1.09–1.52), and in those who developed breast cancer before age 40 (OR = 1.38, CI = 1.11–1.72).[296]

Conclusion

Adding up the benefits of oral contraception, the possible slight increase in risk of breast cancer in young current users is far outweighed by positive effects on our public health. But the impact on public health is of little concern during the private clinician–patient interchange in the office. Here personal risk receives highest priority; fear of cancer is a motivating force, and compliance with effective contraception requires accurate information. For these reasons, we provide the following summary of our assessment of the impact of oral contraceptives on the risk of breast cancer.

SUMMARY: Oral Contraceptives and the Risk of Breast Cancer

- Current and recent use of oral contraceptives may be associated with about a 20% increased risk of early (under age 35) premenopausal breast cancer, essentially limited to localized disease and a very small increase in the actual number of cases (so small, there would be no major impact on incidence figures). This finding may be due to detection/surveillance bias and accelerated growth of already present malignancies, a situation similar to the effects of pregnancy and postmenopausal hormone therapy on the risk of breast cancer. Further comfort can be derived from the fact that the increase in breast cancer in American women was greater in older women from 1973 to 1994, those who did not have the opportunity to use oral contraception.[297] In women under 50 years of age, there was only a slight increase during this same time period. The large American case-control study of women age 35–64 years was totally negative and very reassuring.

- There is no effect of past use or duration of oral contraceptive use (up to 15 years of continuous use) on the risk of breast cancer, and there is no evidence indicating that higher dose oral contraceptives increased the risk of breast cancer.

- Previous oral contraceptive use may be associated with a reduced risk of metastatic breast cancer later in life and possibly with a reduced risk of postmenopausal breast cancer.

- Oral contraceptive use does not further increase the risk of breast cancer in women with positive family histories of breast cancer or in women with proven benign breast disease.

- The clinician should not fail to take every opportunity to direct attention to all factors that affect breast cancer. Breastfeeding and control of alcohol intake are good examples and are components of preventive health care. Especially important is this added motivation to encourage breastfeeding. The protective effect of breast feeding is exerted mainly on premenopausal breast cancer, the cancer of concern to younger women using oral contraception.

Other Cancers

The Walnut Creek study suggested that melanoma was linked to oral contraception; however, the major risk factor for melanoma is exposure to sunlight. More recent and accurate evaluation utilizing both the Royal College General Practitioners and Oxford Family Planning Association prospective cohorts and accounting for exposure to sunlight did not indicate a significant difference in the risk of melanoma comparing users to nonusers.[298, 299] There is no evidence linking oral contraceptive use to kidney cancer, gallbladder cancer, or pituitary tumors.[300] Long-term oral contraceptive use may slightly increase the risk of molar pregnancy.[301–303] A case-control study concluded that oral contraceptives reduce the risk of salivary gland cancer.[304] Although previous studies have not been in agreement, the Nurses' Health Study reported about a 40% reduced risk of colorectal cancer associated with 8 years of previous use of oral contraceptives (most likely higher dose products).[305] A meta-analysis of published studies concluded that there is about a 20% reduction in risk of colorectal cancer in users of oral contraception, with a stronger effect in recent users.[306]

Endocrine Effects

Adrenal Gland

Estrogen increases the cortisol-binding globulin (CBG). It had been thought that the increase in plasma cortisol while on oral contraception was due to increased binding by this globulin and not an increase in free active cortisol. Now it is apparent that free and active cortisol levels are also elevated but only slightly.[307] Estrogen decreases the ability of the liver to metabolize cortisol, and in addition, progesterone and related compounds can displace cortisol from transcortin, and thus contribute to the elevation of unbound cortisol. The effects of these elevated levels over prolonged periods of time are unknown, but no obvious impact has become apparent. To put this into perspective, the increase is not as great as that which occurs in pregnancy, and, in fact, it is within the normal range for nonpregnant women.

The adrenal gland responds to adrenocorticotropic hormone (ACTH) normally in women on oral contraceptives; therefore, there is no suppression of the adrenal gland itself. Initial studies indicated that the response to metyrapone (an 11β-hydroxylase blocker) was abnormal, suggesting that the pituitary was suppressed. However, estrogen accelerates the conjugation of metyrapone by the liver; and, therefore, the drug has less effect, thus explaining the subnormal responses initially reported. The pituitary-adrenal reaction to stress is normal in women on oral contraceptive pills.

Thyroid

Estrogen increases the synthesis and circulating levels of thyroxine-binding globulin, Prior to the introduction of new methods for measuring free thyroxine levels, evaluation of thyroid function was a problem. Measurement of TSH (thyroid-stimulating hormone) and the free thyroxine level in a woman on oral contraception provide an accurate assessment of a patient's thyroid state. Oral contraception affects the total thyroxine level in the blood as well as the amount of binding globulin, but the free thyroxine level is unchanged.[307]

Oral Contraception and Reproduction

The impact of oral contraceptives on the reproductive system is less than initially thought. Early studies that indicated adverse effects have not stood the test of time and the scrutiny of multiple, careful studies. There are two major areas that warrant review: (1) inadvertent use of oral contraceptives during the cycle of conception and during early pregnancy, and (2) reproduction after discontinuing oral contraception.

Inadvertent Use during the Cycle of Conception and during Early Pregnancy

One of the reasons, if not the major reason, why a lack of withdrawal bleeding while using oral contraceptives is such a problem is the anxiety produced in both patient and clinician. The patient is anxious because of the uncertainty regarding pregnancy, and the clinician is anxious because of the concerns stemming from the retrospective studies that indicated an increased risk of congenital malformations among the offspring of women who were pregnant and using oral contraception. Organogenesis does not occur in the first 2 embryonic weeks (first 4 weeks since last menstrual period); however, teratogenic effects are possible between the third and eighth embryonic weeks (5 to 10 weeks since last menstrual period).

Initial positive reports linking the use of contraceptive steroids to congenital malformations have not been substantiated. Many suspect a strong component of recall bias in the few positive studies due to a tendency of patients with malformed infants to recall details better than those with normal children. Other confounding problems have included a failure to consider the reasons for the administration of hormones (e.g., bleeding in an already abnormal pregnancy) and a failure to delineate the exact timing of the treatment (e.g., treatment was sometimes confined to a period of time during which the heart could not have been affected).

An association with cardiac anomalies was first claimed in the 1970s.[308, 309] This link received considerable support with a report from the U.S. Collaborative Perinatal Project; however, subsequent analysis of these data uncovered several methodologic shortcomings.[310] Simpson and Phillips, in a very thorough and critical review in 1990, concluded that there was no reliable evidence implicating sex steroids as cardiac teratogens.[311] In fact, in their review, Simpson and Phillips found no relationship between oral contraception and the following problems: hypospadias, limb reduction anomalies, neural tube defects, and mutagenic effects that would be responsible for chromosomally abnormal fetuses. Even virilization is not a practical consideration because the doses required (e.g., 20–40 mg norethindrone per day) are in excess of anything currently used. These conclusions reflect use of combined oral contraceptives as well as progestins alone.

In the past there was a concern regarding the VACTERL complex. VACTERL refers to a complex of vertebral, anal, cardiac, tracheoesophageal, renal, and limb anomalies. While case-control studies indicated a relationship with oral contraception, prospective studies have failed to observe any connection between sex steroids and the VACTERL complex.[312] Meta-analyses of the studies of the risk of birth defects with oral contraceptive ingestion during pregnancy concluded that there was no increase in risk for major malformations, congenital heart defects, or limb reduction defects.[313, 314]

Women who become pregnant while taking oral contraceptives or women who inadvertently take birth control pills early in pregnancy should be advised that the risk of a significant congenital anomaly is no greater than the general rate of 2–3%. This recommendation can be extended to those pregnant woman who have been exposed to a progestational agent such as medroxyprogesterone acetate or 17-hydroxyprogesterone caproate.[315, 316]

Reproduction after Discontinuing Oral Contraception
Fertility

The early reports from the British prospective studies indicated that former users of oral contraception had a delay in achieving pregnancy. In the Oxford Family Planning Association study, former use had an effect on fertility for up to 42 months in nulligravida women and for up to 30 months in multigravida women.[317] Presumably, the delay is due to lingering suppression of the hypothalamic-pituitary reproductive system.

A later analysis of the Oxford data indicated that the delay was concentrated in women age 30–34 who had never given birth.[318] At 48 months, 82% of these women had given birth compared with 89% of users of other contraceptive methods, not a big difference. No effect was observed in women younger than 30 or in women who had previously given birth. Childless women age 25–29 experienced some delay in return to fertility, but by 48 months, 91% had given birth compared with 92% in users of other methods. After 72 months the proportions of women who remained undelivered were the same in both groups of women.

This delay has been observed in the United States as well. In the Boston area, the interval from cessation of contraception to conception was 13 months or greater for 24.8% of prior oral contraceptive users compared with 10.6% for former users of all other methods (12.4% for intrauterine device, IUD, users, 8.5% for diaphragm uses, and 11.9% for other methods).[319] Oral contraceptive users had a lower monthly percentage of conceptions for the first 3 months, and somewhat lower percentage from 4 to 10 months. It took 24 months for 90% of previous oral contraceptive users to become pregnant, 14 months for IUD users, and 10 months for diaphragm users. Similar findings in Connecticut indicate that this delay lasts at least a year, and the effect is greater with higher dose preparations.[320] Despite this delay, there is no evidence that infertility is increased by the use of oral contraception. In fact, in young women, previous oral contraceptive use is associated with a lower risk of primary infertility.[321] Furthermore, the studies indicating a delay in conception are influenced by older, higher dose products. In a prospective study from the United Kingdom reflecting modern, low-dose oral contraceptives, no delay to conception was found and long-term use was actually associated with greater fertility.[322]

Spontaneous Miscarriage

There is no increase in the incidence of spontaneous miscarriage in pregnancies after the cessation of oral contraception. Indeed, the rate of spontaneous miscarriages and stillbirths is slightly less in former pill users, about 1% less for spontaneous miscarriages and 0.3% less for stillbirths.[323] A protective effect of previous oral contraceptive use against spontaneous miscarriage has been observed to be more apparent in women who become pregnant after age 30.[324]

Pregnancy Outcome

There is no evidence that oral contraceptives cause changes in individual germ cells that would yield an abnormal child at a later time.[311] There is no increase in the number of abnormal children born to former oral contraceptive users, and there is no change in the sex ratio (a sign of sex-linked recessive mutations).[323, 325] These observations are not altered when analyzed for duration of use. Initial observations that women who had previously used oral contraception had an increase in chromosomally abnormal fetuses have not been confirmed. Furthermore, as noted above, there is no increase in the miscarriage rate after discontinuation, something one would expect if oral contraceptives induce chromosomal abnormalities because these are the principal cause of spontaneous miscarriage.

In a 3-year follow-up of children whose mothers used oral contraceptives prior to conception, no differences could be detected in weight, anemia, intelligence, or development.[326] Former pill users have no increased risks for the following: perinatal morbidity or mortality, prematurity, and low birth weight.[327, 328] Dizygous twinning has been observed to be nearly 2-fold (1.6% versus 1.0%) increased in women who conceive soon after cessation of oral contraception.[323] This effect was greater with longer duration of use.

The only reason (and it is a good one) to recommend that women defer attempts to conceive for a month or two after stopping the pill is to improve the accuracy of gestational dating by allowing accurate identification of the last menstrual period.

Breastfeeding

Oral contraception has been demonstrated to diminish the quantity and quality of lactation in postpartum women. Also of concern is the potential hazard of transfer of contraceptive steroids to the infant (a significant amount of the progestational component is transferred into breast milk);[329] however, no adverse effects have thus far been identified. Women who use oral contraception have a lower incidence of breastfeeding after the sixth postpartum month, regardless of whether oral contraception is started at the first, second, or third postpartum month.[330–332]

In adequately nourished breastfeeding women, no impairment of infant growth can be detected; presumably, compensation is achieved either through supplementary feedings or increased suckling.[333–335] In an 8-year follow-up study of children breastfed by mothers using oral contraceptives, no effect could be detected on diseases, intelligence, or psychological behavior.[336] This study also found that mothers on birth control pills lactated a significantly shorter period of time than controls, a mean of 3.7 months versus 4.6 months in controls.

Because the above considerations indicate that oral contraception shortens the duration of breastfeeding, it is worthwhile to consider the contraceptive effectiveness of lactation. The contraceptive effectiveness of lactation, i.e., the length of the interval between births, depends on the level of nutrition of the mother (if low, the longer the contraceptive interval), the intensity of suckling, and the extent to which supplemental food is added to the infant diet. If suckling intensity and/or frequency is diminished, contraceptive effect is reduced. Only amenorrheic women who exclusively breastfeed (full breastfeeding) at regular intervals, including nighttime, during the first 6 months have the contraceptive protection equivalent to that provided by oral contraception (98% efficacy); with menstruation or after 6 months, the chance of ovulation increases.[337, 338] With full or nearly full breastfeeding, approximately 70% of women remain amenorrheic through 6 months and only 37% through 1 year; nevertheless with exclusive breastfeeding, the contraceptive efficacy at 1 year is high, at 92%.[338] Fully breastfeeding women commonly have some vaginal bleeding or spotting in the first 8 postpartum weeks, but this bleeding is not due to ovulation.[339]

Supplemental feeding increases the chance of ovulation (and pregnancy) even in amenorrheic women.[340] Total protection is achieved by the exclusively breastfeeding woman for a duration of only 10 weeks.[339] Half of women studied who are not fully breastfeeding ovulate before the 6th week, the time of the traditional postpartum visit; a visit during the 3rd postpartum week is strongly recommended for contraceptive counseling.

It is apparent that although lactation provides a contraceptive effect, it is variable and not reliable for every woman. Furthermore, because frequent suckling is required to maintain full milk production, women who use oral contraception and who breastfeed less frequently (e.g., because they work outside their home) have two reasons for decreased milk volume. This combination can make it especially difficult to continue nursing.

Initiation of Oral Contraception in the Postpartum Period

The individual woman is in need of contraception early in the postpartum period. In a careful study of 22 postpartum, nonbreastfeeding women, the mean time from delivery to the first menses was 45 ± 10.1 days, and no woman ovulated before 25 days after delivery.[341] A high proportion of the first cycles (81.8%) and the subsequent cycles (37%) were not normal; however, this is certainly not predictable in individual women. Others have documented a mean delay of 7 weeks before resumption of ovulation, but half of the women studied ovulated before the sixth week, the time of the traditional postpartum visit. The obstetrical tradition of scheduling the postpartum visit at 6 weeks should be changed. A 3-week visit would be more productive in avoiding postpartum surprises.

The Rule of 3's:

In the presence of FULL breastfeeding, a contraceptive method should be used beginning in the *3rd postpartum month*.

With PARTIAL breastfeeding or NO breastfeeding, a contraceptive method should begin during the *3rd postpartum week*.

After the termination of a pregnancy of less than 12 weeks, oral contraception can be started immediately. After a pregnancy of 12 or more weeks, oral contraception has traditionally been started 2 weeks after delivery to avoid an increased risk of thrombosis during the initial postpartum period. We believe that oral contraception can be started immediately after a second-trimester abortion or premature delivery.

Because of the concerns regarding the impact of oral contraceptives on breastfeeding, a useful alternative is to combine the contraceptive effect of lactation with the progestin-only minipill. This low dose of progestin has no negative impact on breast milk, and some studies document an increase in milk quantity and nutritional quality.[342] Highly effective (near total) protection can be achieved with the combination of lactation and the minipill. Because of the slight positive impact on lactation, the minipill can be started immediately after delivery.[343] Use of the progestin-only minipill has been reported to be associated with a 3-fold increased risk of diabetes mellitus in overweight, lactating, Latina women with recent gestational diabetes.[176] Women who have experienced gestational diabetes should consider other methods of contraception.

Other Considerations

Prolactin-Secreting Adenomas

Because estrogen is known to stimulate prolactin secretion and to cause hypertrophy of the pituitary lactotrophs, it is appropriate to be concerned over a possible relationship between oral contraception and prolactin-secreting adenomas. Case-control studies have uniformly concluded that no such relationship exists.[344, 345] Data from both the Royal College of General Practitioners and the Oxford Family Planning Association studies indicated no increase in the incidence of pituitary adenomas.[300, 346] Previous use of oral contraceptives is not related to the size of prolactinomas at presentation and diagnosis.[346, 347] Oral contraception can be prescribed to patients with pituitary microadenomas without fear of subsequent tumor growth.[348, 349] *We have routinely prescribed oral contraception to patients with pituitary microadenomas and have never observed evidence of tumor growth.*

Postpill Amenorrhea

The approximate incidence of "postpill amenorrhea" is 0.7–0.8%, which is equal to the incidence of spontaneous secondary amenorrhea,[328, 350, 351] and there is no evidence to support the idea that oral contraception causes secondary amenorrhea. If a cause-and-effect relationship exists between oral contraception and subsequent amenorrhea, one would expect the incidence of infertility to be increased after a given population discontinues use of oral contraception. In those women who discontinue oral contraception in order to get pregnant, 50% conceive by 3 months, and after 2 years, a maximum of 15% of nulliparous women and 7% of parous women fail to conceive,[328] rates comparable with those quoted for the prevalence of spontaneous infertility. Attempts to document a cause-and-effect relationship between oral contraceptive use and secondary amenorrhea have failed.[352] Although patients with this problem come more quickly to our attention because of previous oral contraceptive use and follow-up, there is no cause-and-effect relationship. Women who have not resumed menstrual function within 12 months should be evaluated as any other patient with secondary amenorrhea.

Use During Puberty

Should oral contraception be advised for a young woman with irregular menses and oligo-ovulation or anovulation? The fear of subsequent infertility should not be a deterrent to providing appropriate contraception. Women who have irregular menstrual periods are more likely to develop secondary amenorrhea whether they use oral contraception or not. The possibility of subsequent secondary amenorrhea is less of a risk and a less urgent problem for a young woman than leaving her unprotected. The need for contraception takes precedence.

There is no evidence that the use of oral contraceptives in the pubertal, sexually active girl impairs growth and development of the reproductive system.[321] Again, the most important concern is and should be the prevention of an unwanted pregnancy. For most teenagers, oral contraception, dispensed in the 28-day package for better compliance, is the contraceptive method of choice; however, even better compliance can be achieved with the vaginal and transdermal methods of estrogen-progestin contraception (Chapter 4).

Eye and Ear Diseases

In the 1960s and 1970s, there were numerous anecdotal reports of eye disorders in women using oral contraception. An analysis of the two large British cohort studies (the Royal College of General Practitioners' Study and the Oxford Family Planning Association Study) could find no increase in risk for the following conditions: conjunctivitis, keratitis, iritis, lacrimal disease, strabismus, cataract, glaucoma, and retinal detachment.[353] Retinal vascular lesions were slightly more common in recent users of oral contraception, but this finding did not reach statistical significance. Contact lens may be less well tolerated, requiring more frequent use of wetting solutions.

The Oxford Family Planning Association Study could detect no evidence of any adverse effects of oral contraception on ear disorders.[354]

Multiple Sclerosis

There is no evidence in two cohort studies (the Royal College of General Practitioners' Study and the Oxford Family Planning Association Study) that there is any effect of oral contraceptive use on the risk or course of multiple sclerosis.[355, 356]

Infections and Oral Contraception

Viral STIs

The viral sexually transmitted infections (STIs) include human immuno-deficiency virus (HIV), human papillomavirus (HPV), herpes simplex virus (HSV), and hepatitis B (HBV). At the present time, no known associations exist between oral contraception and the viral STIs. Of course, significant prevention includes barrier methods of contraception. Thus far, most studies have found no association between oral contraceptive use and HIV seropositivity, and some have indicated a protective effect.[357-359] Antiretroviral drugs may decrease oral contraceptive efficacy by affecting drug metabolism or causing diarrhea and vomiting. The degree of clinical impact, if any, is not established. *For women not in a stable, monogamous relationship, a dual approach is recommended, combining the contraceptive efficacy and protection against pelvic inflammatory disease (PID) offered by estrogen-progestin contraception with the use of a barrier method for prevention of viral STIs.*

Bacterial STIs

Sexually transmitted infections (STIs) are one of the most common public health problems in the United States. Pelvic inflammatory disease is usually a consequence of STIs. The best estimate of subsequent tubal infertility is derived from an excellent Swedish report; approximately 12% after one episode of PID, 23% after 2 episodes, and 54% after 3 episodes.[360] Because pelvic infection is the single greatest threat to the reproductive future of a young woman, the now recognized protection offered by oral contraception against PID is highly important.[361-363] *The risk of hospitalization for PID is reduced by approximately 50–60%, but at least 12 months of use are necessary, and the protection is limited to current users.*[361, 364] Furthermore, if a patient does get a pelvic infection, the severity of the salpingitis found at laparoscopy is decreased.[365, 366] The mechanism of this protection remains unknown. Speculation includes thickening of the cervical mucus to prevent movement of pathogens and bacteria-laden sperm into the uterus and tubes and decreased menstrual bleeding, reducing movement of pathogens into the tubes as well as a reduction in "culture medium." This protection probably accounts for the greater fertility rate observed in previous users of oral contraception.[321, 322]

The argument has been made that this protection is limited to gonococcal disease, and chlamydial infections may even be enhanced. Fifteen of 17 published studies by 1985 reported a positive association of oral contraceptives with lower genital tract chlamydial cervicitis.[367] Because lower genital tract infections caused by *Chlamydia* are on the rise (now the most prevalent bacterial STI in the United States) and the rate of hospitalization for PID is also increased, it is worthwhile for both patients and clinicians to be alert for symptoms of cervicitis or salpingitis in women on oral contraception who are at high risk of STI (multiple sexual partners, a history of STI, or cervical discharge). The mechanism for the association between chlamydial cervicitis and oral contraceptives may be the well-recognized extension of the columnar epithelium from the endocervix out over the cervix (ectopia) that occurs with oral contraceptive use.[368] This ectropion may allow a more effective collection of cervical specimens for culture, thus introducing detection bias into the epidemiologic studies. However, large, prospective cohort studies have found no association between oral contraceptive use and either chlamydial or gonorrheal infection, and cervical ectopy did not influence the risk of infection.[369, 370] If the impact of oral contraceptives on the risk of chlamydial infection is real, it is a modest one.

Despite this potential relationship between oral contraception and chlamydial infections, it should be emphasized that there is no evidence for an impact of oral contraceptives increasing the incidence of tubal infertility.[371] In fact, a case-control study indicated that oral contraceptive users with *Chlamydia* infection are protected against symptomatic PID.[372] A case-control study has suggested that oral contraceptive users are more likely to harbor unrecognized endometritis, and that this would explain the discrepancy between the observed rates between lower and upper tract infection.[373] However, this would not explain the lack of an association between oral contraceptive use and tubal infertility. Thus, the influence of oral contraception on the upper reproductive tract may be different than on the lower tract. These observations on fertility are derived mostly, if not totally, from women using oral contraceptives containing 50 μg of estrogen. The continued progestin dominance of the lower dose formulations, however, should produce the same protective impact. Early evidence indicated protection with low-dose oral contraceptives, but a later study failed to find a reduction in upper genital tract disease with either oral contraceptives or barrier methods.[364, 374]

Other Infections

In the British prospective studies of high-dose oral contraceptives, urinary tract infections were increased in users of oral contraception by 20%, and a correlation was noted with estrogen dose. An increased incidence of cervicitis was also reported, an effect related to the progestin dose. The incidence of cervicitis increased with the length of time the pill was used, from no higher after 6 months to 3 times higher by the sixth year of use. A significant increase in a variety of viral diseases, e.g., chickenpox, was observed, suggesting steroid effects on the immune system. The prevalence of these effects with low-dose oral contraception is unknown.

Oral contraception appears to protect against bacterial vaginosis and infections with *Trichomonas*.[375–377] Evidence is lacking to convincingly implicate oral contraception with vaginal infections with *Candida* species;[375] however, clinical experience is sometimes impressive when recurrence and cure repeatedly follow use and discontinuation of oral contraception.

Patient Management

Absolute Contraindications to the Use of Oral Contraception

1. Thrombophlebitis, thromboembolic disorders (including a close family history, parent or sibling, suggestive of an inherited susceptibility for venous thrombosis), cerebral vascular disease, coronary occlusion, or a past history of these conditions, or conditions predisposing to these problems.

2. Markedly impaired liver function. Steroid hormones are contraindicated in patients with hepatitis until liver function tests return to normal.

3. Known or suspected breast cancer.

4. Undiagnosed abnormal vaginal bleeding.

5. Known or suspected pregnancy.

6. Smokers over the age of 35.

7. Severe hypercholesterolemia or hypertriglyceridemia.

8. Elevated blood pressure.

Relative Contraindications Requiring Clinical Judgment and Informed Consent

1. Migraine headaches.
2. Hypertension.
3. Uterine leiomyoma.
4. Gestational diabetes.
5. Diabetes mellitus.
6. Elective surgery.
7. Seizure disorders.
8. Obstructive jaundice in pregnancy.
9. Sickle cell disease or sickle C disease.
10. Gallbladder disease.
11. Mitral valve prolapse.
12. Systemic lupus erythematosus.
13. Hyperlipidemia.
14. Smoking.
15. Hepatic disease.

Clinical Decisions

Surveillance

Many women can be prescribed hormonal contraception without a clinical breast and pelvic examination.[378] Problems requiring further evaluation can be identified with a careful medical history and measurement of blood pressure. Subsequently, in view of the increased safety of low-dose preparations for healthy young women with no risk factors, patients need be seen only every 12 months for exclusion of problems by history, measurement of the blood pressure, urinalysis, breast examination, palpation of the liver, and pelvic examination with Pap smear. Women with risk factors should be seen every 6 months by appropriately trained personnel for screening of problems by history and blood pressure measurement. Breast and pelvic examinations are necessary only yearly. It is worth emphasizing that better continuation is achieved by reassessing new users within 1–2 months. It is at this time that subtle fears and unvoiced concerns need to be confronted and resolved.

Oral contraception is safer than most people think it is, and the low-dose preparations are extremely safe. Health care providers should make a significant effort to get this message to our patients (and our colleagues). We must make sure our patients receive adequate counseling, either from ourselves or our professional staff. The major reason why patients discontinue oral contraception is fear of side effects.[379] Let's take time to put the risks into proper perspective and to emphasize the benefits as well as the risks.

Laboratory surveillance should be used only when indicated. Routine biochemical measurements fail to yield sufficient information to warrant the expense. Assessing the cholesterol-lipoprotein profile and carbohydrate metabolism should follow the same guidelines applied to all patients, users and nonusers of contraception. The following is a useful guide as to who should be monitored with blood screening tests for glucose, lipids, and lipoproteins:

> Young women, at least once.
> Women 35 years or older.
> Women with a strong family history of heart disease, diabetes mellitus, or hypertension.
> Women with gestational diabetes mellitus.
> Women with xanthomatosis.
> Obese women.
> Diabetic women.

Choice of Pill

The therapeutic principle remains: utilize the formulations that give effective contraception and the greatest margin of safety. You and your patients are urged to choose a low-dose preparation containing less than 50 μg of estrogen, combined with low doses of new or old progestins. Current data support the view that there is greater safety with preparations containing less than 50 μg of estrogen. The arguments in this chapter indicate that all patients should begin oral contraception with low-dose products, and that patients on higher dose oral contraception should be changed to the low-dose preparations. Stepping down to a lower dose can be accomplished immediately with no adverse reactions such as increased bleeding or failure of contraception.

The multiphasic preparations do have a reduced progestin dosage compared with some of the existing monophasic products; however, based on currently available information there is little difference between the low-dose monophasics and the multiphasics.

The pharmacologic effects in animals of various formulations have been used as a basis for therapeutic recommendations in selecting the optimal oral contraceptive pill. *These recommendations (tailor-making the pill to the patient) have not been supported by appropriately controlled clinical trials. All too often this leads to the prescribing of a pill of excessive dosage with its attendant increased risk of serious side effects.* It is worth repeating our earlier comments on potency. Oral contraceptive potency (specifically progestin potency) is no longer a consideration when it comes to prescribing birth control pills. The potency of the various progestins has been accounted for by appropriate adjustments of dose. Clinical advice based on potency is an artificial exercise that has not stood the test of time. The biologic effect of the various progestational components in current low-dose oral contraceptives is approximately the same. Our progress in lowering the doses of the steroids contained in oral contraceptives has yielded products with little serious differences.

Pill Taking

Effective contraception is present during the first cycle of pill use, provided the pills are started no later than the fifth day of the cycle and no pills are missed. Thus, starting oral contraception on the first day of menses ensures immediate protection. In the United States, most clinicians and patients prefer the Sunday start packages, beginning on the first Sunday following menstruation. This can be easier to remember, and it usually avoids menstrual bleeding on weekends. It is probable, but not totally certain, that even if a dominant follicle should emerge in occasional patients after a Sunday start, an LH surge and ovulation would still be prevented.[380] Some clinicians prefer to advise patients to use added protection in the first week of use.

The conventional approach to starting oral contraceptives, either with menses or on Sunday, carries with it a delay in achieving contraception for many women. Many clinicians advocate an immediate start on the day the patient receives her prescription, regardless of the patient's day in her cycle.[381] Combined with a backup method for the first week, preferably condoms, an immediate start may avoid unwanted pregnancies occurring during the delay before initiating oral contraception with the conventional methods. In some instances, a sensitive pregnancy test would be a wise precaution. Women who use the immediate start method do not experience an increase in breakthrough bleeding.[382]

Occasionally patients would like to postpone a menstrual period, e.g., for a wedding, holiday, or vacation. This can be easily achieved by omitting the 7-day hormone-free interval. Simply start a new package of pills the next day after finishing the series of 21 pills in the previous package. Remember, when using a 28-pill package, the patient would start a new package after using the 21 active pills.

There is no rationale for recommending a pill-free interval "to rest." The serious side effects are not eliminated by pill-free intervals. This practice all too often results in unwanted pregnancies.

How important is it to take the oral contraceptive at the same time every day? Although not well studied, there is reason to believe precise pill taking minimizes breakthrough bleeding. In addition, compliance is improved by a fixed schedule that is habit-forming.

Avoiding Menstrual Bleeding

More and more women are embracing the idea that fewer menstrual periods provide a welcome relief from bleeding and menstrual symptoms. A regimen (Seasonale) is available that supplies a package containing the number of pills required for 84 days of daily administration, a reduction of menstrual frequency to 4 per year.[383] However, clinicians for years have prescribed unlimited daily oral contraceptives to treat conditions such as endometriosis, bleeding disorders, menstrual seizures, and menstrual migraine headaches, even to avoid bleeding in athletes and busy individuals. Many women do not require the periodic experience of vaginal bleeding to assure themselves they are not pregnant. And of course, modern society is long past the notion that menstrual bleeding is a cleansing event, a detoxification. It is not necessary for women using oral contraceptives to experience any withdrawal bleeding. Monthly bleeding, periodic bleeding, or no bleeding—this is an individual woman's choice. Any combination oral contraceptive can be used on a daily basis; even the lowest estrogen dose formulations provide excellent bleeding and side-effect profiles in a continuous regimen.[384, 385] A further benefit of continuous use is simplification of the pill-taking schedule with the potential of better compliance and a lower failure rate. When breakthrough bleeding occurs, patients can be reassured that it is almost always temporary. When breakthrough bleeding is persistent, a 3–4 day interruption without pill taking has been reported to be helpful.[386]

What To Do When Pills Are Missed

Irregular pill taking is a common occurrence. Using an electronic monitoring device to measure compliance, it was apparent that consistency of pill taking is even worse than what patients report; only 33% of women were documented to have missed no pills in cycle 1, and by cycle 3, about one-third of the women missed 3 or more pills with many episodes of consecutive days of missed pills.[387] These data indicate that women become less careful over time, emphasizing the importance of repeatedly reviewing with patients what to do when pills are missed.

If a woman misses 1 pill, she should take that pill as soon as she remembers and take the next pill as usual. No backup method is needed.

If she misses 2 pills in the first 2 weeks, she should take 2 pills on each of the next 2 days; it is unlikely that a backup method is needed, but the official consensus is to recommend backup for the next 7 days.

If 2 pills are missed in the third week, or if more than 2 active pills are missed at any time, another form of contraception should be used as backup immediately and for 7 days; if a Sunday starter, keep taking a pill every day until Sunday, and on Sunday start a new package; if a non-Sunday starter, start a new package the same day.

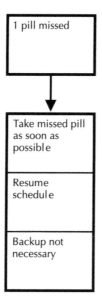

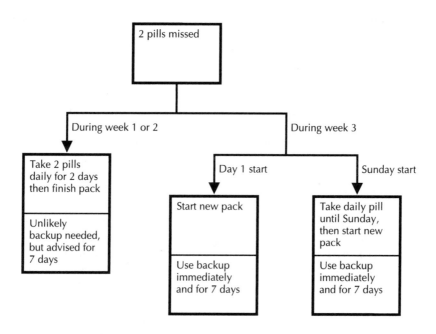

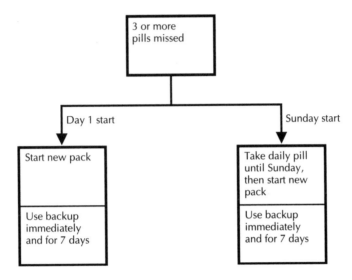

Studies have questioned whether missing pills has an impact on contraception. One study demonstrated that skipping 4 consecutive pills at varying times in the cycle did not result in ovulation.[380] Studies in which women deliberately lengthen their pill-fee interval up to 11 days have failed to show signs of ovulation.[388, 389] So far there is no evidence that moving to lower doses has had an impact on the margin of error. Despite greater follicular activity with the lowest-dose oral contraceptives, ovulation is still effectively prevented.[390]

The studies have involved small numbers of women, and given the large individual variation, it still is possible that some women might be at risk with a small increase in the pill-free interval. However, the progestational effects on endometrium and cervical mucus serve to ensure good contraceptive efficacy.[26] We may well prove that current recommendations are too conservative and that a woman's chance of getting pregnant with missing pills is nearly zero. Nevertheless, this conservative advice is the safest message to convey.

The most prevalent problems that can be identified associated with apparent oral contraceptive failures are vomiting and diarrhea.[30, 31] *Even if no pills have been missed, patients should be instructed to use a backup method for at least 7 days after an episode of gastroenteritis.*

Clinical Problems

Breakthrough Bleeding

A major continuation problem is breakthrough bleeding. Breakthrough bleeding gives rise to fears and concerns; it is aggravating and even embarrassing. Therefore, on starting oral contraception, patients need to be fully informed about breakthrough bleeding.

There are two characteristic breakthrough bleeding problems: irregular bleeding in the first few months after starting oral contraception and unexpected bleeding after many months of use. Effort should be made to manage the bleeding problem in a way that allows the patient to remain on low-dose oral contraception. ***There is no evidence that the onset of bleeding is associated with decreased efficacy, no matter what oral contraceptive formulation is used, even the lowest dose products.*** Indeed, in a careful study, breakthrough bleeding did not correlate with changes in the blood levels of the contraceptive steroids.[391]

The most frequently encountered breakthrough bleeding occurs in the first few months of use. The incidence is greatest in the first 3 months, ranging from 10–30% in the first month to less than 10% in the third. Breakthrough bleeding rates are higher with the lowest dose oral contraceptives but not dramatically.[392, 393] Breakthrough bleeding are higher in women who smoke and in smokers who use formulations with 20 μg ethinyl estradiol.[394] However, the differences among the various formulations currently available are of minimal clinical significance. The basic pattern is the same, highest in the first month and a greater prevalence in smokers, especially in later cycles.

Breakthrough bleeding is best managed by encouragement and reassurance. This bleeding usually disappears by the third cycle in the majority of women. If necessary, even this early pattern of breakthrough bleeding can be treated as outlined below. It is helpful to explain to the patient that this bleeding represents tissue breakdown as the endometrium adjusts from its usual thick state to the relatively thin state allowed by the hormones in oral contraceptives.

Breakthrough bleeding that occurs after many months of oral contraceptive use is a consequence of the progestin-induced decidualization. This endometrium and the blood vessels within the endometrium tend to be fragile and prone to breakdown and asynchronous bleeding.

There are two recognized factors (both preventable) that are associated with a greater incidence of breakthrough bleeding. Consistency of use and smoking increase spotting and bleeding, but inconsistency of pill taking is more important and has a greater effect in later cycles, whereas smoking exerts a general effect at any time.[395] Reinforcement of consistent pill taking can help minimize breakthrough bleeding. Cervical infection can be another cause of breakthrough bleeding; the prevalence of cervical chlamydial infections is higher among oral contraceptive users who report breakthrough bleeding.[396]

If bleeding occurs just before the end of the pill cycle, it can be managed by having the patient stop the pills, wait 7 days, and start a new cycle. If breakthrough bleeding is prolonged or if it is aggravating for the patient, regardless of the point in the pill cycle, control of the bleeding can be achieved with a short course of exogenous estrogen. Conjugated estrogen, 1.25 mg, or estradiol, 2 mg, is administered daily for 7 days when the bleeding is present, no matter where the patient is in her pill cycle. The patient continues to adhere to the schedule of pill taking. Usually, one course of estrogen solves the problem, and recurrence of bleeding is unusual (but if it does recur, another 7-day course of estrogen is effective).

Responding to irregular bleeding by having the patient take 2 or 3 pills is not effective. The progestin component of the pill always dominates; hence, doubling the number of pills also doubles the progestational impact and its decidualizing, atrophic effect on the endometrium and its destabilizing effect on endometrial blood vessels. The addition of extra estrogen while keeping the progestin dose unchanged is logical and effective. This allows the patient to remain on the low-dose formulation with its advantage of greater safety. Breakthrough bleeding, in our view, is not sufficient reason to expose patients to the increased risks associated with higher dose oral contraceptives. Any bleeding that is not handled by this routine requires investigation for the presence of pathology.

There is no evidence that any oral contraceptive formulations that are approximately equivalent in estrogen and progestin dosage are significantly different in the rates of breakthrough bleeding. Clinicians often become impressed that switching to another product effectively stops the breakthrough bleeding. It is more likely that the passage of time is the responsible factor, and bleeding would have stopped regardless of switching and regardless of product.

Amenorrhea

With low-dose pills, the estrogen content is not sufficient in some women to stimulate endometrial growth. The progestational effect dominates to such a degree that a shallow atrophic endometrium is produced, lacking sufficient tissue to yield withdrawal bleeding. It should be emphasized that permanent atrophy of the endometrium does not occur, and resumption of normal ovarian function restores endometrial growth and development. Indeed, there is no harmful, permanent consequence of amenorrhea while on oral contraception.

The major problem with amenorrhea while on oral contraception is the anxiety produced in both patient and clinician because the lack of bleeding may be a sign of pregnancy. The patient is anxious because of the uncertainty regarding pregnancy, and the clinician is anxious because of the medicolegal concerns stemming from the old studies, which indicated an increased risk of congenital abnormalities among the offspring of women who inadvertently used oral contraception in early pregnancy. We reviewed this problem earlier, and emphatically stated that there is no association between oral contraception and an increased risk of congenital malformation, and there is no increased risk of having abnormal children.

The incidence of amenorrhea in the first year of use with low-dose oral contraception is less than 2%. This incidence increases with duration, reaching perhaps 5% after several years of use. It is important to alert patients upon starting oral contraception that diminished bleeding and possibly no bleeding may ensue.

Amenorrhea is a difficult management problem. A pregnancy test allows reliable assessment for pregnancy even at this early stage. However, routine, repeated use of such testing is expensive and annoying and may lead to discontinuation of oral contraception. *A simple test for pregnancy is to assess the basal body temperature during the END of the pill-free week; a basal body temperature less than 98 degrees (36.7°C) is not consistent with pregnancy, and oral contraception can be continued.*

Many women are reassured with an understanding of why there is no bleeding and are able to continue on the pill despite the amenorrhea. Some women cannot reconcile themselves to a lack of bleeding, and this is an indication for trying other formulations (a practice unsupported by any clinical trials, and, therefore, the expectations are uncertain). But again, this problem does not warrant exposing patients to the greater risks of major side effects associated with higher dose products.

Some clinicians have observed that the addition of extra estrogen for 1 month (1.25 mg conjugated estrogens or 2 mg estradiol daily throughout the 21 days while taking the oral contraceptive) rejuvenates the endometrium, and withdrawal bleeding resumes, persisting for many months.

Weight Gain

The complaint of weight gain is frequently cited as a major problem with compliance. Yet, studies of the low-dose preparations fail to demonstrate a significant weight gain with oral contraception, and no major differences among the various products.[193–196, 199, 201] This is obviously a problem of perception, a conclusion supported by finding the weight gain identical in treated and placebo groups. The clinician has to carefully reinforce the lack of association between low-dose oral contraceptives and weight gain and focus the patient on the real culprit: diet and level of exercise. Most women gain a moderate amount of weight as they age, whether they take oral contraceptives or not.

Acne

Low-dose oral contraceptives improve acne regardless of which product is used.[167, 191, 192, 200, 397–400] The low progestin doses (including levonorgestrel formulations) currently used are insufficient to stimulate an androgenic response and provide effective treatment for acne and hirsutism.

Ovarian Cysts

Anecdotal reports suggested that functional ovarian cysts are encountered more frequently and suppress less easily with multiphasic formulations. This observation failed to withstand careful scrutiny.[401, 402] Functional ovarian cysts occurred less frequently in women on higher dose oral contraception.[403] This protection is reduced with the current lower dose products to the point where little effect can be measured.[402, 404–407] Thus, the risk of such cysts is not eliminated; and, therefore, clinicians can encounter such cysts in patients taking any of the oral contraceptive formulations.

Drugs That Affect Efficacy

There are many anecdotal reports of patients who conceived on oral contraceptives while taking antibiotics. There is little evidence, however, that antibiotics such as ampicillin, metronidazole, quinolone, and tetracycline, which reduce the bacterial flora of the gastrointestinal tract, affect oral contraceptive efficacy. Studies indicate that while antibiotics can alter the excretion of contraceptive steroids, plasma levels are unchanged, and there is no evidence of ovulation.[408–411] A review of a large number of patients derived from dermatology practices failed to find an increased rate of pregnancy in women on oral contraceptives and being treated with antibiotics (tetracyclines, penicillins, cephalosporins).[412]

There is good reason to believe that drugs that stimulate the liver's metabolic capacity can affect oral contraceptive efficacy. St. John's wort must be added to this list.[413] On the other hand, a search of a large database failed to discover any evidence that lower dose oral contraceptives are more likely to fail or to have more drug interaction problems when other drugs are used.[414]

To be cautious, patients on medications that affect liver metabolism should choose an alternative contraceptive. A list, which may not be complete, includes the following:

> Carbamazepine (Tegretol).
> Felbamate.
> Nevirapine.
> Oxcarbazepine.
> Phenobarbital.
> Phenytoin (Dilantin).
> Primidone (Mysoline).
> Rifabutin.
> Rifampicin (Rifampin).
> St. John's Wort.
> Topiramate.
> Vigabatrin.
> Possibly ethosuximide, griseofulvin, and troglitazone.

Other Drug Interactions

Although not extensively documented, there is reason to believe that oral contraceptives potentiate the action of diazepam (Valium), chlordiazepoxide (Librium), tricyclic antidepressants, and theophylline.[415] Thus, lower doses of these agents may be effective in oral contraceptive users. Because of an influence on clearance rates, oral contraceptive users may require larger doses of acetaminophen and aspirin.[416]

Migraine Headaches

True migraine headaches are more common in women, while tension headaches (90% of all headaches) occur equally in men and women. There have been no well-done studies to determine the impact of oral contraception on migraine headaches. Patients may report that their headaches are worse or better.

Migraine headaches, especially with aura, are a risk factor for stroke.[417] The risk is greater in women with hypertension, in smokers, with a family history of migraine, and in women with a long history of migraine or with more than 12 attacks per year of migraine with aura.[418, 419] Studies with high-dose pills indicated that migraine headaches were linked to a risk of stroke. More recent studies reflecting the use of low-dose formulations yield mixed results. One failed to find a further increase in stroke in patients with migraine who use oral contraception, another concluded that the use of oral contraception by migraineurs was associated with a 4-fold increase of the already increased risk of ischemic stroke.[420, 421] The World Health Organization case-control study indicated an increased risk in oral contraceptive users who smoked.[418] Because 20–30% of women experience migraine headaches, one would expect the populations in the most recent studies of thrombosis to have included substantial numbers of migraineurs. An adverse effect of low-dose oral contraceptives on stroke risk in migraineurs should have manifested itself in the data. The lack of an increased risk of stroke in these studies is reassuring. Nevertheless, it is believed that migraineurs on oral contraceptives have an increased risk of stroke; the absolute risk in a 20-year-old woman is estimated to be 10 per 100,000 and for a 40-year-old woman, 100 per 100,000.[422]

There are two categories of migraine headaches: common migraine, which is migraine without aura and classic migraine, which is migraine with aura (essentially migraine headaches with visual aura or other neurologic symptoms, occurring in 30% of migraine sufferers). Because of the seriousness of this potential complication, the onset of visual symptoms or severe headaches requires a response. If the patient is at a higher dose, a move to a low-dose formulation may relieve the headaches. Switching to a different brand is worthwhile, if only to evoke a placebo response. True vascular headaches (migraine with aura) are an indication to avoid or discontinue oral contraception. Oral contraceptives should be avoided in women who have migraine with complex or prolonged aura, or if additional stroke factors are present (older age, smoking, hypertension, diabetes mellitus, obesity, family history of arterial disease at a young age).[422] Oral contraceptives can be considered in women under age 35, who have migraine without aura, and who are otherwise healthy and not smokers.

Clues to Migraine with Aura:

- Scotomata or blurred vision.
- Episodes of blindness.
- Numbness, paresthesias.
- Speech difficulties.
- Unilateral symptoms, such as weakness.

In some women, a relationship exists between their fluctuating hormone levels during a menstrual cycle and migraine headaches, with the onset of headaches characteristically coinciding with menses (also seen during the pill-free week of oral contraception). We have had personal success (anecdotal to be sure) alleviating headaches by eliminating the menstrual cycle, either with the use of daily oral contraceptives or the daily administration of a progestational agent (such as 10 mg medroxyprogesterone acetate) or the use of depot-medroxyprogesterone acetate. Some women with migraine headaches have extremely gratifying responses. Women who experience an exacerbation of their headaches with oral contraception should consider one of the progestin-only methods.

Summary: Oral Contraceptive Use and Medical Problems

Migraine Headaches. Some women report an improvement in their headaches with oral contraceptives. Low-dose oral contraception (the lowest estrogen dose formulation) can be tried with careful surveillance in women with migraine headaches without aura. Daily administration can prevent menstrual migraine headaches. Oral contraception is best avoided in women with migraine headaches with aura or if additional stroke risk factors are present (especially older age, smoking, and hypertension).

Hypertension. Low-dose oral contraception can be used in women less than age 35 with hypertension well controlled by medication, and who are otherwise healthy and do not smoke. We recommend the lowest estrogen dose formulations. Nevertheless, a cross-sectional study in Brazil reported worse control of hypertension in users of oral contraceptives.[161] Certainly a woman with controlled hypertension who has additional medical problems or who smokes should not use estrogen-progestin contraceptives (including the transdermal and vaginal methods). In a young woman with controlled hypertension who is otherwise healthy, very frequent and close monitoring of the blood pressure is essential. Myocardial infarction and stroke become more common after age 35, and we believe that combined estrogen-progestin contraception should not be used by women with controlled hypertension after age 35. Progestin-only methods are acceptable.

Pregnancy-Induced Hypertension. Women with pregnancy-induced hypertension can use oral contraception as soon as the blood pressure is normal in the postpartum period.

Uterine Leiomyoma. This is not a contraindication for low-dose oral contraceptives. There is evidence that the risk of leiomyomas was decreased by 31% in women who used higher dose oral contraception for 10 years.[423] However, case-control studies with lower dose oral contraceptives have found neither a decrease nor an increase in risk, although the Nurses' Health Study reported a slightly increased risk when oral contraceptives were first used in early teenage years.[424–426] One case-control study indicated a decreasing risk of uterine fibroids with increasing duration of oral contraceptive use.[427] The administration of low-dose oral contraceptives to women with leiomyomas does not stimulate fibroid growth and is associated with a reduction in menstrual bleeding.[428]

Gestational Diabetes. Low-dose formulations do not produce a diabetic glucose tolerance response in women with previous gestational diabetes, and there is no evidence that combined oral contraceptives increase the incidence of overt diabetes mellitus.[175, 176] We believe that women with previous gestational diabetes can use oral contraception with annual assessment of the fasting glucose level. There is a concern with breastfeeding women using the progestin-only minipill (discussed in Chapter 3).

Diabetes Mellitus. Oral contraception can be used by diabetic women less than 35 years old who do not smoke and are otherwise healthy (especially an absence of diabetic vascular complications). A case-control study could find no evidence that oral contraceptive use by young women with insulin-dependent diabetes mellitus increased the development of retinopathy or nephropathy.[178] In a 1-year study of women with insulin-dependent diabetes mellitus who were using a low-dose oral contraceptive, no deterioration could be documented in lipoprotein or hemostatic biochemical markers for cardiovascular risk.[179] And finally, no effect of oral contraceptives on cardiovascular mortality could be detected in a group of women with diabetes mellitus.[180] Women with diabetes and vascular disease or major cardiovascular risk factors should avoid pharmacologic doses of exogenous estrogen.

Elective surgery. The recommendation that oral contraception should be discontinued 4 weeks before elective major surgery to avoid an increased risk of postoperative thrombosis is based on data derived from high-dose pills. If possible, it is safer to follow this recommendation when a period of immobilization is to be expected. With major surgery and immobilization, prophylactic treatment should be considered for a current or recent user of oral contraceptives. It is prudent to maintain contraception right up to the performance of a sterilization procedure, and this short, outpatient operation carries very minimal, if any, risk.

Seizure Disorders. Oral contraceptives do not exacerbate epilepsy, and in some women, improvement in seizure control has occurred.[429, 430] Antiepileptic drugs that affect liver metabolism, however, may decrease the effectiveness of oral contraception. Some clinicians advocate the use of higher dose (50 μg estrogen) products; however, no studies have been performed to demonstrate that this higher dose is necessary. Another problem is that moving to a higher dose product increases the estrogen dose (and the risk of side effects) but does not significantly change the progestin dose, the component that inhibits ovulation. A wiser course is to consider intrauterine contraception with an IUD, long-acting methods, barrier methods, or sterilization.

Obstructive Jaundice in Pregnancy. Not all patients with this history develop jaundice on oral contraception, especially with the low-dose formulations.

Sickle Cell Disease. Patients with sickle cell trait can use oral contraception. The risk of thrombosis in women with sickle cell disease or sickle C diseases is theoretical (and medicolegal). We believe effective protection against pregnancy in these patients warrants the use of low-dose oral contraception. In the only long-term (10 years) follow-up report of women with sickle cell disease and using oral contraceptives, no apparent adverse effects were observed (at a time when higher dose products were prevalent).[431] A study of erythrocyte deformability in women with sickle cell anemia could detect no adverse effects of contraceptive steroids.[432] Keep in mind that depot-medroxyprogesterone acetate used for contraception is associated with inhibition of sickling and improvement in anemia in patients with sickle cell disease.[433]

Gallbladder Disease. Oral contraception use may precipitate a symptomatic attack in women known to have stones or a positive history for gallbladder disease and, therefore, should either be used very cautiously or not at all.

Mitral Valve Prolapse. Oral contraception use is limited to nonsmoking patients who are asymptomatic (no clinical evidence of regurgitation). There is a small subset of patients with mitral valve prolapse who are at increased risk of thromboembolism. Patients with atrial fibrillation, migraine headaches, or clotting factor abnormalities should consider progestin-only methods or the IUD (prophylactic antibiotics should cover IUD insertion if mitral regurgitation is present).

Systemic Lupus Erythematosus. Oral contraceptive use can exacerbate systemic lupus erythematous, and the vascular disease associated with lupus, when present, represents a contraindication to estrogen-containing contraceptives.[434] The progestin-only methods are a good choice. However, in patients with stable or inactive disease, without renal involvement and high antiphospholipid antibodies, low-dose oral contraception can be considered.[435]

Hyperlipidemia. Because low-dose oral contraceptives have negligible impact on the lipoprotein profile, hyperlipidemia is not an absolute contraindication, with the exception of very high levels of triglycerides (which can be made worse by estrogen). In women with triglyceride levels greater than 250 mg/dL, estrogen should be provided with great caution. If vascular disease is already present, oral contraception should be avoided. If other risk factors are present, especially smoking, oral contraception is not recommended. Dyslipidemic patients who begin oral contraception should have their lipoprotein profiles monitored monthly for a few visits to ensure no adverse impact. If the lipid abnormality cannot be held in control, an alternative method of contraception should be used.[436] Oral contraceptives containing desogestrel, noregestimate, or gestodene can increase HDL levels, but it is not known if this change is clinically significant. If hypertriglyceridemia is the only concern, keep in mind that the triglyceride response to estrogen is rapid. A repeat level should be obtained in 2–4 weeks. A level greater than 750 mg/dL represents an absolute contraindication to estrogen treatment because of the risk of pancreatitis.

Smoking. Oral contraception is absolutely contraindicated in smokers over the age of 35. In patients 35 years old and younger, heavy smoking (15 or more cigarettes per day) is a relative contraindication. The relative risk of cardiovascular events is increased for women of all ages who smoke and use oral contraceptives; however, because the actual incidence of cardiovascular events is so low at a young age, the real risk is very low for young women, although it increases with age. An ex-smoker (for at least 1 year) should be regarded as a nonsmoker. Risk is only linked to active smoking. Is there room for judgment? Given the right circumstances, low-dose oral contraceptives might be appropriate for a light smoker or the user of a nicotine patch. A 20 μg estrogen formulation may be a better choice for smoking women, regardless of age (because this dose of estrogen has no impact on clotting factors and platelet activation).[54, 55]

Hepatic Disease. Oral contraception can be utilized when liver function tests return to normal. Follow-up liver function tests should be obtained after 2–3 months of use.

Hemorrhagic Disorders. Women with hemorrhagic disorders and women taking anticoagulants can use oral contraception. Inhibition of ovulation can avoid the real problem of a hemorrhagic corpus luteum in these patients. A reduction in menstrual blood loss is another benefit of importance.

Obesity. An obese woman who is otherwise healthy can use low-dose oral contraception. However, there are special considerations associated with obesity:

•Obesity is an independent risk factor for venous thrombosis, and case-control studies have indicated this risk adds to that associated with oral contraceptives.[75, 87, 437]

•There is modest evidence that hormonal contraceptive failure is increased in overweight women (over 155 pounds).[438–440] Clinical trials have excluded women with high body weight, and for this reason, the effect of body weight on contraception was not well studied. Selecting a 50 μg estrogen product for over weight women might overcome the failure rate, but this would add the risks associated with a higher dose of estrogen to those already linked with obesity. Keep in mind that the conclusions regarding failure rates and weight were based on differences of only 2 to 4 pregnancies per 100 women per year. Efficacy in overweight women is still greater than that with barrier methods.

Benign Breast Disease. Benign breast disease is not a contraindication for oral contraception; with 2 years of use, the condition may improve.

Congenital Heart Disease or Valvular Heart Disease. Oral contraception is contraindicated only if there is marginal cardiac reserve or a condition that predisposes to thrombosis.

Depression. Low-dose oral contraceptives have minimal, if any, impact on mood.

Polycystic Ovaries and Insulin Resistance. Because older, high-dose oral contraceptives increased insulin resistance, it has been suggested that this treatment should be avoided in anovulatory, overweight women. However, low-dose oral contraceptives have minimal effects on carbohydrate metabolism, and the majority of hyperinsulinemic, hyperandrogenic women can be expected to respond favorably to treatment with oral contraceptives.[441] Insulin and glucose changes with low-dose (less than 50 μg ethinyl estradiol) oral contraceptives are so minimal that it is now believed that they are of no clinical significance.[169] Long-term follow-up studies have failed to detect any increase in the incidence of diabetes mellitus or impaired glucose tolerance (even in past and current users of high-dose pills).[171, 173] Furthermore, there is no evidence of an increase in risk of cardiovascular disease among past users of oral contraceptives.[59, 60] In addition, low-dose oral contraceptives have been administered to women with recent gestational diabetes without an adverse impact, and in women with insulin-dependent diabetes mellitus, low-dose oral contraceptives have not produced deterioration of lipid and biochemical markers for cardiovascular disease or increased the development of retinopathy or nephropathy.[175, 176, 178, 179] The administration of a low-dose oral contraceptive to women with extreme obesity and very severe insulin resistance resulted in only a mild deterioration of glucose tolerance.[442] Impressively, in a follow-up study (about 10 years) of women with polycystic ovaries and hyperinsulinism, comparing oral contraceptive users with nonusers, the metabolic parameters not only did not worsen in the users, but they actually improved, including body weight, glucose tolerance, insulin levels, and

HDL-cholesterol levels, which was in striking contrast to the metabolic worsening observed in the nonusers.[443] This experience supports the safety of estrogen-progestin contraceptive treatment for anovulatory, hyperandrogenic, hyperinsulinemic women.

Eating Disorders. In patients with eating disorders, bone density correlates with body weight. The response to hormone therapy impaired as long as an abnormal weight is maintained.[444] The failure to respond to estrogen treatment with an increase in bone density may be due to the adverse bone effects of the hypercortisolism associated with stress disorders. Furthermore, because the pubertal gain in bone density is so significant, individuals who fail to experience this adolescent increase may continue to have a deficit in bone mass despite hormone treatment. Reduced menstrual function for any reason early in life (even beyond adolescence) may leave a residual deficit in bone density that cannot be totally retrieved with resumption of menses or with hormone treatment.[445, 446]

Pituitary Prolactin-Secreting Adenomas. Low-dose oral contraception can be used in the presence of microadenomas.

Infectious Mononucleosis. Oral contraception can be used as long as liver function tests are normal.

Ulcerative Colitis. There is no association between oral contraception and ulcerative colitis. Women with this problem can use oral contraceptives.[203] Oral contraceptives are absorbed mainly in the small bowel.

Regional Enteritis (Crohn's Disease). In a prospective cohort of women with Crohn's disease, no adverse impact of oral contraceptives could be detected on the clinical course, specifically on flare-ups.[447]

An Alternative Route of Administration

Occasionally, a situation may be encountered when an alternative to oral administration of contraceptive pills is required. For example, patients receiving chemotherapy can either have significant nausea and vomiting, or mucositis, both of which would prevent oral drug administration. The low-dose oral contraceptives can be administered vaginally. Initially, it was claimed that two pills must be placed high in the vagina daily to produce contraceptive steroid blood levels comparable with the oral administration of one pill.[448] However, a large clinical trial has demonstrated typical contraceptive efficacy with one pill administered vaginally per day.[449] In a comparative study, a major reduction in side effects was associated with vaginal administration.[450] Of course, the vaginal and transdermal methods discussed in Chapter 4 should also be considered.

Athletes and Oral Contraception

Because athletes are often amenorrheic and hypoestrogenic, oral contraceptives provide not only confidence against the risk of an unwanted pregnancy but also estrogen support against bone loss. This is a situation where bone density measurements are worthwhile. A low bone density can help motivate an athlete to take hormone therapy, and a subsequent bone density measurement that reveals a failure of response to estrogen can indicate the presence of a hidden eating disorder. The amenorrheic exerciser should be made aware that the hypoestrogenic state is associated with a greater risk of stress fractures.

Competing athletes are often concerned that oral contraceptives could reduce exercise performance. A rationale for the concern can be traced to the physiologic increase in ventilation during pregnancy, mediated by progesterone. Thus, progestin enhancement of ventilatory response could consume energy otherwise available for athletic performance. Indeed, reports have generated conflicting data as measured by laboratory testing. However, experimental studies that simulate athletic events can find no adverse effects on oxygen uptake, respiratory rate, endurance, or isometric exercises.[451, 452] One study documented decreased soreness, both perceived and with palpation, after exercise in women using oral contraceptives.[453] Oral contraceptive use has no effect on prevalence or severity of low back pain, a common problem among female athletes.[454]

Estrogen-progestin contraceptives have a lot to offer with no serious drawbacks for athletes. In athletes who wish to avoid menstrual bleeding, oral contraceptives can be administered on a daily basis, with no breaks, preventing withdrawal bleeding. Continuous administration is also a good choice for women in the military. The vaginal and transdermal methods (Chapter 4) can be used in a similar fashion.

The Noncontraceptive Benefits of Oral Contraception

The noncontraceptive benefits of low-dose oral contraception can be grouped into two main categories: benefits that incidentally accrue when oral contraception is specifically utilized for contraceptive purposes and benefits that result from the use of oral contraceptives to treat problems and disorders.

The noncontraceptive incidental benefits can be listed as follows:

Effective Contraception:
    •**Less need for induced abortion.**
    •**Less need for surgical sterilization.**
Less Endometrial Cancer.
Less Ovarian Cancer.
Fewer Ectopic Pregnancies.
More Regular Menses:
    •**Less flow.**
    •**Less dysmenorrhea.**
    •**Less anemia.**
Less Salpingitis.
Increased Bone Density.
Probably Less Endometriosis.
Possibly Less Benign Breast Disease.
Possibly Less Rheumatoid Arthritis.
Possibly Protection against Atherosclerosis.
Possibly Fewer Fibroids.
Possibly Fewer Ovarian Cysts.

Many of these benefits have been previously discussed. Protection against PID is especially noteworthy and a major contribution to not only preservation of fertility but to lower health care costs. Also important is the prevention of ectopic pregnancies. Ectopic pregnancies have increased in incidence (partly due to an increase in STIs) and represent a major cost for our society and a threat to both fertility and life for individual patients. Of course, prevention of benign and malignant neoplasia is an outstanding feature of oral contraception. High-dose oral contraceptive use decreased the incidence of benign breast disease diagnosed clinically as well as fibrocystic disease and fibroadenomas diagnosed by biopsy; hopefully, the same impact becomes evident with current lower dose formulations. A 40% reduction in ovarian cancer and a 50% reduction in endometrial cancer represent substantial protection.

Studies with higher dose formulations documented in long-term users a 31% reduction in uterine leiomyomas and, in current users, a 78% reduction in corpus luteum cysts and a 49% reduction in functional ovarian cysts.[403] Two case-control studies with low-dose oral contraceptives have found no impact on the risk of uterine fibroids, neither increased nor decreased,[424, 425] and one indicated a decreasing risk with increasing duration of use, reaching a 50% reduction after 7 or more years of use (the effect was limited to current users).[427] Epidemiologic studies have indicated that a progressive decline in the incidence of ovarian cysts is proportional to the steroid doses in oral contraceptives.[404, 405] Current low-dose monophasic and multiphasic formulations provide no protection against functional ovarian cysts.[404-407] This apparent weaker protection afforded by the current low-dose formulations makes it very likely that clinicians will encounter such cysts in their patients on oral contraceptives.

The low-dose contraceptives are as effective as higher dose preparations in reducing menstrual flow and the prevalence and severity of dysmenorrhea.[455-457] The use of oral contraception is associated with a lower incidence of endometriosis, although the protective effect is probably limited to current or recent use.[458-460] These benefits involving two common gynecologic problems have an important, positive impact on compliance.

An Austrian study concluded that osteoporosis occurs later and is less frequent in women who have used long-term oral contraception.[461] Most studies indicate that prior use of oral contraception is associated with higher levels of bone density and that the degree of protection is related to duration of exposure.[462-468] However, other studies reflecting modern use of low-dose products indicate little impact of oral contraceptive use on bone.[469-471] These measurements of bone density are not as important as the clinical outcome: fractures. The available evidence fails to provide a clear-cut picture. Retrospective studies indicated a reduction in fractures in postmenopausal women who had previously used oral contraceptives.[472-475] In the Royal College of General Practitioners Study, the overall risk of fractures in long-time users of oral contraceptives was actually slightly increased.[476] Similar results have been observed in the Oxford Family Planning Association Study.[477] It is likely that the increased risk reflects lifestyle effects among oral contraceptive users, but there was no evidence of a protective effect against fractures. In contrast, a case-control study from Sweden found a reduction in the risk of postmenopausal hip fractures when oral contraceptives (mostly older high-dose products) were used after age 40 by women who were not overweight, with an increasing benefit with increasing duration of use.[478] Previous oral contraceptive users are just now becoming elderly and reaching the age of greatest fracture prevalence. Future studies of postmenopausal women should eventually reveal the accurate relationship between oral contraceptive use and osteoporotic fractures.

The literature on rheumatoid arthritis has been controversial, with studies in Europe finding evidence of protection and studies in North America failing to demonstrate such an effect. An excellent Danish case-control study was designed to answer criticisms of shortcomings in the previous literature.[479] Long-time use of oral contraception reduced the relative risk of rheumatoid arthritis by 60%, and the strongest protection was present in women with a positive family history. One meta-analysis concluded that the evidence consistently indicated a protective effect, but that rather than preventing the development of rheumatoid arthritis, oral contraception may modify the course of disease, inhibiting the progression from mild to severe disease, whereas a later meta-analysis concluded there was no evidence of a protective effect.[480, 481]

Oral contraceptives are frequently utilized to manage the following problems and disorders:

Definitely Beneficial:
- **Dysfunctional uterine bleeding.**
- **Dysmenorrhea.**
- **Mittelschmerz.**
- **Endometriosis prophylaxis.**
- **Acne and hirsutism.**
- **Hormone therapy for hypothalamic amenorrhea.**
- **Prevention of menstrual porphyria.**
- **Control of bleeding (dyscrasias, anovulation).**

Possibly Beneficial:
- **Functional ovarian cysts.**
- **Premenstrual syndrome.**

Oral contraceptives have been a cornerstone for the treatment of anovulatory, dysfunctional uterine bleeding; the only randomized, placebo-controlled trial documented the beneficial impact long recognized by clinicians.[457] For patients who need effective contraception, oral contraceptives are a good choice to provide hormone therapy for amenorrheic patients, as well as to treat dysmenorrhea. Oral contraceptives are also a good choice to provide prophylaxis against the recurrence of endometriosis in a woman who has already undergone more vigorous treatment with surgery or the gonadotropin-releasing hormone (GnRH) analogues. To protect against endometriosis, oral contraceptives should be taken daily, with no break and no withdrawal bleeding. In a prospective series, women with endometriosis who had persistent dysmenorrhea despite cyclic oral contraceptive treatment experienced a significant decrease in symptoms with daily, continuous use.[482] Endometriosis may be associated with a slight increase in the risk of ovarian cancer, and another benefit of treatment with estrogen-progestin contraception is a reduction in this risk comparable to that in women without endometriosis.[483]

The low-dose oral contraceptives are effective in treating acne and hirsutism. Suppression of free testosterone levels is comparable with that achieved with higher dosage.[397, 484] The beneficial clinical effect is the same with low-dose preparations containing levonorgestrel, previously recognized to cause acne at high dosage.[397, 485] Formulations with desogestrel, gestodene, and norgestimate are associated with greater increases in sex hormone-binding globulin and significant decreases in free testosterone levels. Comparison studies with oral contraceptives containing these progestins can detect no differences in effects on various androgen measurements among the various products or compared with older products.[15, 399, 486] Theoretically, these products would be more effective in the treatment of acne and hirsutism; however, this has not been documented by clinical studies. It is likely that all low-dose formulations, through the combined effects of an increase in sex hormone-binding globulin and a decrease in testosterone production, produce an overall similar clinical response, especially over time (a year or more).

Oral contraceptives have long been used to speed the resolution of ovarian cysts, but the efficacy of this treatment has not been established. Randomized trials have been performed with women who develop ovarian cysts after induction of ovulation.[487–489] No advantage for the contraceptive treatment could be demonstrated. The cysts resolved completely and equally fast in both treated and nontreated groups. Of course, these were functional cysts secondary to ovulation induction, and this experience may not apply to spontaneously appearing cysts. Two short-term (5 and 6 weeks) randomized studies could document no greater effect of oral contraceptive treatment on resolution of spontaneous ovarian cysts when compared with expectant management.[490, 491] Clinical experience (untested by studies) leads us to believe that oral contraception does provide protection in women against the recurrent formation of ovarian cysts.

A case-control study indicated a reduced risk for benign ovarian tumors; however, the results did not achieve statistical significance.[492] The impact was limited to endometrioid lesions, an expected result.

Continuation: Failure or Success?

Despite the fact that oral contraception is highly effective, hundreds of thousands of unintended pregnancies (close to 1 million) occur each year in the United States because of the failure of oral contraception. Worldwide, millions of unintended pregnancies result from poor compliance. In general, unmarried, poor, and minority women are more likely to have failures, reaching rates of 10–20%.[493, 494] Overall, the failure rate with actual use is as high as 8%. This difference between the theoretical efficacy and actual use reflects compliance and noncompliance. Noncompliance includes a wide variety of behavior: failure to fill the initial prescription, failure to continue on the medication, and incorrectly taking oral contraception. Compliance (continuation) is an area in which personal behavior, biology, and pharmacology come together. Oral contraceptive continuation reflects the interaction of these influences. Unfortunately, women who discontinue oral contraception often utilize a less effective method or, worse, fail to substitute another method.

There are 3 major factors that affect continuation:

1. The experience of side effects, such as breakthrough bleeding and amenorrhea, and perceived experience of "minor" problems, such as headaches, nausea, breast tenderness, and weight gain. Multiple side effects dramatically and progressively increase the likelihood of discontinuation.[495, 496] Because these complaints respond well even to placebo treatment,[497] it is reasonable to expect a favorable response to sensitive and attentive counseling, as well as changing to a different product.

2. Fears and concerns regarding cancer, cardiovascular disease, and the impact of oral contraception on future fertility.

3. Nonmedical issues, such as inadequate instructions on pill taking, complicated pill packaging, and difficulties arising from the patient package insert.

The information in this chapter is the foundation for good continuation, but the clinician must go beyond the presentation of information and develop an effective means of communicating that information. We recommend the following approach to the clinician–patient encounter as one way to improve continuation with oral contraception.

1. Explain how oral contraception works.

2. Review briefly the risks and benefits of oral contraception, but be careful to put the risks in proper perspective, and to emphasize the safety and noncontraceptive benefits of low-dose oral contraceptives.

3. Show and demonstrate to the patient the package of pills she will use.

4. Explain how to take the pills:
   •When to start.
   •The importance of developing a daily routine to avoid missing pills.
   •What to do if pills are missed (identify a backup method).

5. Review the side effects that can affect continuation: amenorrhea, breakthrough bleeding, headaches, weight gain, nausea, etc., and what to do if one or more occurs.

6. Explain the warning signs of potential problems: abdominal or chest pain, trouble breathing, severe headaches, visual problems, leg pain or swelling.

7. Ask the patient to be sure to call if another clinician prescribes other medications.

8. Ask the patient to repeat critical information to make sure she understands what has been said. Ask if the patient has any questions.

9. Schedule a return appointment in 1–2 months to review understanding and address fears and concerns; a visit at 3 months is too late because most questions and side effects occur early.[496] Inconsistent use of oral contraceptives is more common in women who are new starters.[494]

10. Make sure a line of communication is open to clinician or office personnel. Ask the patient to call for any problem or concern before she stops taking the oral contraceptives.

Concluding Thoughts

In the 1970s, as epidemiologic data first became available, we emphasized in our teaching and in our communication with patients the risks and dangers associated with oral contraceptives. In the 1990s, with better patient screening and epidemiologic data documenting the effects of low-dose products, we appropriately emphasized the benefits and safety of modern oral contraceptives. In the new millennium, we can with confidence promote the idea that the use of oral contraceptives yields an overall improvement in individual health, and from a public health point of view, the collection of effects associated with oral contraceptives leads to a decrease in the cost of health care.

Contraceptive advice is a component of good preventive health care, and the clinician's approach is a key factor. This is an era of informed choice by the patient. Patients deserve to know the facts and need help in dealing with the state of the art and those issues clouded by uncertainty. But there is no doubt that patients are influenced in their choices by their clinician's advice and attitude. Although the role of a clinician is to provide the education necessary for the patient to make proper choices, one should not lose sight of the powerful influence exerted by the clinician in the choices ultimately made. Emphasizing the safety and benefits of oral contraceptives, and the contribution of oral contraceptives to individual and public health, allows a clinician to present oral contraception with a very positive attitude, an approach that makes an important contribution to a patient's ability to make appropriate health choices.

References

1. **Halberstam D,** The Fifties, Ballantine Books, New York, 1993.

2. **Perone N,** The progestins, In: Goldzieher JW, ed. Pharmacology of the Contraceptive Steroids, Raven Press, Ltd., New York, 1994, pp 5–20.

3. **Asbell B,** The Pill: A Biography of the Drug that Changed the World, Random House, New York, 1995.

4. **Planned Parenthood Federation of America,** A history of contraceptive methods, www. plannedparenthood.org, 2002.

5. **Djerassi C,** The Pill, Pygmy Chimps, and Degas' Horse, Basic Books, New York, 1992.

6. **Pincus G,** The Control of Fertility, Academic Press, New York, 1965.

7. **Goldzieher JW,** Selected aspects of the pharmacokinetics and metabolism of ethinyl estrogens and their clinical implications, Am J Obstet Gynecol 163:318, 1990.

8. **Stanczyk FZ, Roy S,** Metabolism of levonorgestrel, norethindrone, and structurally related contraceptive steroids, Contraception 42:67, 1990.

9. **Edgren RA,** Progestagens, In: Givens J, ed. Clinical Uses of Steroids, Yearbook, Chicago, pp 1980, 1–29.

10. **Kuhnz W, Blode H, Maher M,** Systemic availability of levonorgestrel after single oral administration of a noregestimate-containing combination oral contraceptive to 12 young women, Contraception 49:255, 1994.

11. **Stanczyk FZ,** Pharmacokinetics of the new progestogens and influence of gestodene and desogestrel on ethinylestradiol metabolism, Contraception 55:273, 1997.

12. **Hammond GL, Abrams LS, Creasy GW, Natarajan J, Allen JG, Siiteri PK,** Serum distribution of the major metabolites of noregestimate in relation to its pharmacological properties, Contraception 67:93, 2003.

13. **Foster RH, Wilde MI,** Dienogest, Drugs 56:825, 1998.

14. **Speroff L, DeCherney A,** Evaluation of a new generation of oral contraceptives, Obstet Gynecol 81:1034, 1993.

15. **Breitkopf DM, Rosen MP, Young SL, Nagamani M,** Efficacy of second versus third generation oral contraceptives in the treatment of hirsutism, Contraception 67:349, 2003.

16. **Fuhrmann U, Krattenmacher R, Slater EP, Fritzemeier K-H,** The novel progestin drospirenone and its natural counterpart progesterone: biochemical profile and antiandrogenic potential, Contraception 54:243, 1996.

17. **Oelkers W, Helmerhorst FM, Wuttke W, Heithecker R,** Effect of an oral contraceptive containing drospirenone on the renin-angiotensin-aldosterone system in healthy female volunteers, Gynecol Endocrinol 14:204, 2000.

18. **Brown C, Ling F, Wan J,** A new monophasic oral contraceptive containing drospirenone. Effect on premenstrual symptoms, J Reprod Med 47:14, 2002.

19. **Freeman EW, Kroll R, Rapkin A, Pearlstein T, Brown C, Parsey K, Zhang P, Patel H, Foegh M, PMS/PMDD Research Group,** Evaluation of a unique oral contraceptive in the treatment of premenstrual dysphoric disorder, Women's Health Gend Based Med 10:561, 2001.

20. **Foidart JM, Wuttke W, Bouw GM, Gerlinger C, Heithecker R,** A comparative investigation of contraceptive reliability, cycle control and tolerance of two monophasic oral contraceptives containing either drospirenone or desogestrel, Eur J Contracept Reprod Health Care 5:124, 2000.

21. **Rowan JP,** "Estrophasic" dosing: a new concept in oral contraceptive therapy, Am J Obstet Gynecol 180:S302, 1999.

22. **Boyd RA, Zegarac EA, Posvar EL, Flack MR,** Minimal androgenic activity of a new oral contraceptive containing norethindrone acetate and graduated doses of ethinyl estradiol, Contraception 63:71, 2001.

23. **Gilliam M, Elam G, Maloney JM, Flack MR, Sevilla CL,** McLaughlin-Derman R, Acne treatment with a low-dose oral contraceptive, Obstet Gynecol 97(Suppl 1):S9, 2001.

24. **Sullivan H, Furniss H, Spona J, Elstein M,** Effect of 21-day and 24-day oral contraceptive regimens containing gestodene (60 μg) and ethinyl estradiol (15 μg) on ovarian activity, Fertil Steril 72:115, 1999.

25. **Schlaff WD, Lynch AM, Hughes HD, Cedars MI, Smith DL,** Manipulation of the pill-free interval in oral contraceptive users: the effect on follicular suppression, Am J Obstet Gynecol 190:943, 2004.

117

26. **Rossmanith WG, Steffens D, Schramm G,** A comparative randomized trial on the impact of two low-dose oral contraceptives on ovarian activity, cervical permeability, and endometrial receptivity, Contraception 56:23, 1997.

27. **Trussell J, Hatcher RA, Cates Jr W, Stewart FH, Kost K,** A guide to interpreting contraceptive efficacy studies, Obstet Gynecol 76:558, 1990.

28. **Trussell J, Hatcher RA, Cates Jr W, Stewart FH, Kost K,** Contraceptive failure in the United States: an update, Stud Fam Plann 21:51, 1990.

29. **Trussell J, Vaughan B,** Contraceptive failure, method-related discontinuation and resumption of use: results from the 1995 National Survey of Family Growth, Fam Plann Perspect 31:64, 1999.

30. **Sparrow MJ,** Pill method failures, N Z Med J 100:102, 1987.

31. **Hansen TH, Lundvall F,** Factors influencing the reliability of oral contraceptives, Acta Obstet Gynecol Scand 76:61, 1997.

32. **Fu H, Darroch JE, Haas T, Ranjit N,** Contraceptive failure rates: new estimates from the 1995 National Survey of Family Growth, Fam Plann Perspect 31:58, 1999.

33. **Trussell J,** Contraceptive failure in the United States, Contraception 70:89, 2004.

34. **Child TJ, Rees M, MacKenzie IZ,** Pregnancy terminations after oral contraception scare, Lancet 347:1260, 1996.

35. **Skjeldestad FE,** Increased number of induced abortions in Norway after media coverage of adverse vascular events from the use of third-generation oral contraceptives, Contraception 55:11, 1997.

36. **Martinelli I, Sacchi E, Landi G, Taioli E, Duca F, Mannucci PM,** High risk of cerebral-vein thrombosis in carriers of a prothrombin-gene mutation and in users of oral contraceptives, New Engl J Med 338:1793, 1998.

37. **Hajjar KA,** Factor V Leiden: an unselfish gene? New Engl J Med 331:1585, 1994.

38. **Svensson PJ, Dahlbäck B,** Resistance to activated protein C as a basis for venous thrombosis, New Engl J Med 330:517, 1994.

39. **Zöller B, Hillarp A, Berntorp E, Dahlbäck B,** Activated protein C resistance due to a common factor V gene mutation is a major risk factor for venous thrombosis, Ann Rev Med 48:45, 1997.

40. **Vandenbroucke JP, van der Meer FJM, Helmerhorst FM, Rosendaal FR,** Factor V Leiden, Br Med J 313:1127, 1996.

41. **Emmerich J, Rosendaal FR, Cammarata CL, Margaglione M, De Stefano V, Cumming T, Arruda V, Hillarp A, Reny JL,** Combined effect of factor V Leiden and prothrombin 20210A on the risk of venous thromboembolism-pooled analysis of 8 case-control studies including 2310 cases and 3204 controls. Study Group for Pooled-Analysis in Venous Thromboembolism, Thromb Haemost 86:809, 2001.

42. **Sidney S, Petitti DB, Soff GA, Cundiff DL, Tolan KK, Quesenberry CP, Jr.,** Venous thromboembolic disease in users of low-estrogen combined estrogen-progestin oral contraceptives, Contraception 70:3, 2004.

43. **Rees DC, Cox M, Clegg JB,** World distribution of factor V Leiden, Lancet 346:1133, 1995.

44. **Zivelin A, Griffin JH, Xu X, Pabinger I, Samama M, Conard J, Brenner B, Eldor A, Seligsohn U,** A single genetic origin for a common Caucasian risk factor for venous thrombosis, Blood 89:397, 1997.

45. **Poort SR, Rosendaal FR, Reitsma PH, Bertina RM,** A common genetic variation in the 3'-untranslated region of the prothrombin gene is associated with elevated plasma prothrombin levels and an increase in venous thrombosis, Blood 88:3698, 1996.

46. **Rosendaal FR, Doggen CJM, Zivelin A, Arruda VR, Aiach M, Siscovick DS, Hillarp H, Watzke HH, Bernardi F, Cumming AM, Preston FE, Reitsma PH,** Geographic distribution of the 20210 G to A prothrombin variant, Thromb Haemost 79:706, 1998.

47. **Martinelli I, Taioli E, Bucciarelli P, Akhavan S, Mannucci PM,** Interaction between the G20210A mutation of the prothrombin gene and oral contraceptive use in deep vein thrombosis, Arterioscler Thromb Vasc Biol 19:700, 1999.

48. **Legnani C, Cosmi B, Valdre L, Boggian O, Bernardi F, Coccheri S, Palareti G,** Venous thromboembolism, oral contraceptives and high prothrombin levels, J Thromb Haemost 1:112, 2003.

49. **Meade TW,** Oral contraceptives, clotting factors, and thrombosis, Am J Obstet Gynecol 142:758, 1982.

50. **The Oral Contraceptive and Hemostasis Study Group,** The effect of seven monophasic oral contraceptive regimens on hemostatic variables: conclusions from a large randomized multicenter study, Contraception 67:173, 2003.

51. **Jespersen J, Petersen KR, Skouby SO,** Effects of newer oral contraceptives on the inhibition of coagulation and fibrinolysis in relation to dosage and type of steroid, Am J Obstet Gynecol 163:396, 1990.

52. **Notelovitz M, Kitchens CS, Khan FY,** Changes in coagulation and anticoagulation in women taking low-dose triphasic oral contraceptives: a controlled comparative 12-month clinical trial, Am J Obstet Gynecol 167:1255, 1992.

53. **Schlit AF, Grandjean P, Donnez J, Lavenne E,** Large increase in plasmatic 11-dehydro-TXB2 levels due to oral contraceptives, Contraception 51:53, 1995.

54. **Fruzzetti F, Ricci C, Fioretti P,** Haemostasis profile in smoking and nonsmoking women taking low-dose oral contraceptives, Contraception 49:579, 1994.

55. **Basdevant A, Conard J, Pelissier C, Guyene T-T, Lapousterle C, Mayer M, Guy-Grand B, Degrelle H,** Hemostatic and metabolic effects of lowering the ethinyl-estradiol dose from 30 mcg to 20 mcg in oral contraceptives containing desogestrel, Contraception 48:193, 1993.

56. **Winkler UH, Schindler AE, Endrikat J, Düsterberg B,** A comparative study of the effects of the hemostatic system of two monophasic gestodene oral contraceptives containing 20 μg and 30 μg ethinylestradiol, Contraception 53:75, 1996.

57. **Croft P, Hannaford PC,** Risk factors for acute myocardial infarction in women: evidence from the Royal College of General Practitioners' oral contraception study, Br Med J 298:165, 1989.

58. **Rosenberg L, Palmer JR, Lesko SM, Shapiro S,** Oral contraceptive use and the risk of myocardial infarction, Am J Epidemiol 131:1009, 1990.

59. **Stampfer MJ, Willett WC, Colditz GA, Speizer FE, Hennekens CH,** Past use of oral contraceptives and cardiovascular disease: a meta-analysis in the context of the Nurses' Health Study, Am J Obstet Gynecol 163:285, 1990.

60. **Colditz GA, and the Nurses' Health Study Research Group,** Oral contraceptive use and mortality during 12 years of follow-up: the Nurses' Health Study, Ann Intern Med 120:821, 1994.

61. **Beral V, Hermon C, Kay C, Hannaford P, Darby S, Reeves G,** Mortality associated with oral contraceptive use: 25-year follow-up of cohort of 46,000 women from Royal College of General Practitioners' oral contraception study, Br Med J 318:96, 1999.

62. **Vessey M, Painter R, Yeates D,** Mortality in relation to oral contraceptive use and cigarette smoking, Lancet 362:185, 2003.

63. **Böttiger LE, Boman G, Eklund G, Westerholm B,** Oral contraceptives and thromboembolic disease: effects of lowering oestrogen content, Lancet i:1097, 1980.

64. **Gerstman BB, Piper JM, Tomita DK, Ferguson WJ, Stadel BV, Lundin FE,** Oral contraceptive estrogen dose and the risk of deep venous thromboembolic disease, Am J Epidemiol 133:32, 1991.

65. **Vessey M, Mant D, Smith A, Yeates D,** Oral contraceptives and venous thromboembolism: findings in a large prospective study, Br Med J 292:526, 1986.

66. **Helmrich SP, Rosenberg L, Kaufman DW, Strom B, Shapiro S,** Venous thromboembolism in relation to oral contraceptive use, Obstet Gynecol 69:91, 1987.

67. **Thorogood M, Mann J, Murphy M, Vessey M,** Risk factors for fatal venous thromboembolism in young women: a case-control study, Int J Epidemiol 21:48, 1992.

68. **Rosenberg L, Hennekens CH, Rosner B, Belanger C, Rothman KH, Speizer FE,** Oral contraceptive use in relation to nonfatal myocardial infarction, Am J Epidemiol 11:59, 1980.

69. **Royal College of General Practitioners' Oral Contraceptive Study,** Incidence of arterial disease among oral contraceptive users, J Roy Coll Gen Pract 33:75, 1983.

70. **Lidegaard Ø,** Oral contraception and risk of a cerebral thromboembolic attack: results of a case-control study, Br Med J 306:956, 1993.

71. **Lawson DH, Davidson JF, Jick H,** Oral contraceptive use and venous thromboembolism: absence of an effect of smoking, Br Med J ii:729, 1977.

72. **Petitti DB, Wingerd J, Pellegrin F, Ramcharan S,** Oral contraceptives, smoking, and other factors in relation to risk of venous thromboembolic disease, Am J Epidemiol 108:480, 1978.

120

73. **Royal College of General Practitioners, Oral contraceptive study:** Oral contraceptives, venous thrombosis, and varicose veins, J Roy Coll Gen Pract 28:393, 1978.

74. **Porter JB, Hershel J, Walker AM,** Mortality among oral contraceptive users, Obstet Gynecol 70:29, 1987.

75. **WHO Collaborative Study of Cardiovascular Disease and Steroid Hormone Contraception,** Venous thromboembolic disease and combined oral contraceptives: results of international multicentre case-control study, Lancet 346:1575, 1995.

76. **WHO Collaborative Study of Cardiovascular Disease and Steroid Hormone Contraception,** Effect of different progestagens in low oestrogen oral contraceptives on venous thromboembolic disease, Lancet 346:1582, 1995.

77. **Spitzer WO, Lewis MA, Heinemann LAJ, Thorogood M, MacRae KD, on behalf of the Transnational Research Group on Oral Contraceptives and the Health of Young Women,** Third generation oral contraceptives and risk of venous thromboembolic disorders: an international case-control study, Br Med J 312:83, 1996.

78. **Jick H, Jick SS, Gurewich V, Myers MW, Vasilakis C,** Risk of idiopathic cardiovascular death and nonfatal venous thromboembolism in women using oral contraceptives with differing progestagen components, Lancet 348:1589, 1995.

79. **Jick H, Kaye JA, Vasilakis-Scaramozza C, Jick SS,** Risk of venous thromboembolism among users of third generation of oral contraceptives compared with users of oral contraceptives with levonorgestrel before and after 1995: cohort and case-control analysis, Br Med J 321:1190, 2000.

80. **Bloemenkammp KWM, Rosendaal FR, Helmerhorst FM, Büller HR, Vandenbroucke JP,** Enhancement by factor V Leiden mutation of risk of deep-vein thrombosis associated with oral contraceptives containing a third-generation progestagen, Lancet 348:1593, 1995.

81. **Speroff L,** Oral contraceptives and venous thromboembolism, Int J Gynecol Obstet 54:45, 1996.

82. **Lewis MA, Heinemann LAJ, MacRae KD, Bruppacher R, Spitzer WO,** The increased risk of venous thromboembolism and the use of third generation progestagens: role of bias in observational research, Contraception 54:5, 1996.

83. **Lidegaard Ø, Milsom I,** Oral contraceptives and thrombotic diseases: impact of new epidemiologic studies, Contraception 53:135, 1996.

84. **McPherson K,** Third generation oral contraception and venous thromboembolism. The published evidence confirms the Committee on Safety of Medicine's concerns, Br Med J 312:68, 1996.

85. **Vandenbroucke JP, Rosendaal FR,** End of the line for "third-generation-pill" controversy, Lancet 349:1113, 1997.

86. **Lidegaard Ø, Edström B, Kreiner S,** Oral contraceptives and venous thromboembolism. A case-control study, Contraception 5:291, 1998.

87. **Lidegaard Ø, Edström B, Kreiner S,** Oral contraceptives and venous thromboembolism: a five-year national case-control study, Contraception 65:187, 2002.

88. **Farmer RDT, Lawrenson RA, Thompson CR, Kennedy JG, Hambleton IR,** Population-based study of risk of venous thromboembolism associated with various oral contraceptives, Lancet 349:83, 1997.

89. **Farmer RD, Lawrenson RA, Todd JC, Williams TJ, MacRae KD, Tyrer F, Leydon GM,** A comparison of the risks of venous thromboembolic disease in association with different combined oral contraceptives, Br J Clin Pharmacol 49:580, 2000.

90. **Farmer RDT, Todd J-C, Lewis MA, MacRae KD, Williams TJ,** The risks of venous thromboembolic disease among German women using oral contraceptives: a database study, Contraception 57:67, 1998.

91. **Farmer RDT, Williams TJ, Simpson EL, Nightingale AL,** Effect of 1995 pill scare on rates of venous thromboembolism among women taking combined oral contraceptives: analysis of General Practice Research Database, Br Med J 321:477, 2000.

92. **Suissa S, Blais L, Spitzer WO, Cusson J, Lewis M, Heinemann L,** First-time use of newer oral contraceptives and the risk of venous thromboembolism, Contraception 56:141, 1997.

93. **Suissa S, Spitzer WO, Rainville B, Cusson J, Lewis M, Heinemann L,** Recurrent use of newer oral contraceptives and the risk of venous thromboembolism, Hum Reprod 15:817, 2000.

94. **Todd J, Lawrenson R, Farmer RD, Williams TJ, Leydon GM,** Venous thromboembolic disease and combined oral contraceptives: a re-analysis of the MediPlus database, Hum Reprod 14:1500, 1999.

95. **Heinemann LAJ, Lewis MA, Assmann A, Thiel C,** Case-control studies on venous thromboembolism: bias due to design? A methodological study on venous thromboembolism and steroid hormone use, Contraception 65:207, 2002.

96. **Kuhl H, Jung-Hoffman C, Heidt F,** Alterations in the serum levels of gestodene and SHBG during 12 cycles of treatment with 30 micrograms ethinylestradiol and 75 micrograms gestodene, Contraception 38:477, 1988.

97. **Jung-Hoffman C, Kuhl H,** Interaction with the phamacokinetics of ethinylestradiol and progestogens contained in oral contraceptives, Contraception 40:299, 1989.

98. **Hümpel M, Täuber U, Kuhnz W, Pfeffer M, Brill K, Heithecker R, Louton T, Steinberg B, Seifert W, Schütt B,** Protein binding of active ingredients and comparison of serum ethinyl estradiol, sex hormone-binding globulin, corticosteroid-binding globulin, and cortisol levels in women using a combination of gestodene/ethinyl estradiol or a combination of desogestrel/ethinyl estradiol (Marvelon) and single dose ethinyl estradiol bioequivalence from both oral contraceptives, Am J Obstet Gynecol 163:329, 1990.

99. **Dibbelt L, Knuppen R, Jütting G, Heimann S, Klipping CO, Parikka-Olexik H,** Group comparison of serum ethinyl estradiol, SHBG and CBG levels in 83 women using two low-dose oral contraceptives for three months, Contraception 43:1, 1991.

100. **Heinemann LAJ, Lewis MA, Assman A, Gravens L, Guggenmoos-Holzmann I,** Could preferential prescribing and referral behaviour of physicians explain the elevated thrombosis risk found to be associated with third generation oral contraceptives? Pharmacoepidemiol Drug Saf 5:285, 1996.

101. **Jamin C, de Mouzon J,** Selective prescribing of third generation oral contraceptives (OCs), Contraception 54:55, 1996.

102. **Van Lunsen WH,** Recent oral contraceptive use patterns in four European countries: evidence for selective prescribing of oral contraceptives containing third generation progestogens, Eur J Contracept Reprod Health 1:39, 1996.

103. **Sheldon T,** Dutch GPs warned against new contraceptive pill, Br Med J 324:869, 2002.

104. **Farmer RDT, Preston TD,** The risk of venous thromboembolism associated with low estrogen oral contraceptives, J Obstet Gynaecol 15:195, 1995.

105. **Ridker PM, Miletich JP, Hennekens CH, Buring JE,** Ethnic distribution of factor V Leiden in 4047 men and women: implications for venous thromboembolism screening, JAMA 277:1305, 1997.

106. **Vensson PJ, Dahlbäck B,** Resistance to activated protein C as a basis for venous thrombosis, New Engl J Med 330:517, 1994.

107. **Hellgren M, Svensson PJ, Dahlbäck B,** Resistance to activated protein C as a basis for venous thromboembolism associated with pregnancy and oral contraceptives, Am J Obstet Gynecol 173:210, 1995.

108. **Vandenbroucke JP, Koster T, Briët E, Reitsma PH, Bertina RM, Rosendaal FR,** Increased risk of venous thrombosis in oral-contraceptive users who are carriers of factor V Leiden mutation, Lancet 344:1453, 1994.

109. **Spannagl M, Heinemann AJ, Schramm W,** Are factor V Leiden carriers who use oral contraceptives at extreme risk for venous thromboembolism? Eur J Contracept Reprod Health Care 5:105, 2000.

110. **Bloemenkamp KW, Rosendaal FR, Helmerhorst FM, Vandenbroucke JP,** Higher risk of venous thrombosis during early use of oral contraceptives in women with inherited clotting defects, Arch Intern Med 160:49, 2000.

111. **Winkler UH,** Blood coagulation and oral contraceptives. A critical review, Contraception 57:203, 1998.

112. **Lidegaard Ø, Kreiner S,** Cerebral thrombosis and oral contraceptives. A case-control study, Contraception 57:303, 1998.

113. **Lidegaard Ø, Edström B,** Oral contraceptives and myocardial infarction. A case-control study (abstract), Eur J Contracept Reprod Health Care 1(Suppl):72, 1996.

114. **Sidney S, Petitti DB, Quesenberry CP, Klatsky AL, Ziel HK, Wolf S,** Myocardial infarction in users of low-dose oral contraceptives, Obstet Gynecol 88:939, 1996.

115. **Lewis MA, Heinemann LAJ, Spitzer WO, MacRae KD, Bruppacher R, for the Transnational Research Group on Oral Contraceptives and the Health of Young Women,** The use of oral contraceptives and the occurrence of acute myocardial infarction in young women. Results from the Transnational Study on Oral Contraceptives and the Health of Young Women, Contraception 56:129, 1997.

116. **Lewis MA, Spitzer WO, Heinemann LAJ, MacRae KD, Bruppacher R,** Lowered risk of dying of heart attack with third generation pill may offset risk of dying of thromboembolism, Br Med J 315:679, 1997.

117. **Dunn N, Thorogood M, Garagher B, de Caestecker L, MacDonald TM, McCollum C, Thomas S, Mann R,** Oral contraceptives and myocardial infarction: results of the MICA case-control study, Br Med J 318:1579, 1999.

118. **Tanis BC, van den Bosch MA, Kemmeren JM, Cats VM, Helmerhorst FM, Algra A, van der Graaf Y, Rosendaal FR,** Oral contraceptives and the risk of myocardial infarction, New Eng J Med 345:1787, 2001.

119. **Spitzer WO, Faith JM, MacRae KD,** Myocardial infarction and third generation oral contraceptives: aggregation of recent studies, Hum Reprod 17:2307, 2002.

120. **Rosenberg L, Palmer JR, Rao RS, Shapiro S,** Low-dose contraceptive use and the risk of myocardial infarction, Arch Intern Med 161:1065, 2001.

121. **WHO Collaborative Study of Cardiovascular Disease and Steroid Hormone Contraception,** Acute myocardial infarction and combined oral contraceptives: results of an international multicentre case-control study, Lancet 349:1202, 1997.

122. **Petitti DB, Sidney S, Quesenberry CP, Jr., Bernstein A,** Incidence of stroke and myocardial infarction in women of reproductive age, Stroke 28:280, 1997.

123. **Jick H, Porter J, Rothman KJ,** Oral contraceptives and nonfatal stroke in healthy young women, Ann Int Med 89:58, 1978.

124. **Vessey MP, Lawless M, Yeates D,** Oral contraceptives and stroke: findings in a large prospective study, Br Med J 289:530, 1984.

125. **Hannaford PC, Croft PR, Kay CR,** Oral contraception and stroke: evidence from the Royal College of General Practitioners' Oral Contraception Study, Stroke 25:935, 1994.

126. **Petitti DB, Sidney S, Bernstein A, Wolf S, Quesenberry C, Ziel HK,** Stroke in users of low-dose oral contraceptives, New Engl J Med 335:8, 1996.

127. **Heinemann LAJ, Lewis MA, Spitzer WO, Thorogood M, Guggenmoos-Holzmann I, Bruppacher R, and the Transnational Research Group on Oral Contraceptives and the Health of Young Women,** Thromboembolic stroke in young women. A European case-control study on oral contraceptives, Contraception 57:29, 1998.

128. **Kemmeren JM, Tanis BC, van den Bosch MA, Bollen EL, Helmerhorst FM, van der Graaf Y, Rosendaal FR, Algra A,** Risk of arterial thrombosis in relation to oral contraceptives (RATIO) study: oral contraceptives and the risk of ischemic stroke, Stroke 33:1202, 2002.

129. **Schwartz SM, Siscovick DS, Longstreth WT, Jr., Psaty BM, Beverly RK, Raghunathan TE, Lin D, Koepsell TD,** Use of low-dose oral contraceptives and stroke in young women, Ann Intern Med 127:596, 1997.

130. **Schwartz SM, Petitti DB, Siscovick DS, Longstreth NT, Jr., Sidney S, Raghunathan TE, Quesenberry CP, Jr., Kelaghan J,** Stroke and use of low-dose oral contraceptives in young women: a pooled analysis of two US studies, Stroke 29:2277, 1998.

131. **WHO Collaborative Study of Cardiovascular Disease and Steroid Hormone Contraception,** Ischaemic stroke and combined oral contraceptives: results of an international, multicentre case-control study, Lancet 348:498, 1996.

132. **WHO Collaborative Study of Cardiovascular Disease and Steroid Hormone Contraception,** Haemorrhagic stroke, overall stroke risk, and combined oral contraceptives: results of an international, multicentre, case-control study, Lancet 348:505, 1996.

133. **Lidegaard Ø, Kreiner S,** Contraceptives and cerebral thrombosis: a five-year national case-control study, Contraception 65:197, 2002.

134. **Barrett DH, Anda RF, Escobedo LG, Croft JB, Williamson DF, Marks JS,** Trends in oral contraceptive use and cigarette smoking, Arch Fam Med 3:438, 1994.

135. **Wahl P, Walden C, Knopp R, Hoover J, Wallace R, Heiss R, Refkind B,** Effect of estrogen/progestin potency on lipid/lipoprotein cholesterol, New Engl J Med 308:862, 1983.

136. **Burkman RT, Robinson JC, Kruszon-Moran D, Kimball AW, Kwiterovich P, Burford RG,** Lipid and lipoprotein changes associated with oral contraceptive use: a randomized clinical trial, Obstet Gynecol 71:33, 1988.

137. **Patsch W, Brown SA, Grotto AM, Jr., Young RL,** The effect of triphasic oral contraceptives on plasma lipids and lipoproteins, Am J Obstet Gynecol 161:1396, 1989.

138. **Gevers Leuven JA, Dersjant-Roorda MC, Helmerhorst FM, de Boer R, Neymeyer-Leloux A, Havekes L,** Estrogenic effect of gestodene-desogestrel-containing oral contraceptives on lipoprotein metabolism, Am J Obstet Gynecol 163:358, 1990.

139. **Kloosterboer HJ, Rekers H,** Effects of three combined oral contraceptive preparations containing desogestrel plus ethinyl estradiol on lipid metabolism in comparison with two levonorgestrel preparations, Am J Obstet Gynecol 163:370, 1990.

140. **Notelovitz M, Feldmand EB, Gillespy M, Gudat J,** Lipid and lipoprotein changes in women taking low-dose, triphasic oral contraceptives: a controlled, comparative, 12-month clinical trial, Am J Obstet Gynecol 160:1269, 1989.

141. **Young RL, DelConte A,** Effects of low-dose monophasic levonorgestrel with ethinyl estradiol preparation on serum lipid levels: A twenty-four-month clinical trial, Am J Obstet Gynecol 181:S59, 1999.

142. **Adams MR, Clarkson TB, Koritnik DR, Nash HA,** Contraceptive steroids and coronary artery atherosclerosis in cynomolgus macaques, Fertil Steril 47:1010, 1987.

143. **Clarkson TB, Adams MR, Kaplan JR, Shively CA, Koritnik DR,** From menarche to menopause: coronary artery atherosclerosis and protection in cynomolgus monkeys, Am J Obstet Gynecol 160:1280, 1989.

144. **Clarkson TB, Shively CA, Morgan TM, Koritnik DR, Adams MR, Kaplan JR,** Oral contraceptives and coronary artery atherosclerosis of cynomolgus monkeys, Obstet Gynecol 75:217, 1990.

145. **Kushwaha R, Hazzard W,** Exogenous estrogens attenuate dietary hypercholesterolemia and atherosclerosis in the rabbit, Metabolism 30:57, 1981.

146. **Hough JL, Zilversmit DB,** Effect of 17 beta estradiol on aortic cholesterol content and metabolism in cholesterol-fed rabbits, Arteriosclerosis 6:57, 1986.

147. **Henriksson P, Stamberger M, Eriksson M, Rudling M, Diczfalusy U, Berglund L, Angelin B,** Oestrogen-induced changes in lipoprotein metabolism: role in prevention of atherosclerosis in the cholesterol-fed rabbit, Eur J Clin Invest 19:395, 1989.

148. **Engel JH, Engel E, Lichtlen PR,** Coronary atherosclerosis and myocardial infarction in young women — role of oral contraceptives, Eur Heart J 4:1, 1983.

149. **Jugdutt BI, Stevens GF, Zacks DJ, Lee SJK, Taylor RF,** Myocardial infarction, oral contraception, cigarette smoking, and coronary artery spasm in young women, Am Heart J 106:757, 1983.

150. **Victory R, D'Souza C, Diamond MP, McNeely SG, vista-Deck D, Hendrix S,** Adverse cardiovascular disease outcomes are reduced in women with a history of oral contraceptive use: results from the Women's Health Initiative Database (abstract), Fertil Steril 82:S52, 2004.

151. **Kovacs L, Bartfai G, Apro G, Annus J, Bulpitt C, Belsey E, Pinol A,** The effect of the contraceptive pill on blood pressure: a randomized controlled trial of three progestogen-oestrogen combinations in Szeged, Hungary, Contraception 33:69, 1986.

152. **Nichols M, Robinson G, Bounds W, Newman B, Guillebaud J,** Effect of four combined oral contraceptives on blood pressure in the pill-free interval, Contraception 47:367, 1993.

153. **Qifang S, Deliang L, Ziurong J, Haifang L, Zhongshu Z,** Blood pressure changes and hormonal contraceptives, Contraception 50:131, 1994.

154. **Darney P,** Safety and efficacy of a triphasic oral contraceptive containing desogestrel: results of three multicenter trials, Contraception 48:323, 1993.

155. **Chasan-Taber L, Willett WC, Manson JE, Spiegelman D, Hunter DJ, Curhan G, Colditz GA, Stampfer MJ,** Prospective study of oral contraceptives and hypertension among women in the United States, Circulation 94:483, 1996.

156. **Brady WA, Kritz-Silverstein D, Barrett-Connor E, Morales AJ,** Prior oral contraceptive use is associated with higher blood pressure in older women, J Women's Health 7:221, 1998.

157. **Pritchard JA, Pritchard SA,** Blood pressure response to estrogen-progestin oral contraceptives after pregnancy-induced hypertension, Am J Obstet Gynecol 129:733, 1977.

158. **Braken MB, Srisuphan W,** Oral contraception as a risk factor for preeclampsia, Am J Obstet Gynecol 142:191, 1982.

159. **Gratacos E, Torres P, Cararach V, Quinto L, Alonso PL, Fortuny A,** Does the use of contraception reduce the risk of pregnancy-induced hypertension? Hum Reprod 11:2138, 1996.

124

160. **Thadhani R, Stampfer MJ, Chasan-Taber L, Willett WC, Curhan GC,** A prospective study of pregravid oral contraceptive use and risk of hypertensive disorders of pregnancy, Contraception 60:145, 1999.

161. **Lubianca JN, Faccin CS, Fuchs FD,** Oral contraceptives: a risk factor for uncontrolled blood pressure among hypertensive women, Contraception 67:19, 2003.

162. **de Bruijn SFTM, Stam J, Koopman MMW, Vandenbroucke JP, for the Cerebral Venous Sinus Thrombosis Study Group,** Case-control study of risk of cerebral sinus thrombosis in oral contraceptive users who are carriers of hereditary prothrombotic conditions, Br Med J 316:589, 1998.

163. **Cosmi B, Legnani C, Bernardi F, Coccheri S, Palareti G,** Role of family history in identifying women with thrombophilia and higher risk of venous thromboembolism during oral contraception, Arch Intern Med 163:1105, 2003.

164. **Baglin T, Luddington R, Brown K, Baglin C,** Incidence of recurrent venous thromboembolism in relation to clinical and thrombophilic risk factors: prospective cohort study, Lancet 362:523, 2003.

165. **Pabinger I, Schneider B, and the GTH Study Group,** Thrombotic risk of women with hereditary antithrombin III, protein C, and protein S deficiency taking oral contraceptive medication, Thromb Haemost 5:548, 1994.

166. **Godsland IF, Crook D, Simpson R, Proudler T, Gelton C, Lees B, Anyaoku V, Devenport M, Wynn V,** The effects of different formulations of oral contraceptive agents on lipid and carbohydrate metabolism, New Engl J Med 323:1375, 1990.

167. **van der Vange N, Kloosterboer HJ, Haspels AA,** Effect of seven low-dose combined oral contraceptive preparations on carbohydrate metabolism, Am J Obstet Gynecol 156:918, 1987.

168. **Bowes WA, Katta LR, Droegemueller W, Braight TG,** Triphasic randomized clinical trial: Comparison of effects on carbohydrate metabolism, Am J Obstet Gynecol 161:1402, 1989.

169. **Gaspard UJ, Lefebvre PJ,** Clinical aspects of the relationship between oral contraceptives, abnormalities in carbohydrate metabolism, and the development of cardiovascular disease, Am J Obstet Gynecol 163:334, 1990.

170. **Troisi RJ, Cowie CC, Harris MI,** Oral contraceptive use and glucose metabolism in a national sample of women in the United States, Am J Obstet Gynecol 183:389, 2000.

171. **Hannaford PC, Kay CR,** Oral contraceptives and diabetes mellitus, Br Med J 299:315, 1989.

172. **Rimm EB, Manson JE, Stampfer MJ, Colditz GA, Willett WC, Rosner B, Hennekens CH, Speizer FE,** Oral contraceptive use and the risk of type 2 (non-insulin-dependent) diabetes mellitus in a large prospective study of women, Diabetologia 35:967, 1992.

173. **Duffy TJ, Ray R,** Oral contraceptive use: prospective follow-up of women with suspected glucose intolerance, Contraception 30:197, 1984.

174. **Chasan-Taber L, Colditz GA, Willett WC, Stampfer MJ, Hunter DJ, Colditz GA, Spiegelman D, Manson JE,** A prospective study of oral contraceptives and NIDDM among U.S. women, Diabetes Care 20:330, 1997.

175. **Kjos SL, Shoupe D, Douyan S, Friedman RL, Bernstein GS, Mestman JH, Mishell DR, Jr.,** Effect of low-dose oral contraceptives on carbohydrate and lipid metabolism in women with recent gestational diabetes: results of a controlled, randomized, prospective study, Am J Obstet Gynecol 163:1822, 1990.

176. **Kjos SL, Peters RK, Xiang A, Thomas D, Schaefer U, Buchanan TA,** Contraception and the risk of type 2 diabetes in Latino women with prior gestational diabetes, JAMA 280:533, 1998.

177. **Skouby SO, Malsted-Pedersen L, Kuhl C, Bennet P,** Oral contraceptives in diabetic women: metabolic effects of compounds with different estrogen/progestogen profiles, Fertil Steril 46:858, 1986.

178. **Garg SK, Chase HP, Marshall G, Hoops SL, Holmes DL, Jackson WE,** Oral contraceptives and renal and retinal complications in young women with insulin-dependent diabetes mellitus, JAMA 271:1099, 1994.

179. **Petersen KR, Skouby SO, Sidelmann J, Mølsted-Petersen L, Jespersen J,** Effects of contraceptive steroids on cardiovascular risk factors in women with insulin-dependent diabetes mellitus, Am J Obstet Gynecol 171:400, 1994.

180. **Klein BE, Klein R, Moss SE,** Mortality and hormone-related exposures in women with diabetes, Diabetes Care 22:248, 1999.

181. **Hannaford PC, Kay CR, Vessey MP, Painter R, Mant J,** Combined oral contraceptives and liver disease, Contraception 55:145, 1997.

182. **Royal College of General Practitioners' Oral Contraception Study,** Oral contraceptives and gallbladder disease, Lancet ii:957, 1982.

183. **Bennion LJ, Ginsberg RL, Garnick MB, Bennett PH,** Effects of oral contraceptives on the gallbladder bile of normal women, New Engl J Med 294:189, 1976.

184. **Grodstein F, Colditz GA, Hunter DJ, Manson JE, Willett WC, Stampfer MJ,** A prospective study of symptomatic gallstones in women: relation with oral contraceptives and other risk factors, Obstet Gynecol 84:207, 1994.

185. **La Vecchia C, Negri E, D'Avanzo B, Parazzini F, Genitle A, Franceschi S,** Oral contraceptives and noncontraceptive oestrogens in the risk of gallstone disease requiring surgery, J Epidemiol Community Health 46:234, 1992.

186. **Vessey M, Painter R,** Oral contraceptive use and benign gallbladder disease; revisited, Contraception 50:167, 1994.

187. **Cherqui D, Rahmouni A, Charlotte F, Boulahdour H, Metreau JM, Meignan M, Fagniez PL, Zafrani ES, Mathieu D, Dhumeaux C,** Management of focal nodular hyperplasia and hepatocellular adenoma in young women: a series of 41 patients with clinical radiological and pathological correlations, Hepatology 22:1674, 1995.

188. **Côté C,** Regression of focal nodular hyperplasia of the liver after oral contraceptive discontinuation, Clin Nucl Med 9:587, 1997.

189. **Heinemann LA, Weimann A, Gerken G, Thiel C, Schlaud M, Do Minh T,** Modern oral contraceptive use and benign liver tumors: the German Benign Liver Tumor Case-Control Study, Eur J Contracept Reprod Health Care 3:194, 1998.

190. **Scalori A, Tavani A, Gallus S, La Vecchia C, Colombo M,** Oral contraceptives and the risk of focal nodular hyperplasia of the liver: a case-control study, Am J Obstet Gynecol 186:195, 2002.

191. **Lucky AW, Henderson TA, Olson WH, Robisch DM, Lebwohl M, Swinyer LJ,** Effectiveness of norgestimate and ethinyl estradiol in treating moderate acne vulgaris, J Am Acad Dermatol 37:746, 1997.

192. **Redmond GP, Olson WH, Lippman JS, Kafrissen ME, Jones TM, Jorizzo JL,** Norgestimate and ethinyl estradiol in the treatment of acne vulgaris: a randomized, placebo-controlled trial, Obstet Gynecol 89:615, 1997.

193. **Redmond G, Godwin AJ, Olson W, Lippman JS,** Use of placebo controls in an oral contraceptive trial: methodological issues and adverse event incidence, Contraception 60:81, 1999.

194. **Carpenter S, Neinstein LS,** Weight gain in adolescent and young adult oral contraceptive users, J Adolesc Health Care 7:342, 1986.

195. **Reubinoff BE, Wurtman J, Rojansky N, Adler D, Stein P, Schenker JG, Brzezinski A,** Effects of hormone replacement therapy on weight, body composition, fat distribution, and food intake in early postmenopausal women: a prospective study, Fertil Steril 64:963, 1995.

196. **Moore LL, Valuck R, McDougall C, Fink W,** A comparative study of one-year weight gain among users of medroxyprogesterone acetate, levonorgestrel implants, and oral contraceptives, Contraception 52:215, 1995.

197. **Rosenberg M,** Weight change with oral contraceptive use and during the menstrual cycle. Results of daily measurements, Contraception 58:345, 1998.

198. **Risser WL, Gefter L, Barratt MS, Risser JM,** Weight change in adolescents who used hormonal contraception, J Adolesc Health 24:433, 1999.

199. **Gupta S,** Weight gain on the combined pill—is it real? Hum Reprod Update 6:427, 2000.

200. **Thiboutot D, Archer DF, Lemay A, Washenik K, Roberts J, Harrison DD,** A randomized, controlled trial of a low-dose contraceptive containing 20 μg of ethinyl estradiol and 100 μg of levonorgestrel for acne treatment, Fertil Steril 76:461, 2001.

201. **Coney P, Washenik K, Langley RGB, DiGiovanna JJ, Harrison DD,** Weight change and adverse event incidence with a low-dose oral contraceptive: two randomized, placebo-controlled trials, Contraception 63:297, 2001.

202. **Vessey MP, Villard-Mackintosh L, Painter R,** Oral contraceptives and pregnancy in relation to peptic ulcer, Contraception 46:349, 1992.

203. **Lashner BA, Kane SV, Hanauer SB,** Lack of association between oral contraceptive use and ulcerative colitis, Gastroenterology 99:1032, 1990.

126

204. **Milman N, Kirchhoff M, Jorgensen T,** Iron status markers, serum ferritin and hemoglobin in 1359 Danish women in relation to menstruation, hormonal contraception, parity, and postmenopausal hormone treatment, Ann Hematol 65:96, 1992.

205. **Galan P, Yoon HC, Preziosi P, Viteri P, Fieux B, Briancon S, Malvy D, Roussel AM, Favier A, Hercberg S,** Determing factors in the iron status of adult women in the SU.VI.MAX study, Eur J Clin Nutr 52:383, 1998.

206. **Task Force for Epidemiological Research on Reproductive Health, United Nations Development Programme/United Nations Population Fund/World Health Organization/World Bank Special Programme of Research, Develpment and Research Training in Human Reproduction,** Effects of contraceptives on hemoglobin and ferritin, Contraception 58:261, 1998.

207. **Mooij PN, Thomas CMG, Doesburg WH, Eskes TKAB,** Multivitamin supplementation in oral contraceptive users, Contraception 44:277, 1991.

208. **Wendler J, Siegert C, Schelhorn P, Klinger G, Gurr S, Kaufmann J, Aydinlik S, Braunschweig T,** The influence of Microgynon® and Diane-35®, two sub-fifty ovulation inhibitors, on voice function in women, Contraception 52:343, 1995.

209. **The Cancer and Steroid Hormone Study of the CDC and NICHD,** Combination oral contraceptive use and the risk of endometrial cancer, JAMA 257:796, 1987.

210. **Schlesselman JJ,** Oral contraceptives and neoplasia of the uterine corpus, Contraception 43:557, 1991.

211. **Vessey MP, Painte R,** Endometrial and ovarian cancer and oral contraceptives — findings in a large cohort study, Br J Cancer 71:1340, 1995.

212. **Schlesselman JJ,** Risk of endometrial cancer in relation to use of combined oral contraceptives. A practitioner's guide to meta-analysis, Hum Reprod 12:1851, 1997.

213. **Salazar-Martinez E, Lazcano-Ponce EC, Gonzalez Lira-Lira G, Escudero-De los Rios P, Salmeron-Castro J, Hernandez-Avila M,** Reproductive factors of ovarian and endometrial cancer risk in a high fertility population in Mexico, Cancer Res 59:3658, 1999.

214. **Weiderpass E, Adami HO, Baron JA, Magnusson C, Lindgren A, Persson I,** Use of oral contraceptives and endometrial cancer risk (Sweden), Cancer Causes Control 10:277, 1999.

215. **Jick SS, Walker AM, Jick H,** Oral contraceptives and endometrial cancer, Obstet Gynecol 82:931, 1993.

216. **Sherman ME, Sturgeon S, Brinton LA, Potischman N, Kurman RJ, Berman ML, Mortel R, Twiggs LB, Barrett rJ, Wilbanks GD,** Risk factors and hormone levels in patients with serous and endometrioid uterine carcinomas, Mod Pathol 10:963, 1997.

217. **Mant JWF, Vessey MP,** Ovarian and endometrial cancers, Cancer Surveys 19:287, 1994.

218. **Adami HO, Bergstrom R, Persson I, Sparen P,** The incidence of ovarian cancer in Sweden, 1960–1984, Am J Epidemiol 132:446, 1990.

219. **Silva IS, Swerdlow AJ,** Recent trends in incidence of and mortality from breast, ovarian and endometrial cancer in England and Wales and their relation to changing fertility and oral contraceptive use, Br J Cancer 72:485, 1995.

220. **Oriel KA, Hartenbach EM, Remington PL,** Trends in United States ovarian cancer mortality, 1979–1995, Obstet Gynecol 93:30, 1999.

221. **The Cancer and Steroid Hormone Study of the CDC and NICHD,** The reduction in risk of ovarian cancer associated with oral-contraceptive use, New Engl J Med 316:650, 1987.

222. **Hankinson SE, Colditz GA, Hunter DJ, Spencer TL, Rosner B, Stampfer MJ,** A quantitative assessment of oral contraceptive use and risk of ovarian cancer, Obstet Gynecol 80:708, 1992.

223. **Whittemore AS, Harris R, Itnyre J, and the Collaborative Ovarian Cancer Group,** Characteristics relating to ovarian cancer risk: collaborative analysis of 12 US case-control studies. II: Invasive epithelial ovarian cancers in white women, Am J Epidemiol 136:1184, 1992.

224. **Wittenberg L, Cook LS, Rossing MA, Weiss NS,** Reproductive risk factors for mucinous and non-mucinous epithelial ovarian cancer, Epidemiology 10:761, 1999.

225. **Ness RB, Grisso JA, Klapper J, Schlesselman JJ, Silberzweig S, Vergona R, Morgan M, Wheeler JE, and the SHARE Study Group,** Risk of ovarian cancer in relation to estrogen and progestin dose and use characteristics of oral contraceptives, Am J Epidemiol 152:233, 2000.

226. **Royar J, Becher H, Chang-Claude J,** Low-dose oral contraceptives: protective effect on ovarian cancer risk, Int J Cancer 95:370, 2001.

227. Rosenberg L, Palmer JR, Zauber AG, Warshauer ME, Lewis JL, Jr., Strom BL, Harlap S, Shapiro S, A case-control study of oral contraceptive use and invasive epithelial ovarian cancer, Am J Epidemiol 139:654, 1994.

228. Gross TP, Schlesselman JJ, The estimated effect of oral contraceptive use on the cumulative risk of epithelial ovarian cancer, Obstet Gynecol 83:419, 1994.

229. Walker GR, Schlesselman J, Ness RB, Family history of cancer, oral contraceptive use, and ovarian cancer risk, Am J Obstet Gynecol 186:8, 2002.

230. Narod SA, Risch H, Moslehi R, Dørum A, Neuhausen S, Olsson H, Provencher D, Radice P, Evans G, Bishop IS, Brunet J-S, Ponder BAJ, for the Hereditary Ovarian Cancer Clinical Study Group, Oral contraceptives and the risk of hereditary ovarian cancer, New Engl J Med 339:424, 1998.

231. Modan B, Hartge P, Hirsh-Yechezkel G, Chetrit A, Lubin F, Beller U, Ben-Baruch G, Fishman A, Menczer J, Ebbers SM, Tucker MA, Wacholder S, Struewing JP, Friedman E, Piura B, National Israel Ovarian Cancer Study Group, Parity, oral contraceptives, and the risk of ovarian cancer among carriers and noncarriers of a BRCA1 or BRCA2 mutation, New Engl J Med 345:235, 2001.

232. Ness RB, Grisso JA, Vergona R, Klapper J, Morgan M, Wheeler JE, for the Study of Health and Reproduction (SHARE) Study Group, Oral contraceptives, other methods of contraception, and risk reduction for ovarian cancer, Epidemiology 12:307, 2001.

233. Brinton LA, Oral contraceptives and cervical neoplasia, Contraception 43:581, 1991.

234. Delgado-Rodriguez M, Sillero-Arenas M, Martin-Moreno JM, Galvez-Vargas R, Oral contraceptives and cancer of the cervix uteri. A meta-analysis, Acta Obstet Gynecol Scand 71:368, 1992.

235. Gram IT, Macaluso M, Stalsberg H, Oral contraceptive use and the incidence of cervical intraepithelial neoplasia, Am J Obstet Gynecol 167:40, 1992.

236. Irwin KL, Rosero-Bixby L, Oberle MW, Lee NC, Whatley AS, Fortney JA, Bonhomme MG, Oral contraceptives and cervical cancer risk in Costa Rica: detection bias or causal association? JAMA 259:59, 1988.

237. Ye Z, Thomas DB, Ray RM, and the WHO Collaborative Study of Neoplasia and Steroid Contraceptives, Combined oral contraceptives and risk of cervical carcinoma in situ, Int J Epidemiol 24:19, 1995.

238. Ylitalo N, Sorensen P, Josefsson A, Frisch M, Sparen P, Ponten J, Gyllensten U, Melbye M, Adami HO, Smoking and oral contraceptives as risk factors for cervical carcinoma in situ, Int J Cancer 81:357, 1999.

239. Brinton LA, Reeves WC, Brenes MM, Herrero R, de Britton RC, Gaitan E, Tenorio F, Garcia M, Rawls WE, Oral contraceptive use and risk of invasive cervical cancer, Int J Epidemiol 19:4, 1990.

240. Ursin G, Peters RK, Hendeson BE, d'Ablaing G, III., Monroe KR, Pike MC, Oral contraceptive use and adenocarcinoma of cervix, Lancet 344:1390, 1994.

241. Thomas DB, Ray RM, and the World Health Organization Collaborative Study of Neoplasia and Steroid Contraceptives, Oral contraceptives and invasive adenocarcinomas and adenosquamous carcinomas of the uterine cervix, Am J Epidemiol 144:281, 1996.

242. Schwartz SM, Weiss NS, Increased incidence of adenocarcinoma of the cervix in young women in the United States, Am J Epidemiol 124:1045, 1986.

243. Smith JS, Green J, de Gonzalez AB, Appleby P, Peto J, Plummer M, Franceschi S, Beral V, Cervical cancer and use of hormonal contraceptives: a systematic review, Lancet 361:1159, 2003.

244. Moreno V, Bosch FX, Muñoz N, Meijer CJLM, Shah KV, Walboomers JMM, Herrero R, Franceschi S, for the International Agency for Research on Cancer (IARC) Multicentric Cervical Cancer Study Group, Effect of oral contraceptives on risk of cervical cancer in women with human papillomavirus infection: the IARC multicentric case-control study, Lancet 359:1085, 2002.

245. Neuberger J, Forman D, Doll R, Williams R, Oral contraceptives and hepatocellular carcinoma, Br Med J 292:1355, 1986.

246. Palmer JR, Rosenberg L, Kaufman DW, Warshauer ME, Stolley P, Shapiro S, Oral contraceptive use and liver cancer, Am J Epidemiol 130:878, 1989.

247. **WHO Collaborative Study of Neoplasia and Steroid Contraceptives,** Combined oral contraceptives and liver cancer, Int J Cancer 43:254, 1989.

248. **The Collaborative MILTS Project Team,** Oral contraceptives and liver cancer. Results of the Multicentre International Liver Tumor Study (MILTS), Contraception 56:275, 1997.

249. **Mant JWF, Vessey MP,** Trends in mortality from primary liver cancer in England and Wales 1975–92: influence of oral contraceptives, Br J Cancer 72:800, 1995.

250. **Waetjen LE, Grimes DA,** Oral contraceptives and primary liver cancer: temporal trends in three countries, Obstet Gynecol 88:945, 1996.

251. **El-Serag HB, Mason AC,** Rising incidence of hepatocellular carcinoma in the United States, New Engl J Med 340:745, 1999.

252. **Brinton LA, Vessey MP, Flavel R, Yeates D,** Risk factors for benign breast disease, Am J Epidemiol 113:203, 1981.

253. **Franceschi S, La Vecchia C, Parazzini F, Fasoli M, Regallo M, Decarli A, Gallus G, Tognoni G,** Oral contraceptives and benign breast disease: a case-control study, Am J Obstet Gynecol 149:602, 1984.

254. **Rohan TE, L'Abbe KA, Cook MG,** Oral contraceptives and risk of benign proliferative epithelial disorders of the breast, Int J Cancer 50:891, 1992.

255. **Charreau I, Plu-Bureau G, Bachelot A, Contesso G, Guinebretiere JM, L'e MG,** Oral contraceptive use and risk of benign breast disease in a French case-control study of young women, Eur J Cancer Prev 2:147, 1993.

256. **Rohan TE, Miller AB,** A cohort study of oral contraceptive use and risk of benign breast disease, Int J Cancer 82:191, 1999.

257. **Royal College of General Practitioners' Oral Contraceptive Study,** Further analyses of mortality in oral contraceptive users, Lancet i:541, 1981.

258. **Vessey M, Baron J, Doll R, McPherson K, Yeates D,** Oral contraceptives and breast cancer: final report of an epidemiological study, Br J Cancer 47:455, 1982.

259. **Vessey M, McPherson K, Villard-Mackintosh L, Yeates D,** Oral contraceptives and breast cancer: latest findings in a large cohort study, Br J Cancer 59:613, 1989.

260. **Romieu I, Willett WC, Colditz GA, Stampfer MJ, Rosner B, Hennekens CH, Speizer FE,** Prospective study of oral contraceptive use and risk of breast cancer in women, J Natl Cancer Inst 81:1313, 1989.

261. **Ramcharan S, Pellegrin FA, Ray RM, Hsu J-P,** The Walnut Creek Contraceptive Drug Study. A prospective study of the side effects of oral contraceptives, J Reprod Med 25:360, 1980.

262. **McPherson K, Neil A, Vessey MP,** Oral contraceptives and breast cancer, Lancet ii:414, 1983.

263. **La Vecchia C, Decarli A, Fasoli M, Franceschi S, Gentile A, Negri E, Parazzini F, Tognomi G,** Oral contraceptives and cancers of the breast and of the female genital tract. Interim results from a case-control study, Br J Cancer 54:311, 1986.

264. **Meirik O, Dami H, Christoffersen T, Lund E, Bergstrom R, Bergsjo P,** Oral contraceptive use and breast cancer in young women, Lancet ii:650, 1986.

265. **Kay CR, Hannaford PC,** Breast cancer and the pill — further report from the Royal College of General Practitioners' oral contraceptive study, Br J Cancer 58:675, 1988.

266. **Miller DR, Rosenberg L, Kaufman DW, Stolley P, Warshauer ME, Shapiro S,** Breast cancer before age 45 and oral contraceptive use: new findings, Am J Epidemiol 129:269, 1989.

267. **UK National Case-Control Study Group,** Oral contraceptive use and breast cancer risk in young women, Lancet i:973, 1989.

268. **WHO Collaborative Study of Neoplasia and Steroid Contraceptives,** Breast cancer and combined oral contraceptives: results from a multinational study, Br J Cancer 61:110, 1990.

269. **La Vecchia C, Negri E, Franceschi S, Talamini R, Amadori D, Filiberti R, Conti E, Montella M, Veronesi A, Parazzini F, Ferraroni M, Decarli A,** Oral contraceptives and breast cancer: a cooperative Italian study, Int J Cancer 60:163, 1995.

270. **Rosenberg L, Palmer JR, Rao RS, Zauber AG, Strom BL, Warshauer ME, Harlap S, Shapiro S,** Case-control study of oral contraceptive use and risk of breast cancer, Am J Epidemiol 143:25, 1996.

271. **Hennekens CH, Speizer FE, Lipnik RJ, Rosner B, Bain C, Belanger C, Stampfer MJ, Willett W, Peto R,** Case-control study of oral contraceptive use and breast cancer, J Natl Cancer Inst 72:39, 1984.

128

272. Rosenberg L, Miller DR, Kaufman DW, Helmrich SP, Stolley PD, Schoffenfeld D, Shapiro S, Breast cancer and oral contraceptive use, Am J Epidemiol 119:167, 1984.

273. Stadel BV, Rubin GL, Webster LA, Schlesselmann JJ, Wingo PA, Oral contraceptives and breast cancer in young women, Lancet ii:970, 1985.

274. Pike MC, Krailo MD, Henderson BE, Duke A, Roy S, Breast cancer in young women and use of oral contraceptives: possible modifying effect of formulation and age at use, Lancet ii:926, 1983.

275. Wingo PA, Lee NC, Ory HW, Beral V, Peterson HB, Rhodes P, Age-specific differences in the relationship between oral contraceptive use and breast cancer, Obstet Gynecol 78:161, 1991.

276. Ursin G, Aragaki CC, Paganini-Hill A, Siemiatycki J, Thompson WD, Haile RW, Oral contraceptives and premenopausal bilateral breast cancer: a case-control study, Epidemiology 3:414, 1992.

277. Rookus MA, Leeuwen FE, for the Netherlands Oral Contraceptives and Breast Cancer Study Group, Oral contraceptives and risk of breast cancer in women aged 20–54 years, Lancet 344:844, 1994.

278. White E, Malone KE, Weiss NS, Daling JR, Breast cancer among young U.S. women in relation to oral contraceptive use, J Natl Cancer Inst 86:505, 1994.

279. Brinton LA, Daling JR, Liff JM, Schoenberg JB, Malone KE, Stanford JL, Coates RJ, Gammon MD, Hanson L, Hoover RN, Oral contraceptives and breast cancer risk among younger women, J Natl Cancer Inst 87:827, 1995.

280. Cancer and Steroid Hormone Study, CDC and NICHD, Oral contraceptive use and the risk of breast cancer, New Engl J Med 315:405, 1986.

281. Schlesselman JJ, Stadel BV, Murray P, Shenghan L, Breast cancer risk in relation to type of estrogen contained in oral contraceptives, Contraception 36:595, 1987.

282. Stanford JL, Brinton LA, Hoover RN, Oral contraceptives and breast cancer: results from an expanded case-control study, Br J Cancer 60:375, 1989.

283. Murray P, Schlesselman JJ, Stadel BV, Shenghan L, Oral contraceptives and breast cancer risk in women with a family history of breast cancer, Am J Obstet Gynecol 73:977, 1989.

284. Schildkraut JM, Hulka BS, Wilkinson WE, Oral contraceptives and breast cancer: a case-control study with hospital and community controls, Obstet Gynecol 76:395, 1990.

285. Collaborative Group on Hormonal Factors in Breast Cancer, Breast cancer and hormonal contraceptives: collaborative reanalysis of individual data on 53,297 women with breast cancer and 100,239 women without breast cancer from 54 epidemiological studies, Lancet 347:1713, 1996.

286. Collaborative Group on Hormonal Factors in Breast Cancer, Breast cancer and hormonal contraceptives: further results, Contraception 54:1S, 1996.

287. Lambe M, Hsieh C, Trichopoulos D, Ekbom A, Pavia M, Adami H-O, Transient increase in the risk of breast cancer after giving birth, New Engl J Med 331:5, 1994.

288. Guinee VF, Olsson H, Moller T, Hess KR, Taylor SH, Fahey T, Gladikov JV, van den Blink JW, Bonichon F, Dische S, et al., Effect of pregnancy on prognosis for young women with breast cancer, Lancet 343:1587, 1994.

289. Kroman N, Wohlfart J, Andersen KW, Mouriudsen HT, Westergaard U, Melbye M, Time since childbirth and prognosis in primary breast cancer: population based study, Br Med J 315:851, 1997.

290. Rosenberg L, Palmer JR, Clarke EA, Shapiro S, A case-control study of the risk of breast cancer in relation to oral contraceptive use, Am J Epidemiol 136:1437, 1992.

291. Magnusson CM, Persson IR, Baron JA, Ekbom A, Bergström R, Adami H-O, The role of reproductive factors and use of oral contraceptives in the aetiology of breast cancer in women aged 50 to 74 years, Int J Cancer 80:231, 1999.

292. Marchbanks PA, McDonald JA, Wilson HG, Folger SG, Mandel MG, Daling JR, Bernstein L, Malone KE, Ursin G, Strom BL, Norman SA, Wingo PA, Burkman RT, Berlin JA, Simon JS, Spirtas R, Weiss LK, Oral contraceptives and the risk of breast cancer, New Engl J Med 346:2025, 2002.

293. Victory R, D'Souza C, Diamond MP, McNeely SG, Vista-Deck D, Hendrix S, Reduced cancer risks in oral contraceptive users: results from the Women's Health Initiative (abstract), Fertil Steril 82:S104, 2004.

294. **Grabrick DM, Hartmann LC, Cerhan JR, Vierkant RA, Therneau TM, Vachon CM, Olson JE, Couch FJ, Anderson KE, Pankratz VS, Sellers TA,** Risk of breast cancer with oral contraceptive use in women with a family history of breast cancer, JAMA 284:1791, 2000.

295. **Ursin G, Henderson BE, Haile RW, Pike MC, Zhou N, Diep A, Bernstein L,** Does oral contraceptive use increase the risk of breast cancer in women with BRCA1/BRCA2 mutations more than in other women? Cancer Res 57:3678, 1997.

296. **Narod S, Dube MP, Klijn J, Lubinski J, Lynch HT, Ghadirian P, Provencher D, et al.,** Oral contraceptives and the risk of breast cancer in BRCA1 and BRCA2 mutation carriers, J Natl Cancer Inst 94:1773, 2002.

297. **American Cancer Society, Breast Cancer Facts & Figures 2003–2004,** http://www.cancer.org/downloads/STT/CAFF2003BrFPWSecured.pdg, 2004.

298. **Green A,** Oral contraceptives and skin neoplasia, Contraception 43:653, 1991.

299. **Hannaford PC, Villard-Mackintosh L, Vessey MP, Kay CR,** Oral contraceptives and malignant melanoma, Br J Cancer 63:430, 1991.

300. **Milne R, Vessey M,** The association of oral contraception with kidney cancer, colon cancer, gallbladder cancer (including extrahepatic bile duct cancer) and pituitary tumors, Contraception 43:667, 1991.

301. **Berkowitz RS, Bernstein MR, Harlow BL, Rice LW, Lage JM, Goldstein DP, Cramer DW,** Case-control study of risk factors for partial molar pregnancy, Am J Obstet Gynecol 173:788, 1995.

302. **Palmer JR, Driscoll SG, Rosenberg L, Berkowitz RS, Lurain JR, Soper J, Twiggs LB, Gershenson DM, Kohorn EI, Berman M, Shapiro S, Rao RS,** Oral contraceptive use and risk of gestational trophoblastic tumors, J Natl Cancer Inst 91:635, 1999.

303. **Parazzini F, Cipriani S, Mangili G, Garavaglia E, Guarnerio P, Ricci E, Benzi G, Salerio B, Polverino G, La Vecchia C,** Oral contraceptives and risk of gestational trophoblastic disease, Contraception 65:425, 2002.

304. **Horn-Ross PL, Morrow M, Ljung BM,** Menstrual and reproductive factors for salivary gland cancer risk in women, Epidemiology 10:528, 1999.

305. **Martinez ME, Grodstein F, Giovannucci E, Colditz GA, Speizer FE, Hennekens C, Rosner B, Willett WC, Stampfer MJ,** A prospective study of reproductive factors, oral contraceptive use, and risk of colorectal cancer, Cancer Epidemiol Biomarkers Prev 6:1, 1997.

306. **Fernandez E, La Vecchia C, Balducci A, Chatenoud L, Franceschi S, Negri E,** Oral contraceptives and colorectal cancer risk: a meta-analysis, Br J Cancer 84:722, 2001.

307. **Wiegratz I, Kutschera E, Lee JH, Moore C, Mellinger U, Winkler UH, Kuhl H,** Effect of four oral contraceptives on thyroid hormones, adrenal and blood pressure parameters, Contraception 67:361, 2003.

308. **Janerich DT, Dugan JM, Standfast SJ, Strite L,** Congenital heart disease and prenatal exposure to exogenous sex hormones, Br Med J i:1058, 1977.

309. **Nora JJ, Nora AH, Blu J, Ingram J, Foster D,** Exogenous progestogen and estrogen implicated in birth defects, JAMA 240:837, 1978.

310. **Heinonen OP, Slone D, Monson RR, Hook ER, Shapiro S,** Cardiovascular birth defects in antenatal exposure to female sex hormones, New Engl J Med 296:67, 1976.

311. **Simpson JL, Phillips OP,** Spermicides, hormonal contraception and congenital malformations, Adv Contraception 6:141, 1990.

312. **Michaelis J, Michaelis H, Gluck E, Koller S,** Prospective study of suspected associations between certain drugs administered during early pregnancy and congenital malformations, Teratology 27:57, 1983.

313. **Bracken MB,** Oral contraception and congenital malformations in offspring: a review and meta-analysis of the prospective studies, Obstet Gynecol 76:552, 1990.

314. **Raman-Wilms L, Tseng AL, Wighardt S, Einarson TR, Koren G,** Fetal genital effects of first trimester sex hormone exposure: a meta-analysis, Obstet Gynecol 85:141, 1995.

315. **Ressequie LJ, Hick JF, Bruen JA, Noller KL, O'Fallon WM, Kurland LT,** Congenital malformations among offspring exposed in utero to progestins, Olsted County, Minnesota, 1936-1974, Fertil Steril 43:514, 1985.

316. **Katz Z, Lancet M, Skornik J, Chemke J, Mogilemer B, Klinberg M,** Teratogenicity of progestogens given during the first trimester of pregnancy, Obstet Gynecol 65:775, 1985.

317. **Vessey MP, Wright NH, McPherson K, Wiggins P,** Fertility after stopping different methods of contraception, Br Med J i:265, 1978.

318. **Vessey MP, Smith MA, Yates D,** Return of fertility after discontinuation of oral contraceptives: influence of age and parity, Br J Fam Plann 11:120, 1986.

319. **Linn S, Schoenbaum SC, Monson RR, Rosner B, Ryan KJ,** Delay in conception for former 'pill' users, JAMA 247:629, 1982.

320. **Bracken MB, Hellenbrand KG, Holford TR,** Conception delay after oral contraceptive use: the effect of estrogen dose, Fertil Steril 53:21, 1990.

321. **Bagwell MA, Coker AL, Thompson SJ, Baker ER, Addy CL,** Primary infertility and oral contraceptive steroid use, Fertil Steril 63:1161, 1995.

322. **Farrow A, Hull MGR, Northstone K, Taylor H, Ford WCL, Golding J,** Prolonged use of oral contraception before a planned pregnancy is associated with a decreased risk of delayed conception, Hum Reprod 17:2754, 2002.

323. **Rothman KJ,** Fetal loss, twinning, and birth weight after oral-contraceptive use, New Engl J Med 297:468, 1977.

324. **Ford JH, MacCormac L,** Pregnancy and lifestyle study: the long-term use of the contraceptive pill and the risk of age-related miscarriage, Hum Reprod 10:1397, 1995.

325. **Rothman KJ, Liess J,** Gender of offspring after oral-contraceptive use, New Engl J Med 295:859, 1976.

326. **Magidor S, Poalti H, Harlap S, Baras M,** Long-term follow-up of children whose mothers used oral contraceptives prior to contraception, Contraception 29:203, 1984.

327. **Vessey M, Doll R, Peto R, Johnson B, Wiggins P,** A long-term follow-up study of women using different methods of contraception — an interim report, J Biosoc Sci 8:373, 1976.

328. **Royal College of General Practitioners,** The outcome of pregnancy in former oral contraceptive users, Br J Obstet Gynaecol 83:608, 1976.

329. **Betrabet SS, Shikary ZK, Toddywalla VS, Toddywalla SP, Patel D, Saxena BN,** Transfer of norethisterone (NET) and levonorgestrel (LNG) from a single tablet into the infant's circulation through the mother's milk, Contraception 35:517, 1987.

330. **Diaz S, Peralta O, Juez G, Herreros C, Casado ME, Salvatierra AM, Miranda P, Durn E, Croxatto HB,** Fertility regulation in nursing women: III. Short-term influence of a low-dose combined oral contraceptive upon lactation and infant growth, Contraception 27:1, 1982.

331. **Croxatto HB, Diaz S, Peralta O, Juez G, Herreros C, Casado ME, Salvatierra AM, Miranda P, Durn E,** Fertility regulation in nursing women: IV. Long-term influence of a low-dose combined oral contraceptive initiated at day 30 postpartum upon lactation and child growth, Contraception 27:13, 1983.

332. **Peralta O, Diaz S, Juez G, Herreros C, Casado ME, Salvatierra AM, Miranda P, Durn E, Croxatto HB,** Fertility regulation in nursing women: V. Long-term influence of a low-dose combined oral contraceptive initiated at day 90 postpartum upon lactation and infant growth, Contraception 27:27, 1983.

333. **WHO, Special Programme of Research, Development, and Research Training in Human Reproduction, Task Force on Oral Contraceptives,** Effects of hormonal contraceptives on milk volume and infant growth, Contraception 30:505, 1984.

334. **WHO Task Force for Epidemiological Research on Reproductive Health, Special Programme of Research, Development and Research Training in Human Reproduction,** Progestogen-only contraceptives during lactation. I. Infant growth, Contraception 50:35, 1994.

335. **WHO Task Force for Epidemiological Research on Reproductive Health, Special Programme of Research, Development and Research Training in Human Reproduction,** Progestogen-only contraceptives during lactation. II. Infant development, Contraception 50:55, 1994.

336. **Nilsson S, Melbin T, Hofvander Y, Sundelin C, Valentin J, Nygren KG,** Long-term follow-up of children breast-fed by mothers using oral contraceptives, Contraception 34:443, 1986.

337. **Campbell OM, Gray RH,** Characteristics and determinants of postpartum ovarian function in women in the United States, Am J Obstet Gynecol 169:55, 1993.

338. **Labbok MH, Hight-Laukaran V, Peterson AE, Fletcher V, von Hertzen H, Van Look PFA,** Multicenter study of the lactational amenorrhea method (LAM): I. Efficacy, duration, and implications for clinical application, Contraception 55:327, 1997.

339. **Visness CM, Kennedy KI, Gross BA, Parenteau-Carreau S, Flynn AM, Brown JB,** Fertility of fully breast-feeding women in the early postpartum period, Obstet Gynecol 89:164, 1997.

340. **Diaz S, Aravena R, Cardenas H, Casado ME, Miranda P, Schiappacasse V, Croxatto HB,** Contraceptive efficacy of lactational amenorrhea in urban Chilean women, Contraception 43:335, 1991.

341. **Gray RH, Campbell OM, Zacur HA, Labbok MH, MacRae SL,** Postpartum return of ovarian activity in nonbreastfeeding women monitored by urinary assays, J Clin Endocrinol Metab 64:645, 1987.

342. **McCann MF, Moggia AV, Hibbins JE, Potts M, Becker C,** The effects of a progestin-only oral contraceptive (levonorgestrel 0.03 mg) on breast-feeding, Contraception 40:635, 1989.

343. **Halderman LD, Nelson AL,** Impact of early postpartum administration of progestin-only hormonal contraceptives compared with nonhormonal contraceptives on short-term breast-feeding patterns, Am J Obstet Gynecol 186:1250, 2002.

344. **Pituitary Adenoma Study Group,** Pituitary adenomas and oral contraceptives: a multicenter case-control study, Fertil Steril 39:753, 1983.

345. **Shy FKK, McTiernan AM, Daling JR, Weiss NS,** Oral contraceptive use and the occurrence of pituitary prolactinomas, JAMA 249:2204, 1983.

346. **Wingrave SJ, Kay CR, Vessey MP,** Oral contraceptives and pituitary adenomas, Br Med J 280:685, 1980.

347. **Hulting A-L, Werner S, Hagenfeldt K,** Oral contraceptives do not promote the development or growth of prolactinomas, Contraception 27:69, 1983.

348. **Corenblum B, Donovan L,** The safety of physiological estrogen plus progestin replacement therapy and oral contraceptive therapy in women with pathological hyperprolactinemia, Fertil Steril 59:671, 1993.

349. **Testa G, Vegetti W, Motta T, Alagna F, Bianchedi D, Carlucci C, Bianchi M, Parazzini F, Crosignani PG,** Two-year treatment with oral contraceptives in hyperprolactinemic patients, Contraception 58:69, 1998.

350. **Furuhjelm M, Carlstrom K,** Amenorrhea following use of combined oral contraceptives, Acta Obstet Gynecol Scand 52:373, 1973.

351. **Shearman RP, Smith ID,** Statistical analysis of relationship between oral contraceptives, secondary amenorrhea and galactorrhea, J Obstet Gynaecol Br Commonw 79:654, 1972.

352. **Jacobs HS, Knuth UA, Hull MGR, Franks S,** Post "pill" amenorrhea — cause or coincidence? Br Med J ii:940, 1977.

353. **Vessey MP, Hannaford P, Mant J, Painter R, Frith P, Chappel D,** Oral contraception and eye disease: findings in two large cohort studies, Br Med J 82:538, 1998.

354. **Vessey M, Painter R,** Oral contraception and ear disease: findings in a large cohort study, Contraception 63:61, 2001.

355. **Villard-Mackintosh L, Vessey MP,** Oral contraceptives and reproductive factors in multiple sclerosis incidence, Contraception 47:161, 1993.

356. **Thorogood M, Hannaford PC,** The influence of oral contraceptives on the risk of multiple sclerosis, Br J Obstet Gynaecol 105:1296, 1998.

357. **Costello Daly C, Helling-Giese GE, Mati JK, Hunter DJ,** Contraceptive methods and the transmission of HIV: implications for family planning, Genitourin Med 70:110, 1994.

358. **Taneepanichskul S, Phuapradit W, Chaturachinda K,** Association of contraceptives and HIV-1 infection in Thai female commercial sex workers, Aust N Z J Obstet Gynaecol 37:86, 1997.

359. **Kapiga SH, Lyamuya EF, Lwihula GK, Hunter DJ,** The incidence of HIV infection among women using family planning methods in Dar-es-Salaam, Tanzania, AIDS 12:75, 1998.

360. **Westrom I,** Incidence, prevalence, and trends of acute pelvic inflammatory disease and its consequences in industrialized countries, Am J Obstet Gynecol 138:880, 1980.

361. **Eschenbach DA, Harnisch JP, Holmes KK,** Pathogenesis of acute pelvic inflammatory disease: role of contraception and other risk factors, Am J Obstet Gynecol 128:838, 1977.

362. **Rubin GL, Ory WH, Layde PM,** Oral contraceptives and pelvic inflammatory disease, Am J Obstet Gynecol 140:630, 1980.

363. **Senanayake P, Kramer DG,** Contraception and the etiology of pelvic inflammatory diseases: new perspectives, Am J Obstet Gynecol 138:852, 1980.

364. **Panser LA, Phipps WR,** Type of oral contraceptive in relation to acute, initial episodes of pelvic inflammatory disease, Contraception 43:91, 1991.

365. **Svensson L, Westrom L, Mardh P,** Contraceptives and acute salpingitis, JAMA 251:2553, 1984.

366. **Wolner-Hanssen P,** Oral contraceptive use modifies the manifestations of pelvic inflammatory disease, Br J Obstet Gynaecol 93:619, 1986.

367. **Cates Jr W, Washington AE, Rubin GL, Peterson HB,** The pill, chlamydia and PID, Fam Plann Perspect 17:175, 1985.

368. **Critchlow CW, Wölner-Hanssen P, Eschenbach DA, Kiviat NB, Koutsky LA, Stevens CE, Holmes KK,** Determinants of cervical ectopia and of cervicitis: age, oral contraception, specific cervical infection, smoking, and douching, Am J Obstet Gynecol 173:534, 1995.

369. **Jacobson DL, Peralta L, Farmer M, Graham NM, Gaydos C, Zenilman J,** Relationship of hormonal contraception and cervical ectopy as measured by computerized planimetry to chlamydial infection in adolescents, Sex Transm Dis 27:313, 2000.

370. **Morrison CS, Bright P, Wong EL, Kwok C, Yacobson I, Gaydos CA, Tucker HT, Blumenthal PD,** Hormonal contraceptive use, cervical ectopy, and the acquisition of cervical infections, Sex Transm Dis 31:561, 2004.

371. **Cramer DW, Goldman MB, Schiff I, Belisla S, Albrecht B, Stadel B, Gibson M, Wilson E, Stillman R, Thompson I,** The relationship of tubal infertility to barrier method and oral contraceptive use, JAMA 257:2446, 1987.

372. **Wolner-Hanssen P, Eschenbach DA, Paavonen J, Kiviat N, Stevens CE, Critchlow C, DeRouen T, Holmes KK,** Decreased risk of symptomatic chlamydial pelvic inflammatory disease associated with oral contraceptive use, JAMA 263:54, 1990.

373. **Ness RB, Keder LM, Soper DE, Amortegui AJ, Gluck J, Wiesenfeld H, Sweet RL, Rice PA, Peipert JF, Donegan SP, Kanbour-Shakir A,** Oral contraception and the recognition of endometritis, Am J Obstet Gynecol 176:580, 1997.

374. **Ness RB, Soper DE, Holley RL, Peipert J, Randall H, Sweet RL, Sondheimer SJ, et al, for the PID Evaluation and Clinical health (PEACH) Study Investigators,** Hormonal and barrier contraception and risk of upper genital tract disease in the PID Evaluation and Clinical Health (PEACH) study, Am J Obstet Gynecol 185:121, 2001.

375. **Barbone F, Austin H, Louv WC, Alexander WJ,** A follow-up study of methods of contraception, sexual activity, and rates of trichomoniasis, candidiasis, and bacterial vaginosis, Am J Obstet Gynecol 163:510, 1990.

376. **Shoubnikova M, Hellberg D, Nilsson S, Mårdh P-A,** Contraceptive use in women with bacterial vaginosis, Contraception 55:355, 1997.

377. **Baeten JM, Nyange PM, Richardson BA, Lavreys L, Chohan B, Martin HL, Jr, Mandaliya K, Ndinya-Achola JO, Bwayo JJ, Kreiss JK,** Hormonal contraception and risk of sexually transmitted disease acquisition: results from a prospective study, Am J Obstet Gynecol 185:380, 2001.

378. **Stewart FH, Harper CC, Ellertson CE, Grimes DA, Sawaya GF, Trussell J,** Clinical breast and pelvic examination requirements for hormonal contraception. Current practice vs evidence, JAMA 285:2231, 2001.

379. **Milsom I, Sundell G, Andersch B,** A longitudinal study of contraception and pregnancy outcome in a representative sample of young Swedish women, Contraception 43:111, 1991.

380. **Letterie GS, Chow GE,** Effect of "missed" pills on oral contraceptive effectiveness, Obstet Gynecol 79:979, 1992.

381. **Westhoff CL, Kerns J, Morroni C, Tiezzi L, Aikins-Murphy P,** Quick-start: a novel oral contraceptive initiation method, Contraception 66:141, 2002.

382. **Westhoff C, Morroni C, Kerns J, Murphy PA,** Bleeding patterns after immediate vs. conventional oral contraceptive initiation: a randomized, controlled trial, Fertil Steril 79:322, 2003.

383. **Anderson FD, Hait H, the Seasonale-301 Study Group,** A multicenter, randomized study of an extended cycle oral contraceptive, Contraception 68:89, 2003.

384. **Kwiecien M, Edelman A, Nichols MD, Jensen JT,** Bleeding patterns and patient acceptability of standard or continuous dosing regimens of a low-dose oral contraceptive: a randomized trial, Contraception 67:9, 2003.

385. **Miller L, Hughes JP,** Continuous combination oral contraceptive pills to eliminate withdrawal bleeding: a randomized trial, Obstet Gynecol 101:653, 2003.

386. **Sulak PJ, Carl J, Gopalakrishnan I, Coffee A, Kuehl TJ,** Outcomes of extended oral contraceptive regiments with a shortened hormone-free interval to manage breakthrough bleeding, Contraception 70:281, 2004.

387. **Potter L, Oakley D, de Leon-Wong E, Cañamar R,** Measuring compliance among oral contraceptive users, Fam Plann Perspect 28:154, 1996.

388. **Killick SR, Bancroft K, Oelbaum S, Morris J, Elstein M,** Extending the duration of the pill-free interval during combined oral contraception, Adv Contracept 6:33, 1990.

389. **Elomaa K, Rolland R, Brosens I, Moorrees M, Deprest J, Tuominen J, Lähteenmäki P,** Omitting the first oral contraceptive pills of the cycle does not automatically lead to ovulation, Am J Obstet Gynecol 179:41, 1998.

390. **van Heusden AM, Fauser BCJM,** Activity of the pituitary-ovarian axis in the pill-free interval during use of low-dose combined oral contraceptives, Contraception 59:237, 1999.

391. **Jung-Hoffman C, Kuhl H,** Intra- and interindividual variations in contraceptive steroid levels during 12 treatment cycles: no relation to irregular bleedings, Contraception 42:423, 1990.

392. **Endrikat J, Müller U, Düsterberg B,** A twelve-month comparative clinical investigation of two low-dose oral contraceptives containing 20 μg ethinylestradiol/75 μg gestodene and 30 μg ethinylestradiol/75 μg gestodene, with respect to efficacy, cycle control, and tolerance, Contraception 55:131, 1997.

393. **Rosenberg MJ, Meyers A, Roy V,** Efficacy, cycle control, and side effects of low- and lower-dose oral contraceptives: a randomized trial of 20 micrograms and 35 micrograms estrogen preparations, Contraception 60:321, 1999.

394. **Rosenberg MJ, Waugh MS, Stevens CM,** Smoking and cycle control among oral contraceptive users, Am J Obstet Gynecol 174:628, 1996.

395. **Rosenberg MJ, Waugh MS, Higgins JE,** The effect of desogestrel, gestodene, and other factors on spotting and bleeding, Contraception 53:85, 1996.

396. **Krettek SE, Arkin SI, Chaisilwattana P, Monif GR,** *Chlamydia trachomatis* in patients who used oral contraceptives and had intermenstrual spotting, Obstet Gynecol 81:728, 1993.

397. **Lemay A, Dewailly SD, Grenier R, Huard J,** Attenuation of mild hyperandrogenic activity in postpubertal acne by a triphasic oral contraceptive containing low doses of ethynyl estradiol and d,l-norgestrel, J Clin Endocrinol Metab 71:8, 1990.

398. **Mango D, Ricci S, Manna P, Miggiano GAD, Serra GB,** Clinical and hormonal effects of ethinyl estradiol combined with gestodene and desogestrel in young women with acne vulgaris, Contraception 53:163, 1996.

399. **Thorneycroft IH, Stanczyk FZ, Bradshaw KD, Ballagh SA, Nichols M, Weber ME,** Effect of low-dose oral contraceptives on androgenic markers and acne, Contraception 60:255, 1999.

400. **Rosen MP, Breitkopf DM, Nagamani M,** A randomized controlled trial of second- versus third-generation oral contraceptives in the treatment of acne vulgaris, Am J Obstet Gynecol 188:1158, 2003.

401. **Grimes DA, Hughes JM,** Use of multiphasic oral contraceptives and hospitalizations of women with functional ovarian cysts in the United States, Obstet Gynecol 73:1037, 1989.

402. **Holt VL, Cushing-Haugen KL, Daling JR,** Oral contraceptives, tubal sterilization, and functional ovarian cyst risk, Obstet Gynecol 102:252, 2003.

403. **Vessey M, Metcalfe A, Wells C, McPherson K, Westhoff C, Yeates C,** Ovarian neoplasms, functional ovarian cysts, and oral contraceptives, Br Med J 294:1518, 1987.

404. **Lanes SF, Birmann B, Walker AM, Singer S,** Oral contraceptive type and functional ovarian cysts, Am J Obstet Gynecol 166:956, 1992.

405. **Holt VL, Daling JR, McKnight B, Moore D, Stergachis A, Weiss NS,** Functional ovarian cysts in relation to the use of monophasic and triphasic oral contraceptives, Obstet Gynecol 79:529, 1992.

406. **Young RL, Snabes MC, Frank ML, Reilly M,** A randomized, double-blind, placebo-controlled comparison of the impact of low-dose and triphasic oral contaceptives on follicular development, Am J Obstet Gynecol 167:678, 1992.

407. **Grimes DA, Godwin AJ, Rubin A, Smith JA, Lacarra M,** Ovulation and follicular development associated with three low-dose oral contraceptives: a randomized controlled trial, Obstet Gynecol 83:29, 1994.

408. **Neely JL, Abate M, Swinker M, D'Angio R,** The effect of doxycycline on serum levels of ethinyl estradiol, norethindrone, and endogenous progesterone, Obstet Gynecol 77:416, 1991.

409. **Murphy AA, Zacur HA, Charache P, Burkman RT,** The effect of tetracycline on levels of oral contraceptives, Am J Obstet Gynecol 164:28, 1991.

410. **Back DJ, Tija J, Martin C, Millar E, Mant T, Morrison P, Orme P,** The lack of interaction between temafloxacin and combined oral contraceptive steroids, Contraception 43:317, 1991.

411. **Csemiczky G, Alvendal C, Landgren BM,** Risk for ovulation in women taking a low-dose oral contraceptive (Microgynon) when receiving antibacterial treatment with a fluoroquinolone (ofloxacin), Adv Contracep 12:101, 1996.

412. **Helms SE, Bredle DL, Zajic J, Jarjoura D, Brodell RT, Krishnarao I,** Oral contraceptive failure rates and oral antibiotics, J Am Acad Dermatol 36:705, 1997.

413. **Markowitz JS, Donovan JL, DeVane CL, Taylor RM, Ruan Y, Wang J-S, Chavin KD,** Effect of St John's Wort on drug metabolism by induction of cytochrome P450 3A4 enzyme, JAMA 290:1500, 2003.

414. **Szoka PR, Edgren RA,** Drug interactions with oral contraceptives: compilation and analysis of an adverse experience report database, Fertil Steril 49(Suppl):31S, 1988.

415. **Mitchell MC, Hanew T, Meredith CG, Schenker S,** Effects of oral contraceptive steroids on acetaminophen metabolism and elimination, Clin Pharmacol Ther 34:48, 1983.

416. **Gupta KC, Joshi JV, Hazari K, Pohujani SM, Satoskjar RS,** Effect of low estrogen combination oral contraceptives on metabolism of aspirin and phenylbutazone, Int J Clin Pharmacol Ther Toxicol 20:511, 1982.

417. **Tietjen GE,** The relationship of migraine and stroke, Neuroepidemiology 19:13, 2000.

418. **Chang CL, Donaghy M, Poulter N,** Migraine and stroke in young women: case-control study, Br Med J 318:13, 1999.

419. **Donaghy M, Chang CL, Poulter N,** Duration, frequency, recency, and type of migraine and the risk of ischaemic stroke in women of childbearing age, J Neurol Neurosurg Psychiatry 73:747, 2002.

420. **Tzourio C, Tehindrazanarierelo A, Iglésias S, Alpérovitch A, Chgedru F, d'Anglejan-Chatillon J, Bousser M-G,** Case-control study of migraine and risk of ischaemic stroke in young women, Br Med J 310:830, 1995.

421. **Lidegaard Ø,** Oral contraceptives, pregnancy and the risk of cerebral thromboembolism: the influence of diabetes, hypertension, migraine and previous thrombotic disease, Br J Obstet Gynaecol 102:153, 1995.

422. **Curtis KM, Chrisman CE, Peterson HB,** Contraception for women in selected circumstances, Obstet Gynecol 99:1100, 2002.

423. **Ross RK, Pike MC, Vessey MP, Bull D, Yeates D, Casagrande JT,** Risk factors for uterine fibroids: Reduced risk associated with oral contraceptives, Br Med J 293:359, 1986.

424. **Parazzini F, Negri E, La Vecchia C, Fedele L, Rabaiotti M, Luchini L,** Oral contraceptive use and risk of uterine fibroids, Obstet Gynecol 79:430, 1992.

425. **Samadi AR, Lee NC, Flanders D, Boring JR, III., Parris EB,** Risk factors for self-reported uterine fibroids: a case-control study, Am J Public Health 86:858, 1996.

426. **Marshall LM, Spiegelman D, Goldman MB, Manson JE, Colditz GA, Barbieri RL, Stampfer MJ, Hunter DJ,** A prospective study of reproductive factors and oral contraceptive use in relation to the risk of uterine leiomyomata, Fertil Steril 70:432, 1998.

427. **Chiaffarino F, Parazzini F, La Vecchia C, Marsico S, Surace M, Ricci E,** Use of oral contraceptives and uterine fibroids: results from a case-control study, Br J Obstet gynaecol 106:857, 1999.

428. **Friedman AJ, Thomas PP,** Does low-dose combination oral contraceptive use affect uterine size or menstrual flow in premenopausal women with leiomyomas? Obstet Gynecol 85:631, 1995.

429. **Mattson RH, Cramer JA, Darney PD, Naftolin F,** Use of oral contraceptives by women with epilepsy, JAMA 256:238, 1986.

430. **Vessey M, Painter R, Yeates D,** Oral contraception and epilepsy: findings in a large cohort study, Contraception 66:77, 2002.

431. **Lutcher CL, Milner PF,** Contraceptive-induced vascular occlusive events in sickle cell disorders — fact or fiction? (abstract), Clin Res 34:217A, 1986.

432. **Yoong WC, Tuck SM, Yardumian A,** Red cell deformability in oral contraceptive pill users with sickle cell anemia, Br J Haematol 104:868, 1999.

433. **DeCeular K, Gruber C, Hayes R, Serjeant GR,** Medroxyprogesterone acetate and homozygous sickle-cell disease, Lancet ii:229, 1982.

434. **Jungers P, Dougados M, Pelissier L, Kuttenn F, Tron F, Lesavre P, Bach JF,** Influence of oral contraceptive therapy on the activity of systemic lupus erythematosus, Arthritis Rheum 25:618, 1982.

435. **Petri M, Robinson C,** Oral contraceptives and systemic lupus erythematosus, Arthritis Rheum 40:797, 1997.

436. **Knopp RH, LaRosa JC, Burkman RT, Jr.,** Contraception and dyslipidemia, Am J Obstet Gynecol 168:1994, 1993.

437. **Abdollahi M, Cushman M, Rosendaal FR,** Obesity: risk of venous thromboembolism and the interaction with coagulation factor levels and oral contraceptive use, Thromb Haemost 89:493, 2003.

438. **Holt VL, Cushing-Haugen KL, Daling JR,** Body weight and risk of oral contraceptive failure, Obstet Gynecol 99:820, 2002.

439. **Zieman M, Guillebaud J, Weisberg E, Shangold GA, Fisher AC, Creasy GW,** Contraceptive efficacy and cycle control with the Ortho Evra™/Evra™ transdermal system: the analysis of pooled data, Fertil Steril 77(Suppl 2):S13, 2002.

440. **Norris PM, Kamat A, Estes C,** Contraceptive failure in overweight patients taking combination oral contraceptive pills, Contraception 68:Abstract 16, 2003.

441. **Azziz R,** The hyperandrogenic-insulin-resistant acanthosis nigricans syndrome: therapeutic response, Fertil Steril 61:570, 1994.

442. **Nader S, Riad-Gabriel MG, Saad M,** The effect of a desogestrel-containing oral contraceptive on glucose tolerance and leptin concentrations in hyperandrogenic women, J Clin Endocrinol Metab 82:3074, 1997.

443. **Pasquali R, Gambineri A, Anconetani B, Vicennati V, Colitta D, Caramelli E, Casimirri F, Morselli-Labate AM,** The natural history of the metabolic syndrome in young women with the polycystic ovary syndrome and the effect of long-term oestrogen-progestogen treatment, Clin Endocrinol 50:517, 1999.

444. **Klibanski A, Biller BMK, Schoenfeld DA, Herzog DB, Saxe VC,** The effects of estrogen administration on trabecular bone loss in young women with anorexia nervosa, J Clin Endocrinol Metab 80:898, 1995.

445. **Drinkwater BL, Bruemmer B, Chesnut III CH,** Menstrual history as a determinant of current bone density in young athletes, JAMA 263:545, 1990.

446. **Jonnavithula S, Warren MP, Fox RP, Lazaro MI,** Bone density is compromised in amenorrheic women despite return of menses: a 2-year study, Obstet Gynecol 81:669, 1993.

447. **Cosnes J, Carbonnel F, Carrat F, Beaugerie L, Gendre JP,** Oral contraceptive use and the clinical course of Crohn's disease: a prospective cohort study, Gut 45:218, 1999.

448. **Sullivan-Nelson M, Kuller JA, Zacur HA,** Clinical use of oral contraceptives administered vaginally: a case report, Fertil Steril 52:864, 1989.

449. **Coutinho EM, de Souza JC, da Silva AR, de Acosta OM, Flores JG, Gu ZP, Ladipo OA, Adekunle AO, Otolorin EO, Shaaban MM, Abul Oyoom M, et al.,** Comparative study on the efficacy and acceptability of two contraceptive pills administered by the vaginal route: an international multicenter clinical trial, Clin Pharmacol Ther 53:65, 1993.

450. **Ziaei S, Rajaei L, Faghihzadeh S, Lamyian M,** Comparative study and evaluation of side effects of low-dose contraceptive pills administered by the oral and vaginal route, Contraception 65:329, 2002.

451. **Bryner RW, Toffle RC, Ullrich IH, Yeater RA,** Effect of low dose oral contraceptives on exercise performance, Br J Sports Med 30:36, 1996.

452. **Rickenlund A, Carlstrom K, Ekblom B, Brismar TB, Von Schoultz B, Hirschberg AL,** Effects of oral contraceptives on body composition and physical performance in female athletes, J Clin Endocrinol Metab 89:4364, 2004.

453. **Thompson HS, Hyatt JP, De Souza MJ, Clarkson PM,** The effects of oral contraceptives on delayed onset muscle soreness following exercise, Contraception 56:59, 1997.

454. **Brynhildsen J, Lennartsson H, Klemetz M, Dahlquist P, Hedin B, Hammar M,** Oral contraceptive use among female elite athletes and age-matched controls and its relation to low back pain, Acta Obstet Gynecol Scand 76:873, 1997.

455. **Milsom I, Sundell G, Andersch B,** The influence of different combined oral contraceptives on the prevalence and severity of dysmenorrhea, Contraception 42:497, 1990.

456. **Larsson G, Milsom I, Lindstedt G, Rybo G,** The influence of a low-dose combined oral contraceptive on menstrual blood loss and iron status, Contraception 46:327, 1992.

457. **Davis A, Goodwin A, Lippman J, Olson W, Kafrissen M,** Triphasic norgestimate-ethinyl estradiol for treating dysfunctional uterine bleeding, Obstet Gynecol 96:913, 2000.

458. **Vessey MP, Villard-Mackintosh L, Painter R,** Epidemiology of endometriosis in women attending family-planning clinics, Br Med J 306:182, 1993.

459. **Parazzini F, Ferraroni M, Bocciolone L, Tozzi L, Rubessa S, La Vecchia C,** Contraceptive methods and risk of pelvic endometriosis, Contraception 49:47, 1994.

460. **Sangi-Haghpeykar H, Poindexter AN, 3rd,** Epidemiology of endometriosis among parous women, Obstet Gynecol 85:983, 1995.

461. **Enzelsberger H, Metka M, Heytmanek G, Schurz B, Kurz C, Kusztrich M,** Influence of oral contraceptive use on bone density in climacteric women, Maturitas 9:375, 1988.

462. **Lindsay R, Tohme J, Kanders B,** The effect of oral contraceptive use on vertebral bone mass in pre- and post-menopausal women, Contraception 34:333, 1986.

463. **Enzelberger H, Metka M, Heytmanek G, Schurz B, Kurz C, Kusztrich M,** Influence of oral contraceptive use on bone density in climacteric women, Maturitas 9:375, 1988.

464. **Kleerekoper M, Brienza RS, Schultz LR, Johnson CC,** Oral contraceptive use may protect against low bone mass, Arch Intern Med 151:1971, 1991.

465. **Kritz-Silverstein D, Barrett-Connor E,** Bone mineral density in postmenopausal women as determined by prior oral contraceptive use, Am J Public Health 83:100, 1993.

466. **Tuppurrainen M, Kröger H, Saarikoski S, Honkanen R, Alhava E,** The effect of previous oral contraceptive use on bone mineral density in perimenopausal women, Osteoporosis Int 4:93, 1994.

467. **Gambacciani M, Spinetti A, Taponeco F, Cappagli B, Piaggesi L, Fioretti P,** Longitudinal evaluation of perimenopausal vertebral bone loss: effects of a low-dose oral contraceptive preparation on bone mineral density and metabolism, Obstet Gynecol 83:392, 1994.

468. **Pasco JA, Kotowicz MA, Henry MJ, Panahi S, Seeman E, Nicholson GC,** Oral contraceptives and bone mineral density: a population-based study, Am J Obstet Gynecol 182:265, 2000.

469. **Mais V, Fruzzetti F, Aiossa S, Paoletti AM, Guerriero S, Melis GB,** Bone metabolism in young women taking a monophasic pill containing 20 mg ethinylestradiol, Contraception 48:445, 1993.

470. **Polatti F, Perotti F, Filippa N, Gallina D, Nappi RE,** Bone mass and long-term monophasic oral contraceptive treatment in young women, Contraception 51:221, 1995.

471. **Hartard M, Bottermann P, Bartenstein P, Jeschke D,** Schwaiger M, Effects on bone mineral density of low-dosed oral contraceptives compared to and combined with physical activity, Contraception 55:87, 1997.

472. **Mallmin H, Ljunghall S, Persson I, Bergstrom R,** Risk factors for fractures of the distal forearm: a population-based case-control study, Osteoporosis Int 4:97, 1994.

473. **Johansson C, Mellström D,** An earlier fracture as a risk factor for new fracture and its association with smoking and menopausal age in women, Maturitas 24:97, 1996.

474. **O'Neill TW, Marsden D, Adams JE, Silman AJ,** Risk factors, falls, and fracture of the distal forearm in Manchester, UK, J Epidemiol Community Health 50:288, 1996.

475. **O'Neill TW, Silman AJ, Naves Diaz M, Cooper C, Kanis J, Felsenberg D,** Influence of hormonal and reproductive factors on the risk of vertebral deformity in European women, Osteoporosis Int 7:72, 1997.

476. **Cooper C, Hannaford P, Croft P, Kay CR,** Oral contraceptive pill use and fractures in women: a prospective study, Bone 14:41, 1993.

477. **Vessey M, Mant J, Painter R,** Oral contraception and other factors in relation to hospital referral for fracture. Findings in a large cohort study, Contraception 57:231, 1998.

478. **Michaëlsson K, Baron JA, Farahmand BY, Persson I, Ljunghall S,** Oral contraceptive use and risk of hip fracture: a case-control study, Lancet 353:1481, 1999.

479. **Hazes JMW, Dijkmans BAC, Vandenbroucke JP, De Vries RRP, Cats A,** Reduction of the risk of rheumatoid arthritis among women who take oral contraceptives, Arthritis Rheum 33:173, 1990.

480. **Spector TD, Hochberg MC,** The protective effect of the oral contraceptive pill on rheumatoid arthritis: an overview of the analytical epidemiological studies using meta-analysis, J Clin Epidemiol 43:1221, 1990.

481. **Pladevall-Vila M, Delclos GL, Varas C, Guyer H, Brugués-Tarradellas J, Anglada-Arisa A,** Controversy of oral contraceptives and risk of rheumatoid arthritis: meta-analysis of conflicting studies and review of conflicting meta-analyses with special emphasis on analysis of heterogeneity, Am J Epidemiol 144:1, 1996.

482. Vercellini P, Frontino G, De Giorgi O, Pietropaolo G, Pasin R, Crosignani PG, Continuous use of an oral contraceptive for endometriosis-associated recurrent dysmenorrhea that does not respond to a cyclic pill regimen, Fertil Steril 80:560, 2003.

483. Modugno F, Ness RB, Allen GO, Schildkraut JM, Davis FG, Goodman MT, Oral contraceptive use, reproductive history, and risk of epithelial ovarian cancer in women with and without endometriosis, Am J Obstet Gynecol 191:733, 2004.

484. van der Vange N, Blankenstein MA, Kloosterboer HJ, Haspels AA, Thijssen JHH, Effects of seven low-dose combined oral contraceptives on sex hormone binding globulin, corticosteroid binding globulin, total and free testosterone, Contraception 41:345, 1990.

485. Palatsi R, Hirvensalo E, Liukko P, Malmiharju T, Mattila L, Riihiluoma P, Ylöstalo P, Serum total and unbound testosterone and sex hormone binding globulin (SHBG) in female acne patients treated with two different oral contraceptives, Acta Derm Venereol 64:517, 1984.

486. Coenen CMH, Thomas CMG, Borm GF, Rolland R, Changes in androgens during treatment with four low-dose contraceptives, Contraception 53:171, 1996.

487. Steinkampf MP, Hammond KR, Blackwell RE, Hormonal treatment of functional ovarian cysts: a randomized, prospective study, Fertil Steril 54:775, 1990.

488. Ben-Ami M, Geslevich Y, Battino S, Matilsky M, Shalev E, Management of functional ovarian cysts after induction of ovulation. A randomized prospective study, Acta Obstet Gynecol Scand 72:396, 1993.

489. MacKenna A, Fabres C, Alam V, Morales V, Clinical management of functional ovarian cysts: a prospective and randomized study, Hum Reprod 15:2567, 2000.

490. Turan C, Zorlu CG, Ugur M, Ozcan T, Kaleli B, Gokmen O, Expectant management of functional ovarian cysts: an alternative to hormonal therapy, Int J Gynaecol Obstet 47:257, 1994.

491. Nezhat CH, Nezhat F, Borhan S, Seidman DS, Nezhat CR, Is hormonal treatment efficacious in the management of ovarian cysts in women with histories of endometriosis? Hum Reprod 11:874, 1996.

492. Westhoff C, Britton JA, Gammon MD, Wright T, Kelsey JL, Oral contraceptive and benign ovarian tumors, Am J Epidemiol 152:242, 2000.

493. Jones EF, Forrest JD, Contraceptive failure in the United States: revised estimates from the 1982 National Survey of Family Growth, Fam Plann Perspect 21:103, 1989.

494. Peterson LS, Oakley D, Potter LS, Darroch JE, Women's efforts to prevent pregnancy: consistency of oral contraceptive use, Fam Plann Perspect 30:19, 1998.

495. Rosenberg MJ, Waugh MS, Meehan TE, Use and misuse of oral contraceptives: risk indicators for poor pill taking and discontinuation, Contraception 51:283, 1995.

496. Rosenberg MJ, Waugh MS, Oral contraceptive discontinuation: a prospective evaluation of frequency and reasons, Am J Obstet Gynecol 179:577, 1998.

497. Villegas-Salas E, Ponce de León R, Juárez-Perez MA, Grubb GS, Effect of vitamin B6 on the side effects of a low-dose combined oral contraceptive, Contraception 55:245, 1997.

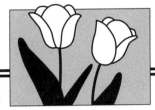

3

Special Uses of Oral Contraception:
Emergency Contraception
The Progestin-Only Minipill

Oral contraception is a phrase that appropriately denotes a vast body of knowledge (Chapter 2) pertaining to the combined estrogen-progestin "birth control pill." However, there are two special types of oral contraception that deserve separate consideration, emergency contraception and the progestin-only minipill.

Emergency Postcoital Contraception

The use of large doses of estrogen to prevent implantation was pioneered by Morris and van Wagenen at Yale in the 1960s. The initial work in monkeys led to the use of high doses of diethylstilbestrol (25–50 mg/day) and ethinyl estradiol in women.[1] It was quickly appreciated that these extremely large doses of estrogen were associated with a high rate of gastrointestinal side effects. Albert Yuzpe developed a method utilizing a combination oral contraceptive, resulting in an important reduction in dosage.[2] The following treatment regimens have been documented to be effective:

> Ovral: 2 tablets followed by 2 tablets 12 hours later.
> Alesse: 5 tablets followed by 5 tablets 12 hours later.
> Lo Ovral, Nordette, Levlen, Triphasil, Trilevlen: 4 tablets followed by 4 tablets 12 hours later.

Levonorgestrel in a dose of 0.75 mg given twice, 12 hours apart, is more successful and better tolerated than the combination oral contraceptive method.[3,4] In many countries, special packages of 0.75 mg levonorgestrel

(Plan B, Norlevo, Vikela) are available for emergency contraception. Greater efficacy and fewer side effects make low-dose levonorgestrel the treatment of choice.

In the United States, a kit (Preven) is available containing 4 tablets, each containing 50 μg ethinyl estradiol and 0.250 mg levonorgestrel, to be used in the usual fashion, 2 tablets followed by 2 tablets 12 hours later. A package (Plan B) containing only levonorgestrel (two 0.75 mg tablets) is also available, one tablet taken within 72 hours of intercourse and the second 12 hours later. **The two tablets can be combined into a single, one-time dose of 1.5 mg levonorgestrel with no loss of efficacy or increase in side effects.[5, 6] This is the strongly recommended choice for drug and schedule of treatment.**

This method has been commonly called postcoital contraception, or the "morning after" treatment. Emergency contraception is a more accurate and appropriate name, indicating the intention to be one-time protection. It is an important option for patients and should be considered when condoms break, sexual assault occurs, if diaphragms or cervical caps dislodge, or with the lapsed use of any method.

It has been argued that the use of emergency contraception would reduce the rates of induced abortions; indeed, in the United States, it is estimated that emergency contraception could annually prevent 1.7 million unintended pregnancies and the number of induced abortions would decrease by about 40%.[7] However, studies do not agree. In two studies at abortion units, it was concluded that 50–60% of the patients would have been suitable for emergency contraception and would have used it if readily available.[8, 9] On the other hand, the advance provision of emergency contraception had no effect on the abortion rates in Scotland or San Francisco.[10–12] It is possible that the sample sizes in these studies were not adequate to detect an effect that would still be of considerable impact. Likewise, widespread public access could also yield a meaningful reduction in the rates of unintended pregnancies.

Many women do not know of this method, and it has been difficult to obtain.[9, 13] Even if women are aware of this method, accurate and detailed knowledge is lacking.[14] A favorable attitude toward this method requires knowledge and availability. Women who have used emergency contraception are very satisfied with the method and, most importantly, do not express an intention to substitute this method for regular contraception.[15]

Information for patients and clinicians, including the latest available products, can be obtained from the web site and hot line maintained by the Office of Population Research at Princeton University:

> http://ec.princeton.edu
> Telephone hotline: 1-888-NOT-2-LATE (1-888-668-2528)

Clinicians should consider providing emergency contraceptive kits to patients (a kit can be a simple envelope containing instructions and the appropriate number of oral contraceptives) to be taken when needed. It would be a major contribution to our efforts to avoid unwanted pregnancies for all patients without contraindications to oral contraceptives to have emergency contraception available for use when needed. In our view, this would be much more effective in reducing the need for abortion than waiting for patients to call. In studies of advanced provision and self-administration, adult women in Scotland and Honk Kong and younger women in San Francisco, Pittsburgh, and Mexico increased the use of emergency contraception without adverse effects such as increasing unprotected sex or changing the use of other contraceptive methods.[10, 12, 16–20]

Progestin-only emergency contraception is now available without a prescription in many countries.[21] In the United States, some states have made progress toward this objective, and eventually approval at the federal level is expected. Women are able to use this nonprescription access effectively and do not develop a reliance on emergency contraception as a regular method.[21] Nevertheless, in some communities, the requirement to go through pharmacists or clinics may be a barrier that limits use,[12] and individual clinicians will continue to play an important role in making emergency contraception available for women.

Mechanism and Efficacy

The mechanism of action is not known with certainty, but it is believed with justification that this treatment combines delay of ovulation with a local effect on the endometrium and prevention of fertilization.[22–27] How much a postfertilization effect contributes to efficacy is not known, but it is not believed to be the primary mechanism.[25, 28] Indeed, an experiment in monkeys could detect no effect of a high dose of levonorgestrel administrated postcoitally once fertilization had occurred.[29] *Clinicians, pharmacists, and patients can be reassured that treatment with emergency contraception is not an abortifacient.*

Efficacy has been confirmed in large clinical trials and summarized in complete reviews of the literature.[30–32] Treatment with high doses of estrogen or with levonorgestrel yields a failure rate of approximately 1%, and

141

with the combination oral contraceptive, about 2–3%. The failure rate is lowest with high doses of ethinyl estradiol given within 72 hours (0.1%), but the side effects make this a poor choice. In general clinical use, the method with oral contraceptives can reduce the risk of pregnancy by about 75%; this degree of reduction in probability of conception (given the relatively low chance, about 8%, for pregnancy associated with one act of coitus[33]) yields the 2% failure rate measured in clinical studies.[34–36]

Results with levonorgestrel are even better, about an 85% reduction in the risk of pregnancy; in the worldwide World Health Organization study, the risk of pregnancy was 60% lower with the levonorgestrel-only method compared with the oral contraceptive method, with less than half as much nausea and vomiting.[4]

Treatment Method

Treatment should be initiated as soon after exposure as possible, and the standard recommendation is that it be no later than 72 hours. Careful assessment of the reported experience with emergency contraception indicated that the method is equally effective when started on the first, second, or third day after intercourse (which would allow user-friendly scheduling), and that efficacy might extend beyond 72 hours.[37, 38] Data from the World Health Organization randomized, clinical trial, however, support the importance of timing, finding a reduction in efficacy after 72 hours, and the greatest protection occurring when the medication is taken within 24 hours of intercourse.[39] Postponing the dose by 12 hours raises the chance of pregnancy by almost 50%. For this reason, the treatment should be initiated as soon as possible after sexual exposure, an important argument in favor of advance provision.

We should emphasize, in case the patient is already pregnant, that there is no evidence that exposure to the amounts of estrogen and progestin in oral contraceptives is teratogenic.[40–42] Furthermore, emergency contraception is ineffective in the presence of an established pregnancy. The earlier in the menstrual cycle that emergency contraception is taken, the more likely the following menstrual period will be early, but administration later in the cycle does not delay the return to menses.[43] A delay in menses after treatment warrants testing for pregnancy and consideration for the possibility of an ectopic pregnancy.

When using oral contraceptives for emergency contraception, it is worth adding an antiemetic, oral or suppository, to the treatment; a long-acting nonprescription agent, 25 or 50 mg meclizine (Bonine, Dramamine II, Antivert) is recommended, to be taken one hour before the emergency contraception treatment. Side effects reflect the high doses used: nausea (50%), vomiting (20%), breast tenderness, headache, and dizziness. If a patient vomits within an hour after taking pills, additional pills must be administered as soon as possible. Nausea and vomiting are experienced at such a lower rate with the levonorgestrel-only method that an antiemetic is not necessary.

It should be noted that an analysis of the U.K. General Practice Research Database could find no evidence for an increased risk of venous thromboembolism with the short-term use of oral contraceptives for emergency contraception (indeed, no cases were found for as long as 60 days after use in more than 100,000 episodes of use).[44] Although short-term treatment with combined oral contraceptives has been documented to have no effect on clotting factors, in our view the usual contraindications for oral contraception apply to this use.[45] *Because of the high dose of estrogen, emergency contraception with combined oral contraceptives should not be provided to women with either a personal or close family history (parent or sibling) of idiopathic thrombotic disease.* For women with a contraindication to exogenous estrogen, the progestin-only method with levonorgestrel should be used for emergency contraception. The levonorgestrel-only method is the treatment of choice anyway because of greater efficacy and fewer side effects.

A 3-week follow-up visit should be scheduled to assess the result and to counsel for routine contraception.

Could other combination oral contraceptive products be used? A norethindrone-ethinyl estradiol combination was found to be equally effective to the levonorgestrel-ethinyl estradiol formulation, and it is likely that any combination oral contraceptive would be successful.[46] However, this is a moot point because the levonorgestrel-only method is now the treatment of choice.

The 3 major problems with the available methods of emergency contraception are the high rate of side effects, the need to start treatment within 72 hours after intercourse, and the small, but important, failure rate. Mifepristone in a single oral dose of 600 mg is associated with markedly less nausea and vomiting and an efficacy rate of nearly 100%.[47, 48] In randomized trials, 10 mg mifepristone was as effective as 25 mg, 50 mg, or 600 mg, preventing about 80–85% of expected pregnancies (the same efficacy as with the levonorgestrel method), with a slight decrease in efficacy when treatment was delayed to 5 days after intercourse.[5, 49, 50] Because the next menstrual cycle is delayed after mifepristone, contraception should be initiated immediately after treatment. Ironically, mifepristone, around which swirls the abortion controversy, can make an effective contribution to preventing unwanted pregnancies and induced abortions.

Another method of emergency contraception is the insertion of a copper IUD, anytime during the preovulatory phase of the menstrual cycle and up to 5 days after ovulation. The failure rate (in a small number of studies) is very low, 0.1%.[30, 31] This method definitely prevents implantation, but it is not suitable for women who are not candidates for intrauterine contraception, e.g., women with multiple sexual partners, or rape victims.

The use of danazol for emergency contraception is not effective.[47]

The Progestin-Only Minipill

The minipill contains a small dose of a progestational agent and must be taken daily, in a continuous fashion.[51, 52] There is no evidence for any major differences in clinical behavior among the available minipill products.

Minipills available worldwide:

1. Micronor, Nor-QD, Noriday, Norod ----------------- 0.350 mg norethindrone
2. Microval, Noregeston, Microlut ---------------------- 0.030 mg levonorgestrel
3. Ovrette, Neogest -------------------------------------- 0.075 mg norgestrel (equivalent to 0.0375 mg levonorgestrel)
4. Exluton -- 0.500 mg lynestrenol
5. Femulen -- 0.500 mg ethynodiol diacetate
6. Cerazette -- 0.075 mg desogestrel

Mechanism of Action

After taking a progestin-only minipill, the small amount of progestin in the circulation (about 25% of that in combined oral contraceptives) has a significant impact only on those tissues very sensitive to the female sex steroids, estrogen and progesterone. The contraceptive effect is more dependent on endometrial and cervical mucus effects, because gonadotropins are not consistently suppressed. The endometrium involutes and becomes hostile to implantation, and the cervical mucus becomes thick and impermeable. Approximately 40% of patients ovulate normally.[53, 54] Tubal physiology may also be affected, but this is speculative. The progestin-only minipill containing 0.075 mg desogestrel appears to be slightly more effective, perhaps because it may exert a greater inhibition of ovulation.[55]

144

Because of the low dose, the minipill must be taken every day at the same time of day. The change in the cervical mucus requires 2–4 hours to take effect, and, most importantly, the impermeability diminishes 22 hours after administration, and by 24 hours sperm penetration is essentially unimpaired.

Ectopic pregnancy is not prevented as effectively as intrauterine pregnancy. Although the overall incidence of ectopic pregnancy is not increased (it is still much lower than the incidence in women not using a contraceptive method), when pregnancy occurs, the clinician must suspect that it is more likely to be ectopic. A previous ectopic pregnancy should not be regarded as a contraindication to the minipill.

There are no significant metabolic effects (lipid levels, carbohydrate metabolism, and coagulation factors remain unchanged),[56-59] and there is an immediate return to fertility on discontinuation (unlike the delay seen with the combination oral contraceptive). Only one disturbing observation has been reported; progestin-only oral contraception was associated with about a 3-fold increased risk of diabetes mellitus in lactating women with recent gestational diabetes, an observation that is difficult to explain.[60] Because this increased risk is not observed with the use of combined oral contraceptives, the low levels of estrogen associated with breastfeeding may allow an unimpeded progestin effect on insulin resistance.

Efficacy

Failure rates have been documented to range from 1.1 to 9.6 per 100 women in the first year of use.[61] The failure rate is higher in younger women (3.1 per 100 woman-years) compared with women over age 40 (0.3 per 100 woman-years).[62] In motivated women, the failure rate is comparable to the rate (less than 1 per 100 woman-years) with combination oral contraception.[63, 64]

Pill Taking

The minipill should be started on the first day of menses, and a backup method must be used for the first 7 days because some women (very few) ovulate as early as 7–9 days after the onset of menses. The pill should be keyed to a daily event to ensure regular administration at the same time of the day. If pills are forgotten or gastrointestinal illness impairs absorption, the minipill should be resumed as soon as possible, and a backup method should be used immediately and until the pills have been resumed for at least 2 days. If 2 or more pills are missed in a row and there is no menstrual bleeding in 4–6 weeks, a pregnancy test should be obtained. *If more than 3 hours late in taking a pill, a backup method should be used for 48 hours.*

Problems

In view of the unpredictable effect on ovulation, it is not surprising that irregular menstrual bleeding is the major clinical problem. The daily progestational impact on the endometrium also contributes to this problem. Patients can expect to have normal, ovulatory cycles (40–50%), short, irregular cycles (40%), or a total lack of cycles ranging from irregular bleeding to spotting and amenorrhea (10%). This is the major reason why women discontinue the minipill method of contraception.[64]

Women on progestin-only contraception develop more functional, ovarian follicular cysts.[65, 66] Nearly all, if not all, regress. This is not a clinical problem of any significance. Women who have experienced frequent ovarian cysts would be happier with methods that effectively suppress ovulation (combined oral contraceptives and depot-medroxyprogesterone acetate).

The levonorgestrel minipill may be associated with acne. The mechanism is similar to that seen with Norplant. The androgenic activity of levonorgestrel decreases the circulating levels of sex hormone-binding globulin (SHBG).[67] Therefore free steroid levels (levonorgestrel and testosterone) are increased despite the low dose. This is in contrast to the action of combined oral contraception where the effect of the progestin is countered by the estrogen-induced increase in SHBG.

The incidence of the other minor side effects is very low, probably at the same rate that would be encountered with a placebo.

Clinical Decisions

There are two situations in which excellent efficacy, probably near-total effectiveness, is achieved: lactating women and women over age 40. In lactating women, the contribution of the minipill is combined with prolactin-induced suppression of ovulation, adding up to very effective protection.[68] As noted, in breastfeeding, overweight, Latina women with prior gestational diabetes, the progestin-only minipill was associated with a 3-fold increased risk of non–insulin dependent diabetes mellitus.[60] It is not known whether this might be a risk in all women who have experienced gestational diabetes; a prudent course would be to advise other methods for this special group of women. In women over age 40, reduced fecundity adds to the minipill's effects.

There is another reason why the minipill is a good choice for the breastfeeding woman. There is no evidence for any adverse effect on breastfeeding as measured by milk volume and infant growth and development.[69–71] In fact, there is a modest positive impact; women using the minipill breastfeed longer and add supplementary feeding at a later time.[72] Because of the slight positive impact on lactation, the minipill can be started immediately after delivery. A study investigating the impact of early initiation found no adverse effects on breastfeeding.[73]

The minipill is a good choice in situations where estrogen is contraindicated, such as patients with serious medical conditions (diabetes with vascular disease, severe systemic lupus erythematosus,[74] cardiovascular disease). It should be noted that the freedom from estrogen effects, although likely, is presumptive. Substantial data, for example on associations with vascular disease, blood pressure, and cancer, are not available because relatively small numbers have chosen to use this method of contraception. On the other hand, it is logical to conclude that any of the progestin effects associated with the combination oral contraceptives can be related to the minipill according to a dose-response curve; all effects should be reduced. Both the World Health Organization case-control study and the Transnational case-control study could find no indication for increased risks of stroke, myocardial infarction, or venous thromboembolism with oral progestin-only contraceptives.[75, 76] No impact can be measured on the coagulation system.[56, 77] The minipill can probably be used in women with previous episodes of thrombosis, and the package insert in the United States was revised, eliminating vascular disease as a contraindication.

The minipill is a good alternative for the occasional woman who reports diminished libido on combination oral contraceptives, presumably due to decreased androgen levels. The minipill should also be considered for the few patients who report minor side effects (gastrointestinal upset, breast tenderness, headaches) of such a degree that the combination oral contraceptive is not acceptable.

Because of the relatively low doses of progestin administered, patients using medications that increase liver metabolism should avoid this method of contraception. These drugs include the following:

> Carbamazepine (Tegretol)
> Felbamate
> Nevirapine
> Oxcarbazepine
> Phenobarbital
> Phenytoin (Dilantin)
> Primidone (Mysoline)
> Rifabutin
> Rifampicin (Rifampin)
> Topiramate
> St. John's Wort
> Vigabatrin
> Possibly ethosuximide, griseofulvin, and troglitazone

Do the noncontraceptive benefits associated with combination oral contraception apply to the minipill? Studies are unable to help us with this issue, again because of the relatively small numbers of users. However, the progestin impact on cervical mucus, endometrium, and ovulation leads one to think the benefits will be present (reduced risks of pelvic infection, endometrial cancer, and ovarian cancer). Although limited by small numbers, one case-control study indicated that protection against endometrial cancer was even greater with progestin-only pills than with combination oral contraceptives.[78]

Good efficacy with the minipill requires regularity, taking the pill at the same time each day. There is less room for forgetting, and, therefore, the minipill is probably not a good choice for a disorganized adult or for the average adolescent.

References

1. **Morris JM, van Wagenen G,** Compounds interfering with ovum implantation and development. III. The role of estrogens, Am J Obstet Gynecol 96:804, 1966.

2. **Yuzpe AA, Smith RP, Rademaker AW,** A multicenter clinical investigation employing ethinyl estradiol combined with dl-norgestrel as a postcoital contraceptive agent, Fertil Steril 37:508, 1982.

3. **Ho PC, Kwan MSW,** A prospective randomized comparison of levonorgestrel with the Yuzpe regimen in post-coital contraception, Hum Reprod 8:389, 1993.

4. **Task Force on Postovulatory Methods of Fertility Regulation,** Randomised controlled trial of levonorgestrel versus the Yuzpe regimen of combined oral contraceptives for emergency contraception, Lancet 352:428, 1998.

5. **von Hertzen H, Piaggio G, Ding J, Chen J, Song S, Bartfai G, Ng E, Gemzell-Danielsson K, Oyunbileg A, Wu S, Cheng W, Ludicke F, Pretnar-Darovec A, Kirkman R, Mittal S, Khomassuridze A, Apter D, Peregoudov A, WHO Research Group on Post-Ovulatory Methods of Fertility Regulation,** Low dose mifepristone and two regimens of levonorgestrel for emergency contraception: a WHO multicentre randomised trial, Lancet 360:1803, 2002.

6. **Arowojoulu AO, Okewole IA, Adekunie AO,** Comparative evaluation of the effectiveness and safety of two regimens of levonorgestrel for emergency contraception in Nigerians, Contraception 66:269, 2002.

7. **Harper CC, Ellerton CE,** The emergency contraceptive pill: a survey of knowledge and attitudes among students at Princeton, Am J Obstet Gynecol 173:1438, 1995.

8. **Burton R, Savage W, Reader F,** The "morning after pill." Is this the wrong name for it? Br J Fam Plann 15:119, 1990.

9. **Young L, McCowan LM, Roberts HE, Farquhar CM,** Emergency contraception — why women don't use it, N Z Med J 108:145, 1995.

10. **Jackson RD, Bimla Schwarz E, Freedman L, Darney P,** Advance supply of emergency contraception: effect on use and usual contraception—a randomized trial, Obstet Gynecol 102:8, 2003.

11. **Glasier A, Fairhurst K, Wyke S, Ziebland S, Seaman P, Walker J, Lakha F,** Advanced provision of emergency contraception does not reduce abortion rates, Contraception 69:361, 2004.

12. **Raine TR, Harper CC, Rocca CH, Fischer R, Padian N, Klausner JD, Darney PD,** Randomized trial of increased access to emergency contraception: impact on pregnancy and sexually transmitted infections, JAMA in press, 2004.

13. **Delbanco SF, Mauldon J, Smith MD,** Little knowledge and limited practice: emergency contraceptive pills, the public, and the obstetrician-gynecologist, Obstet Gynecol 89:1006, 1997.

14. **Trussell J, Stewart F, Guest F, Hatcher RA,** Emergency contraceptive pills: a simple proposal to reduce unintended pregnancies, Fam Plann Perspect 24:269, 1992.

15. **Harvey SM, Beckman LJ, Sherman C, Petitti D,** Women's experience and satisfaction with emergency contraception, Fam Plann Perspect 31:237, 1999.

16. **Glasier A, Baird D,** The effects of self-administering emergency contraception, New Engl J Med 339:1, 1998.

17. **Raine T, Harper C, Leon K, Darney P,** Emergency contraception: advance provision in a young, high-risk clinic population, Obstet Gynecol 96:1, 2000.

18. **Gold MA, Wolford JE, Smith KA, Parker AM,** The effects of advance provision of emergency contraception on adolescent women's sexual and contraceptive behaviors, J Pediatr Adolesc Gynecol 17:87, 2004.

19. **Walker DM, Torres P, Gtutierrez JP, Flemming K, Bertozzi SM,** Emergency contraception use is correlated with increased condom use among adolescents: results from Mexico, J Adolesc Health 35:329, 2004.

20. **Lo SS, Fan SY, Glasier AF,** Effect of advanced provision of emergency contraception on women's contraceptive behaviour: a randomized controlled trial, Hum Reprod 19:2404, 2004.

21. **Gainer E, Blum J, Toverud E-L, Portugal N, Tyden T, Nesheim B-I, Larsson M, Vilar D, Nymoen P, Aneblom G, Lutwick A, Winikoff B,** Bringing emergency contraception over the counter: experiences of nonprescription users in France, Norway, Sweden and Portugal, Contraception 68:117, 2003.

22. **Young DC, Wiehle RD, Joshi SG, Poindexter AN, III.,** Emergency contraception alters progesterone-associated endometrial protein in serum and uterine luminal fluid, Obstet Gynecol 84:266, 1994.

23. **Swahn ML, Westlund P, Johannisson E, Bygdeman M,** Effect of postcoital contraceptive methods on the endometrium and the menstrual cycle, Acta Obstet Gynecol Scand 75:738, 1996.

24. **Trussell J, Raymond EG,** Statistical evidence about the mechanism of action of the Yuzpe regimen of emergency contraception, Obstet Gynecol 93:872, 1999.

25. **Marions L, Hultenby K, Lindell I, Sun X, Stabi B, Gemzell Danielsson K,** Emergency contraception with mifepristone and levonorgestrel: mechanism of action, Obstet Gynecol 100:65, 2002.

26. **Croxatto HB, Fuentealba B, Brache V, Salvatierra AM, Alvarez G, Massai R, Cochon L, Faundes A,** Effects of the Yuzpe regimen, given during the follicular phase, on ovarian function, Contraception 65:121, 2002.

27. **Durand M, Cravioto MCR, E G, Durán-Sanchez O, Cruz-Hinojosa ML, Castell-Rodriguez A, Schiavon R, Larrea F,** On the mechanisms of action of short-term levonorgestrel administration in emergency contraception, Contraception 64:227, 2001.

28. **Trussell J, Ellertson C, Dorflinger L,** Effectiveness of the Yuzpe regimen of emergency contraception by cycle day of intercourse: implications for mechanism of action, Contraception 67:167, 2003.

29. **Ortiz ME, Ortiz RE, Fuentes MA, Parraguez VH, Croxatto HB,** Post-coital administration of levonorgestrel does not interfere with post-fertilization events in the new-world monkey *Cebus apella*, Hum Reprod 19:1352, 2004.

30. **Fasoli M, Parazzini F, Cecchetti G, La Vecchia C,** Post-coital contraception: an overview of published studies, Contraception 39:459, 1989.

31. **Haspels AA,** Emergency contraception: a review, Contraception 50:101, 1994.

32. **Glasier A,** Emergency postcoital contraception, New Engl J Med 337:1058, 1997.

33. **Wilcox AJ, Weinberg CR, Baird DD,** Timing of sexual intercourse in relation to ovulation. Effects on the probability of conception, survival of the pregnancy, and sex of the baby, New Engl J Med 333:1517, 1995.

34. **Trussell J, Ellertson C, Stewart F,** The effectiveness of the Yuzpe regimen of emergency contraception, Fam Plann Perspect 28:58, 1996.

35. **Trussell J, Rodríguez G, Ellertson C,** New estimates of the effectiveness of the Yuzpe regimen of emergency contraception, Contraception 57:363, 1998.

36. **Trussell J, Rodríguez C, Ellertson C,** Updated estimates of the effectiveness of the Yuzpe regimen of emergency contraception, Contraception 59:147, 1999.

37. **Trussell J, Ellertson C, Rodriguez G,** The Yuzpe regimen of emergency contraception: how long after the morning after? Obstet Gynecol 88:150, 1996.

38. **Rodrigues I, Grou F, Joly J,** Effectiveness of emergency contraceptive pills between 72 and 120 hours after unprotected sexual intercourse, Am J Obstet Gynecol 184:531, 2001.

39. **Piaggio G, von Hertzen H, Grimes DA, Van Look PFA, on behalf of the Task Force on Postovulatory Methods of Fertility Regulation,** Timing of emergency contraception with levonorgestrel or the Yuzpe regimen, Lancet 353:721, 1999.

40. **Simpson JL, Phillips OP,** Spermicides, hormonal contraception and congenital malformations, Adv Contraception 6:141, 1990.

41. **Bracken MB,** Oral contraception and congenital malformations in offspring: a review and meta-analysis of the prospective studies, Obstet Gynecol 76:552, 1990.

42. **Raman-Wilms L, Tseng AL, Wighardt S, Einarson TR, Koren G,** Fetal genital effects of first trimester sex hormone exposure: a meta-analysis, Obstet Gynecol 85:141, 1995.

43. **Webb A, Shochet T, Bigrigg A, Loftus-Granberg B, Tyrer A, Gallagherl J, Hesketh C,** Effect of hormonal emergency contraception on bleeding patterns, Contraception 69:133, 2004.

44. **Vasilakis C, Jick SS, Jick H,** The risk of venous thromboembolism in users of postcoital contraceptive pills, Contraception 59:79, 1999.

45. **Webb A, Taberner D,** Clotting factors after emergency contraception, Adv Contracept 9:75, 1993.

46. **Ellertson C, Webb A, Blanchard K, Bigrigg A, Haskell S, Shochet T, Trussell J,** Modifying the Yuzpe regimen of emergency contraception: a multicenter randomized controlled trial, Obstet Gynecol 101:1160, 2003.

47. **Webb AMC, Russell J, Elstein M,** Comparison of Yuzpe regimen, danazol, and mifepristone (RU486) in oral postcoital contraception, Br Med J 305:927, 1992.

48. **Glasier A, Thong KJ, Dewar M, Mackie M, Baird DT,** Mifepristone (RU 486) compared with high-dose estrogen and progestogen for emergency postcoital contraception, New Engl J Med 327:1041, 1992.

49. **Task Force on Postovulatory Methods of Fertility Regulation,** Comparison of three single doses of mifepristone as emergency contraception: a randomised trial, Lancet 353:697, 1999.

50. **Xiao BL, von Hertzen H, Zhao H, Piaggio G,** A randomized double-blind comparison of two single doses of mifepristone for emergency contraception, Hum Reprod 17:3084, 2002.

51. **Chi I,** The safety and efficacy issues of progestin-only oral contraceptives — an epidemiologic perspective, Contraception 47:1, 1993.

52. **McCann MF, Potter LS,** Progestin-only oral contraception: a comprehensive review, Contraception 50(Suppl 1):S9, 1994.

53. **Moghissi KS, Marks C,** Effects of microdose progestogens on endogenous gonadotrophic and steroid hormones, cervical mucus properties, vaginal cytology and endometrium, Fertil Steril 22:424, 1971.

54. **Moghissi KS, Syner FN, McBride LC,** Contraceptive mechanism of microdose norethindrone, Obstet Gynecol 4:585, 1973.

55. **Collaborative Study Group on the Desogestrel-Containing Progestogen-Only Pill,** A double-blind study comparing the contraceptive efficacy, acceptability and safety of two progestogen-only pills containing desogestrel 75 micrograms/day or levonorgestrel 30 micrograms/day, Eur J Contracept Reprod Health Care 3:169, 1998.

56. **Fotherby K,** The progestogen-only pill and thrombosis, Br J Fam Plann 15:83, 1989.

57. **Godsland IF, Crook D, Simpson R, Proudler T, Gelton C, Lees B, Anyaoku V, Devenport M, Wynn V,** The effects of different formulations of oral contraceptive agents on lipid and carbohydrate metabolism, New Engl J Med 323:1375, 1990.

58. **Ball MJ, Gillmer AE,** Progestagen-only oral contraceptives: comparison of the metabolic effects of levonorgestrel and norethisterone, Contraception 44:223, 1991.

59. **Winkler UH,** Blood coagulation and oral contraceptives. A critical review, Contraception 57:203, 1998.

60. **Kjos SL, Peters RK, Xiang A, Thomas D, Schaefer U, Buchanan TA,** Contraception and the risk of type 2 diabetes in Latino women with prior gestational diabetes, JAMA 280:533, 1998.

61. **Trussell J, Kost K,** Contraceptive failure in the United States: a critical review of the literature, Stud Fam Plann 18:237, 1987.

62. **Vessey MP, Lawless M, Yeates D, McPherson K,** Progestogen-only contraception: findings in a large prospective study with special reference to effectiveness, Br J Fam Plann 10:117, 1985.

63. **Bisset AM, Dingwall-Fordyce I, Hamilton MJK,** The efficacy of the progestogen-only pill as a contraceptive method, Br J Fam Plann 16:84, 1990.

64. **Broome M, Fotherby K,** Clinical experience with the progestogen-only pill, Contraception 42:489, 1990.

65. **Tayob Y, Adams J, Jacobs HS, Guillebaud J,** Ultrasound demonstration of increased frequency of functional ovarian cysts in women using progestogen-only oral contraception, Br J Obstet Gynaecol 92:1003, 1985.

66. **Vessey M, Metcalfe A, Wells C, McPherson K, Westhoff C, Yeates C,** Ovarian neoplasms, functional ovarian cysts, and oral contraceptives, Br Med J 294:1518, 1987.

67. **Pakarinen P, Lahteenmaki P, Rutanen EM,** The effect of intrauterine and oral levonorgestrel administration on serum concentrations of sex hormone-binding globulin, insulin and insulin-like growth factor binding protein-1, Acta Obstet Gynecol Scand 78:423, 1999.

68. **Dunson TR, McLaurin VL, Grubb GS, Rosman AW,** A multicenter clinical trial of a progestin-only oral contraceptive in lactating women, Contraception 47:23, 1993.

69. **WHO, Special Programme of Research, Development, and Research Training in Human Reproduction, Task Force on Oral Contraceptives,** Effects of hormonal contraceptives on milk volume and infant growth, Contraception 30:505, 1984.

70. **WHO Task Force for Epidemiological Research on Reproductive Health, Special Programme of Research, Development and Research Training in Human Reproduction,** Progestogen-only contraceptives during lactation. I. Infant growth, Contraception 50:35, 1994.

71. **WHO Task Force for Epidemiological Research on Reproductive Health, Special Programme of Research, Development and Research Training in Human Reproduction,** Progestogen-only contraceptives during lactation. II. Infant development, Contraception 50:55, 1994.

72. **McCann MF, Moggia AV, Hibbins JE, Potts M, Becker C,** The effects of a progestin-only oral contraceptive (levonorgestrel 0.03 mg) on breast-feeding, Contraception 40:635, 1989.

73. **Halderman LD, Nelson AL,** Impact of early postpartum administration of progestin-only hormonal contraceptives compared with nonhormonal contraceptives on short-term breast-feeding patterns, Am J Obstet Gynecol 186:1250, 2002.

74. **Mintz G, Gutierrez G, Deleze M, Rodriguez E,** Contraception with progestogens in systemic lupus erythematosus, Contraception 30:29, 1984.

75. **World Health Organization Collaborative Study of Cardiovascular Disease and Steroid Hormone Contraception,** Cardiovascular disease and use of oral and injectable progestogen-only contraceptives and combined injectable contraceptives. Results of an international, multicenter, case-control study, Contraception 57:315, 1998.

76. **Heinemann LA, Assmann A, Do Minh T, Garbe E,** Oral progestogen-only contraceptives and cardiovascular risk: results from the Transnational Study on Oral Contraceptives and the Health of Young Women, Eur J Contracept Reprod Health Care 4:67, 1999.

77. **Winkler UH, Howie H, Bühler K, Korver T, Geurts TBP, Coelingh Bennink HJT,** A randomized controlled double-blind study of the effects on hemostasis of two progestogen-only pills containing 75 mg desogestrel or 30 mg levonorgestrel, Contraception 57:385, 1998.

78. **Weiderpass E, Adami HO, Baron JA, Magnusson C, Bergstrom R, Lindgren A, Correia N, Persson I,** Risk of endometrial cancer following estrogen replacement with and without progestins, J Natl Cancer Inst 91:1131, 1999.

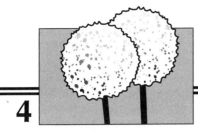

4

Vaginal and Transdermal Estrogen-Progestin Contraception

There are potential advantages in avoiding the first pass through the liver that is associated with the oral intake of steroid hormones. For example, the impact on blood clotting may be reduced, even negligible, because acute stimulation of liver protein synthesis is avoided. Whether vaginal and transdermal administration of steroid hormones is safer must await future epidemiologic assessment, but this remains a theoretical possibility. Another important advantage of vaginal and transdermal steroid contraception is an improvement in compliance achieved by the elimination of a daily regimen of treatment. The more options available for contraception, the more effective family planning is within a society. Vaginal and transdermal steroid contraception will surely appeal to some women unsatisfied with other methods.

Vaginal Estrogen-Progestin Contraception

The vaginal mucosa provides an excellent delivery site for steroid contraception. Like subcutaneous, intramuscular, transdermal, and intrauterine contraceptive systems, the vaginal route avoids gastrointestinal absorption and the first-pass liver effect. Absorption from the gastrointestinal tract can be unpredictable and may be compromised by vomiting, drug-drug interference, or decreased intestinal absorption capacity. The gastrointestinal lumen and the liver are sites of elimination for many compounds, and avoidance of the first-pass effect is particularly advantageous for compounds that undergo a high degree of hepatic metabolism; orally administered natural estrogens for example, are 95% metabolized by the liver. Oral administration results in marked fluctuations of contraceptive steroid serum concentrations that may lead to side effects like irregular bleeding and nausea. These daily changes are lower with vaginal than with oral or transdermal administration and lowest with implant and intrauterine methods.[1, 2]

The vagina provides an ideal site for contraceptive steroid absorption. The stratified squamous epithelium, unlike the skin, is not cornified, permitting easier steroid penetration to the underlying lamina propria, made of collagen and elastin, which is richly vascularized. A muscular layer under the epithelium has smooth muscle fibers running in both circular and longitudinal directions. The final layer of areolar connective tissue contains a second vascular plexus. There are no fat cells, glands (secretions are transudates, not glandular), or hair follicles to interfere with drug absorption.[2]

Vaginal contraceptive rings have been studied for 30 years. Six progestin-only and seven different progestin-estrogen (combined) vaginal contraceptive rings have been designed to provide one week to one year of contraception with weaker progestins like progesterone and medroxyprogesterone in short-acting rings (one week) and more potent levonorgestrel and nesterone in long-acting ones (up to a year). Only the NuvaRing vaginal combined steroid contraceptive is approved and available in the United States It is a flexible, soft, transparent ring made of ethylene vinyl acetate copolymer in which are contained crystals of etonogestrel (the biologically active metabolite of desogestrel, previously known as 3-ketodesogestrel) and ethinyl estradiol. This ring is covered with a 2-micron-thick membrane of ethylene vinyl acetate. The ring is available in only one size, 4 mm in thickness and 54 mm in diameter (smaller than a diaphragm), that fits all women. The NuvaRing releases 15 μg ethinyl estradiol and 120 μg etonogestrel per day.[3] Because the progestin and estrogen are mixed in the ethylene vinyl acetate core, in the unlikely event of damage to the ring, leakage or higher release of the hormones does not occur. Circulating estrogen and progestin levels reach target concentrations within 24 hours. The circulating estrogen levels reach a maximum level after 2–3 days; etonogestrel reaches maximum level after 7 days, and remains stable for 35 days.[1] The ring is inserted by the patient and worn for 3 weeks. Routine use requires the insertion of a new ring every 4 weeks to allow for withdrawal bleeding, but continuous use is obviously an appropriate option.

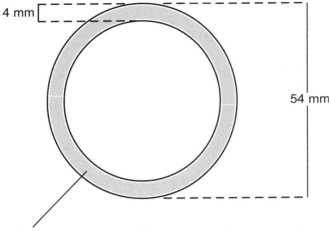

Ethinyl Estradiol- and Etonogestrel-Containing Core

155

The ring produces circulating progestin and estrogen levels that are only 40% and 30%, respectively, of the peak levels associated with an oral contraceptive containing 150 μg desogestrel and 30 μg ethinyl estradiol.[1] These levels effectively inhibit ovulation, providing pregnancy rates of less than 1% in clinical trials.[3-5] Indeed, the ring contains enough steroid hormone to inhibit ovulation for at least 5 weeks.[4] If the vaginal ring is removed and not replaced within 3 hours, the manufacturer recommends backup contraception until the ring has been in place for 7 days.

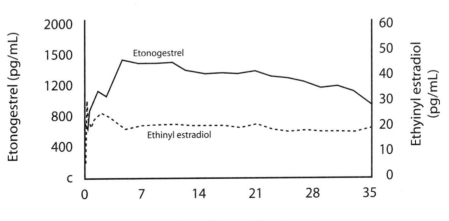

Number of Days After Insertion

Taking into account bioavailability as influenced by protein binding, systemic exposure to etonogestrel is similar comparing the vaginal ring to an oral contraceptive containing 150 μg desogestrel; however, the systemic exposure to ethinyl estradiol is about 50% of that of an oral contraceptive containing 30 μg ethinyl estradiol.[1] This may explain the low incidence of estrogen-related side effects such as nausea and breast tenderness.[3,5] Breakthrough bleeding and spotting rates are lower (around 6%) when compared with an oral contraceptive containing 30 μg of ethinyl estradiol and much lower than with 15 or 20 μg pills.[5,6] The low serum steroid concentrations do not produce significant changes in LDL or HDL levels but do increase triglycerides substantially and sex hormone-binding globulin levels markedly.[7] There are no clinically significant changes in clotting parameters.

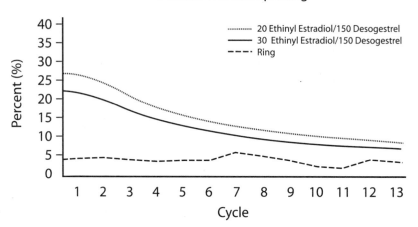

Percent Women Spotting

Legend:
- 20 Ethinyl Estradiol/150 Desogestrel
- 30 Ethinyl Estradiol/150 Desogestrel
- Ring

Y-axis: Percent (%); X-axis: Cycle

It is not necessary to place the vaginal ring in a specific position; it need only be in contact with vaginal mucosa and need not surround the cervix. The vaginal ring is intended to be placed in a normal vagina; infections and anatomic abnormalities are reasons for clinicians and patients to consider other methods. The most common reasons for discontinuation (about 2–4% in the clinical trials) have been vaginal discomfort, unwanted awareness of the ring's presence, coital problems, or expulsion (during a year of use about 2–3% of women experience spontaneous expulsion). Women report that the ring is easy to insert and remove, and, although about 15% of women and 30% of partners report feeling the ring during intercourse, this is not a common reason for discontinuation.[5,8] Removal for sexual intercourse is not recommended, but efficacy is maintained if the ring is replaced within 3 hours. Cervical cytology and the vaginal flora are not affected by the presence of the ring.[5, 9, 10] Despite no change in inflammatory vaginal flora, one well-done study reported that ring users have reported slightly more vaginal wetness (not sufficient to cause discontinuation), perhaps due to an increase in lactobacilli.[11]

The spermicide nonoxynol-9 has no effect on the release and absorption of the hormones in NuvaRing, as assessed by the measurement of serum levels of ethinyl estradiol and etonogestrel.[12] Combining a barrier method that contains nonoxynol-9 should not affect the contraceptive efficacy of the ring. Vaginally applied antifungal agents (miconazole) likewise have no effect on absorption of contraceptive steroids released by NuvaRing nor does the use of tampons.[5, 12, 13]

Vaginal steroid contraception shares the same advantages associated with the transdermal method: avoidance of the first-pass liver effect, more stable circulating levels of hormones, and elimination of daily and rigid schedules of treatment—creating the potential for greater safety and improved compliance. Vaginal administration is associated with the lowest exposure to serum concentrations of ethinyl estradiol according to data based on area under the curve.

Transdermal Estrogen-Progestin Contraception

The transdermal contraceptive patch (Ortho-Evra) has an area of 20 cm² (4.5 cm x 4.5 cm) and three layers in a matrix-type arrangement. The backing outer polyester layer provides support for the middle layer that contains the adhesive and the hormones, and the inner layer is a polyester liner that is removed from the adhesive layer just before application. The size is that required to deliver an effective dose of the steroid hormones. The patch contains 750 μg ethinyl estradiol and 6.0 mg of norelgestromin and delivers 20 μg ethinyl estradiol and 150 μg norelgestromin each day when applied to discrete locations on the lower abdomen, upper outer arm, the buttock, or the upper torso (excluding the breast). Norelgestromin is the primary active metabolite of orally administered norgestimate and was previously known as 17-deacetylnorgestimate. Norelgestromin still undergoes liver metabolism with transdermal application; however, the resulting metabolite, levonorgestrel, is highly bound to sex hormone-binding globulin, limiting its biologic impact. About 97% of norelgestromin is bound to albumin and 3% is unbound.[14]

Blood Level Ethinyl Estradiol

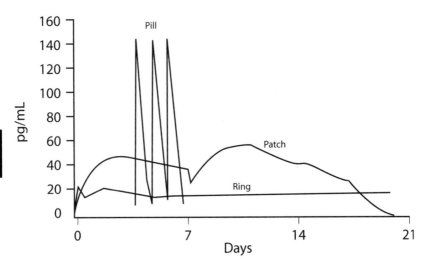

The patch is applied on the same day, but not on the exact same site, once each week for 3 weeks, followed by a week without use of the patch. Timing on the day of application need not be precise; the patch is very forgiving. Instructions for first-day starts or Sunday starts of oral contraception are also recommended for the patch (backup contraception for 7 days unless the starting day is also day 1 of the menstrual period). Application should be chosen with care to avoid contact with tight clothing, and pressure should be applied for at least 10 seconds, making sure that the edges stick. The skin should be clear, clean, and dry, and free of irritation or creams and lotions. The patches are stored in their protective pouches at room temperature. Remaining adhesive on the skin after detachment can be easily removed with the use of a small amount of baby oil or acetone-free nail polish remover. As with oral contraceptives, patient and clinician may choose to use the contraceptive patch continuously, eliminating withdrawal bleeding.

Detachment occurs with about 5% of patches, and about half occur in cycle 1 with inexperienced patients.[15, 16] In studies of at least a year's duration, about 2–5% of patches were replaced.[17, 18] Use of the patch requires common sense; anything other than a secure adhesion deserves a conservative approach. If the patch seems loose or has been partially or totally off for less than 24 hours, the same patch can be reapplied or replaced with a new patch (the patch change day remains the same). Single extra patches are provided for this purpose by pharmacies and clinics if the clinician writes a separate prescription for an extra patch along with the regular prescription.

If the patch has been detached for more than 24 hours, a new patch is applied initiating a new cycle and new change day (backup contraception for 7 days is recommended). Delay of a new patch cycle requires a new start with the usual 7-day backup. A delay within the patch cycle of no more than 2 days has no risk and does not change the cycle, but a delay more than 2 days also requires the initiation of a new cycle and change day with backup. However, in a study that compared 3 treatment-free days in oral contraceptive and patch users, ovulation occurred significantly less with the patch compared with oral contraception.[19]

Serum hormonal concentrations are achieved rapidly after application: an average of about 0.7 ng/mL, with a range of 0.6 to 1.2 ng/mL for norelgestromin, and an average of about 50 pg/mL, with a range of 25 to 75 pg/mL for ethinyl estradiol. These are ranges that are maintained by an oral formulation containing 250 μg norelgestromin and 35 μg ethinyl estradiol.[20, 21] However, the kinetics are not identical to orally administered hormones; daily fluctuations are avoided. These blood levels allow maintenance of contraceptive efficacy if patch replacement is delayed up to 2 days.[22] Gonadotropin levels return to baseline values by 6 weeks after discontinuation.[19] Daily use has been well studied, and activities such as exercise, bathing, swimming, and the use of a sauna or hot tub do not cause detachment or changes in the blood levels of the hormones.[23]

Transdermal contraception produces the same spectrum of actions associated with oral contraceptives, achieving the same high level of efficacy in clinical trials. Therefore, the same considerations reviewed in the chapter on oral contraception apply to transdermal contraception (as well as the vaginal ring), including the same contraindications and noncontraceptive benefits. The avoidance of the liver first-pass effect offers the potential for less interaction with other drugs, but this is not known, and patients on medications that affect liver metabolism should choose an alternative contraceptive. Tetracycline administration does not affect the blood concentrations of the steroid hormones with transdermal contraception, a neutral impact as seen with oral contraceptives.[24]

Recommendations for Patch Detachment

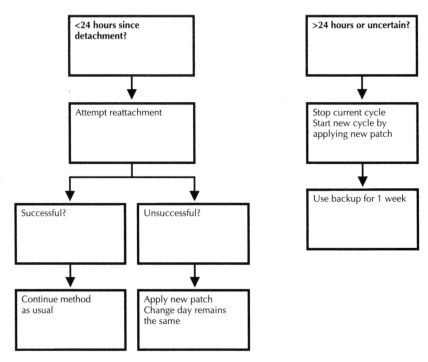

Recommendations for Patch Detachment

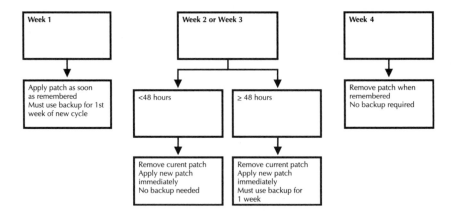

Transdermal administration has effects on clotting proteins and lipoproteins like those seen with low-dose oral contraceptives. There are no clinically significant changes in coagulation parameters; triglycerides increase modestly, and the LDL/HDL ratio declines slightly.[25] As with oral contraceptives, women who are at high risk of thrombosis due to genetic effects like Factor V-Leiden or protein C or S deficiencies or have very high triglycerides should consider hormonal contraceptives that do not contain estrogen.

Clinical Responses. Ovulation suppression is comparable to that achieved with oral contraception, and failure rates in clinical studies are less than 1.0%.[15, 17, 18, 26] Breakthrough bleeding and spotting rates with the transdermal method in randomized trials were comparable to one monophasic and two triphasic formulations, except for a slightly higher incidence of spotting in the first two cycles.[15, 17]

It is now well demonstrated that modern steroid contraception does not cause weight gain. The transdermal method is not an exception; body weight changes were identical in a randomized trial comparing the contraceptive patch with an identical placebo patch.[25] There were 15 pregnancies in the contraceptive patch clinical trials, and 5 of these were among women with body weights greater than 198 pounds (90 kg).[26] This is consistent with the greater failure rate reported in obese women on oral contraceptives.[27] However, a high rate of overall contraceptive efficacy is still achieved in heavy women because only a 10–20% variability in hormone levels can be attributed to increased body weight.[26]

Poor compliance is a major contributor to the typical failure rate associated with oral contraception. The once-a-week schedule with transdermal contraception is simpler and less susceptible to delays and omissions. In randomized trials ranging from 4 cycles to 13 cycles, about 10–20% more of the participants demonstrated good compliance with the transdermal method compared with oral contraception.[15, 17] In the clinical trials with transdermal contraception, lower overall pregnancy rates with the patch compared to oral contraception have been attributed to better compliance. Most importantly, young women, especially those younger than age 20, demonstrated greater compliance with transdermal contraception compared with oral contraceptives than did older women.[28]

About 20% of patients experience some degree of skin reaction at the application site, and about 2% discontinue the method for this reason.[15, 17, 18, 25] Breast discomfort is experienced during the first few months by 20% of users, more often with transdermal contraception compared with oral contraceptives, but it is usually not severe and has led to discontinuation in only 1% of users.[25]

Many women are bothered by the "dirt" ring that forms around the edges of transdermal patches. In our experience, this problem can be eliminated by lightly dusting talcum powder ("baby" powder) around the edges after application. If a ring does form, it is easily removed with mineral oil ("baby" oil).

References

1. **Timmer CJ, Mulders TM,** Pharmacokinetics of etonogestrel and ethinylestradiol released from a combined contraceptive vaginal ring, Clin Pharmacokinet 39:233, 2000.

2. **Alexander NJ, Baker E, Kaptein M, Karck U, Miller L, Zampaglione E,** Why consider vaginal drug administration? Fertil Steril 82:1, 2004.

3. **Roumen FJME, Apter D, Mulders TMT, Dieben TOM,** Efficacy, tolerability and acceptability of a novel contraceptive vaginal ring releasing etonogestrel and ethinyl estradiol, Hum Reprod 16:469, 2001.

4. **Mulders TM, Dieben TO,** Use of the novel combined contraceptive vaginal ring NuvaRing for ovulation inhibition, Fertil Steril 75:865, 2001.

5. **Dieben TOM, Roumen FJME, Apter D,** Efficacy, cycle control, and user acceptability of a novel combined contraceptive vaginal ring, Obstet Gynecol 100:585, 2002.

6. **Bjarnadóttir RI, Tuppurainen M, Killick SR,** Comparison of cycle control with a combined vaginal ring and oral levonorgestrel/ethinyl estradiol, Am J Obstet Gynecol 186:389, 2002.

7. **Tuppurainen M, Klimscheffskij R, Venhola M, Dieben TO,** The combined contraceptive ring (NuvaRing) and lipid metabolism: a comparative study, Contraception 69:389, 2004.

8. **Szarewski A,** High acceptability and satisfaction with NuvaRing use, Eur J Contracept Reprod Health Care 7:31, 2002.

9. **Roumen FJME, Boon ME, van Velzen D, Dieben TOM, Coelingh Bennink HJT,** The cervico-vaginal epithelium during 20 cycles' use of a combined contraceptive vaginal ring, Hum Reprod 11:2443, 1996.

10. **Davies GC, Feng LX, Newton JR, Dieben TO, Coelingh Benink HJ,** The effects of a combined contraceptive vaginal ring releasing ethinyloestradiol and 3-keto-desogestrel on vaginal flora, Contraception 45:511, 1992.

11. **Veres S, Miller L, Burington B,** A comparison between the vaginal ring and oral contraceptives, Obstet Gynecol 104:555, 2004.

12. **Haring T, Mulders TMT,** The combined contraceptive ring NuvaRing® and spermicide co-medication, Contraception 67:271, 2003.

13. **Verhoeven CHJ, Dieben TOM,** The combined contraceptive vaginal ring, NuvaRing, and tampon co-usage, Contraception 69:197, 2004.

14. **Hammond GL, Abrams LS, Creasy GW, Natarajan J, Allen JG, Siiteri PK,** Serum distribution of the major metabolites of noregestimate in relation to its pharmacological properties, Contraception 67:93, 2003.

15. **Dittrich R, Parker L, Rosen JB, Shangold G, Creasy GW, Fisher AC, for the Ortho Evra/Evra 001 Study Group,** Transdermal contraception: evaluation of three transdermal norelgestromin/ethinyl estradiol doses in a randomized multicenter, dose-response study, Am J Obstet Gynecol 186:15, 2002.

16. **Zacur HA, Hedon B, Mansour D, Shangold GA, Fisher AC, Creasy GW,** Integrated summary of Ortho™/Evra™ contraceptive patch adhesion in varied climates and conditions, Fertil Steril 77(Suppl 2):S32, 2002.

17. **Audet M-C, Moreau M, Koltun WD, Waldbaum AS, Shangold G, Fisher AC, Creasy GW, for the ORTHO EVRA/EVRA 004 Study Group,** Evaluation of contraceptive efficacy and cycle control of a transdermal contraceptive patch vs an oral contraceptive. A randomized controlled trial, JAMA 285:2347, 2001.

18. **Smallwood GH, Meador ML, Lenihan JP, Jr., Shangold GA, Fisher AC, Creasy GW, for the ORTHO EVRA/EVRA 002 Study Group,** Efficacy and safety of a transdermal contraceptive system, Obstet Gynecol 98:799, 2001.

19. **Pierson RA, Archer DF, Moreau M, Shangold GA, Fisher AC, Creasy GW, for the Ortho Evra™/Evra™ 008 Study Group,** Ortho Evra™/Evra™ versus oral contraceptives: follicular development and ovulation in normal cycles and after an intentional dosing error, Fertil Steril 80:34, 2003.

20. **Abrams LS, Skee DM, Natarajan J, Wong FA, Lasseter KC,** Multiple-dose pharmacokinetics of a contraceptive patch in healthy women participants, Contraception 64:287, 2001.

21. **Abrams LS, Skee DM, Natarajan J, Wong FA, Anderson BD,** Pharmacokinetics of a contraceptive patch (Evra/Ortho Evra) containing norelgestromin and ethinyloestradiol at four application sites, Br J Clin Pharmacol 53:141, 2002.

163

22. **Abrams LS, Skee DM, Wong FA, Anderson NJ, Leese PT,** Pharmacokinetics of norelgestromin and ethinyl estradiol from two consecutive contraceptive patches, J Clin Pharmacol 41:1232, 2001.

23. **Abrams LS, Skee DM, Natarajan J, Wong FA, Leese PT, Creasy GW, Shangold MM,** Pharmacokinetics of norelgestromin and ethinyl estradiol delivered by a contraceptive patch (Ortho Evra/Evra) under conditions of heat, humidity, and exercise, J Clin Pharmacol 41:1301, 2001.

24. **Abrams LS, Skee DM, Natarajan J, Wong FA,** Pharmacokinetic overview of Ortho Evra™/Evra™, Fertil Steril 77(Suppl 2):S3, 2002.

25. **Sibai BM, Odlind V, Meador ML, Shangold GA, Fisher AC, Creasy GW,** A comparative and pooled analysis of the safety and tolerability of the contraceptive patch (Ortho Evra™/Evra™), Fertil Steril 77(Suppl 2):S19, 2002.

26. **Zieman M, Guillebaud J, Weisberg E, Shangold GA, Fisher AC, Creasy GW,** Contraceptive efficacy and cycle control with the Ortho Evra™/Evra™ transdermal system: the analysis of pooled data, Fertil Steril 77(Suppl 2):S13, 2002.

27. **Holt VL, Cushing-Haugen KL, Daling JR,** Body weight and risk of oral contraceptive failure, Obstet Gynecol 99:820, 2002.

28. **Archer DF, Bigrigg A, Smallwood GH, Shangold GA, Creasy GW, Fisher AC,** Assessment of compliance with a weekly contraceptive patch (Ortho Evra™/Evra™) among North American women, Fertil Steril 77(Suppl 2):S27, 2002.

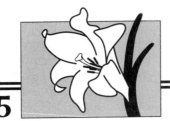

Implant Contraception

5

The high rate of unintended pregnancies and the relatively high failure rates with the typical use of reversible methods of contraception are strong indications of a need for long-acting contraceptive methods that are easier to use. Implantable, subdermal capsules that release progestins for several years are a response to this need.

Implant Systems

Norplant is a "sustained-release" system using silastic tubing permeable to steroid molecules to provide stable circulating levels of synthetic progestin over years of use. The Norplant system consists of 6 capsules, each measuring 34 mm in length with a 2.4-mm outer diameter and containing 36 mg crystalline levonorgestrel. The capsules are made of flexible, medical-grade silastic (polydimethylsiloxane and methylvinyl siloxane copolymer) tubing that is sealed shut with silastic medical adhesive (polydimethylsiloxane). The 6 capsules contain a total of 216 mg levonorgestrel, which is very stable and has remained unchanged in capsules examined after more than 9 years of use. Norplant is no longer sold in the United States In other countries, it has been mostly replaced by a two-rod system (Jadelle or Norplant 2) in which the levonorgestrel is dispersed in silastic and wrapped with a thin silastic membrane. This system is approved by the U.S. Federal Drug Administration, but is yet to be marketed.

Implanon is a single flexible rod 4 cm long and 2 mm in diameter that contains 68 mg of 3-keto desogestrel (etonogestrel, the active metabolite of desogestrel) dispersed in a core of ethylene vinyl acetate wrapped with a 0.6 mm thick membrane of the same material. There is no evidence that either ethylene vinyl acetate or silastic have toxic effects when implanted.[1] The hormone is released at an initial rate of about 67 μg per day decreasing to 30 μg after 2 years; concentrations that inhibit ovulation are achieved within 8 hours of insertion.[2] A steady state is achieved after 4 months after which there is a gradual decline.[2] Implanon, placed subdermally with a disposable inserter, suppresses ovulation for 2.5 years and provides effective contraception for at least 3 years. Side effects are similar to those with Norplant, except for less bleeding and a higher rate of amenorrhea with Implanon.[3-6]

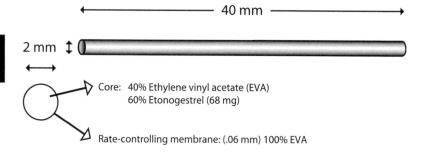

40 mm

2 mm

Core: 40% Ethylene vinyl acetate (EVA)
60% Etonogestrel (68 mg)

Rate-controlling membrane: (.06 mm) 100% EVA

Indications

Contraceptive implants are a good choice for women of reproductive age who are sexually active and desire long-term, continuous contraception. Implants should be considered for women who:

1. Want to delay the next pregnancy for at least 2–3 years.
2. Desire a highly effective, long-term method of contraception.
3. Experience serious or minor estrogen-related side effects with estrogen-progestin contraception.
4. Have difficulty remembering to take pills every day, have contraindications or difficulty using IUDs, or desire a non coitus-related method of contraception.
5. Have completed their childbearing but are not yet ready to undergo permanent sterilization.
6. Have a history of anemia with heavy menstrual bleeding.
7. Intend to breastfeed for a year or two.
8. Have chronic illnesses, in which health is threatened by pregnancy.

Absolute Contraindications

Implant use is contraindicated in women who have:

1. *ACTIVE* thrombophlebitis or thromboembolic disease.
2. Undiagnosed genital bleeding.
3. *ACUTE* liver disease.
4. Benign or malignant liver tumors.
5. Known or suspected breast cancer.

Relative Contraindications

Based on clinical judgment and appropriate medical management, Implants *MAY BE USED* by women with a history of or current diagnosis of the following conditions:

1. Heavy cigarette smoking (15 or more daily) in women older than 35 years.
2. History of ectopic pregnancy.
3. Diabetes mellitus. Because multiple studies have failed to observe a significant impact on carbohydrate metabolism, Implants, in our view, are particularly well suited for diabetic women.
4. Hypercholesterolemia.
5. Hypertension.
6. History of cardiovascular disease, including myocardial infarction, cerebral vascular accident, coronary artery disease, angina, or a previous thromboembolic event. Patients with artificial heart valves.
7. Gallbladder disease.
8. Chronic disease, such as immunocompromised patients.

Implants are not contraindicated in the following situations, but other methods are preferable:

1. Severe acne.
2. Severe vascular or migraine headaches.
3. Severe depression.
4. Concomitant use of medications that induce microsomal liver enzymes:
    Carbamazepine (Tegretol)
    Felbamate
    Nevirapine
    Oxcarbazepine
    Phenobarbital
    Phenytoin (Dilantin)
    Primidone (Mysoline)
    Rifabutin
    Rifampicin (Rifampin)
    St. John's Wort
    Topiramate
    Vigabatrin
    Possibly ethosuximide, griseofulvin, and troglitazone.

We do not recommend the use of implants with any of the previously listed drugs because of a likely increased risk of pregnancy due to lower blood levels of the progestin.[7-9]

Mechanism of Action

The release rate of the contraceptive implants is determined by total surface area and the density of the implant in which the progestin is contained. The progestin diffuses from the implant into the surrounding tissues where it is absorbed by the circulatory system and distributed systemically, avoiding an initial high level in the circulation as with oral or injected steroids. Within 8 hours after insertion of Implanon, plasma concentrations of etonogestrel are about 300 ng/mL, high enough to prevent ovulation;[10] however, a study of cervical mucus changes with Norplant indicates that a backup method should be used for 3 days after insertion: this does not appear to be necessary when Implanon is inserted as directed.[11, 12] Progestin concentrations are much more variable with Norplant than with Implanon.[10]

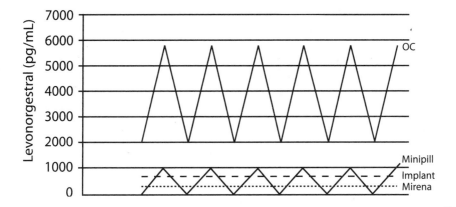

The Implanon rod releases 60 μg of etonogestrel per 24 hours at 3 months of use. This rate declines gradually to 40–50 μg daily by 12 months and 30 μg per day by 2 years of use. The 85 μg of hormone released by Norplant during the first few months of use is about equivalent to the daily dose of levonorgestrel delivered by the progestin-only, minipill oral contraceptive, and 25–50% of the dose delivered by low-dose combined oral contraceptives. After 6 months of use, daily levonorgestrel concentrations are about 0.35 ng/mL; at 2.5 years, the levels decrease to 0.25–0.35 ng/mL. Until the 8-year mark, mean levels remain above 0.25 ng/mL.[13] Mean plasma concentrations below 0.2 ng/mL are associated with increased pregnancy rates for Norplant (lower levels are more likely in heavier women).

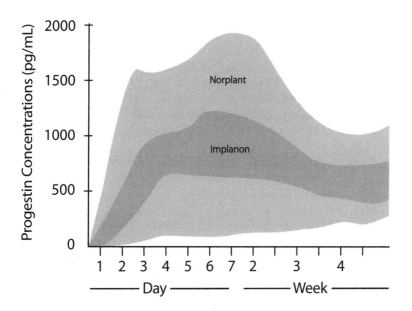

Body weight affects the circulating levels of levonorgestrel; the greater the weight of the user, the lower the levonorgestrel concentrations at any time during Norplant use. The greatest decrease over time occurs in women weighing more than 70 kg (154 pounds), but even for heavy women, the release rate is high enough to prevent pregnancy at least as reliably as oral contraceptives. In Implanon users, etonogestrel concentrations are affected very little by body weight, and failure rates do not increase with increasing body weight. ***Implanon is a good contraceptive choice for obese women.***

Levonorgestrel levels can also be affected by the circulating levels of sex hormone–binding globulin (SHBG). Levonorgestrel has a higher affinity for SHBG than does etonogestrel. In the week after Norplant insertion, SHBG levels decline rapidly and then return to approximately half of preinsertion levels by 1 year of use. This effect on SHBG is not uniform and may account for some of the individual variations in circulating progestin concentrations.[10, 14]

Implants are highly effective contraceptives. There are 3 probable modes of action, which are similar to those attributed to the contraceptive effect of the progestin-only minipills, but because daily dosing is not required, implants are more effective than oral methods.

1. The progestin suppresses, at both the hypothalamus and the pituitary, the luteinizing hormone (LH) surge necessary for ovulation. As determined by progesterone levels in many users over several years, approximately one-third of all cycles in Norplant users are ovulatory.[13, 15] During the first 2 years of use, only about 10% of women are ovulatory, but by 5 years of use, more than 50% are. In those cycles that are ovulatory, there is a high incidence of luteal insufficiency. Implanon inhibits ovulation throughout a 3-year period, accounting for almost all of the contraceptive effect.[16] However, follicular development does occur, avoiding the problem of clinically significant hypoestrogenemia, and in the last 6 months of the 3-year period, there is an occasional ovulation.[17, 18]

2. The steady release of progestin has a prolonged effect on the cervical mucus. The mucus thickens and decreases in amount, forming a barrier to sperm penetration.[11, 17, 19]

3. The progestin suppresses the estradiol-induced cyclic maturation of the endometrium and eventually causes atrophy. These changes could prevent implantation should fertilization occur; however, no evidence of fertilization can be detected in Norplant users.[20]

Advantages

Implants are a safe, highly effective, continuous method of contraception that requires little user effort and, unlike long-acting injectable contraception, is rapidly reversible. Because this is a progestin-only method, it can be used by women who have contraindications for the use of estrogen-containing contraceptives. The sustained release of low doses of progestin avoids the high initial dose delivered by injectables and the daily hormone surge associated with oral contraceptives. Implants are an excellent choice for a breastfeeding woman and can be inserted immediately postpartum. There are no effects on breast milk quality or quantity, and infants grow normally.[21–23] Another advantage of the implant method is that it allows women to plan their pregnancies precisely; return of fertility after removal is prompt, in contrast to the 6- to 18-month delay in ovulation that can follow depot-medroxyprogesterone acetate injections.[18, 24–26]

In breastfeeding, overweight, Latina women with prior gestational diabetes, the progestin-only oral minipill is associated with a 3-fold increased risk of noninsulin dependent diabetes mellitus.[27] It is not known whether this might be a risk in all women who have experienced gestational diabetes or with all progestin-only methods; a prudent course would be to advise other methods for this special group of women.

One of the major advantages of sustained-release methods is the high degree of efficacy, nearly equivalent to the theoretical effectiveness. In couples for whom elective abortion is unacceptable in the event of an unplanned pregnancy, the high efficacy rate is especially important. There are no forgotten pills, broken condoms, lost diaphragms, or missed injections. For women who are at high risk of medical complications should they become pregnant, sustained-release implants present a significant safety advantage. Users should be reassured that implant use has not been associated with changes in carbohydrate or lipid metabolism, coagulation, liver or kidney function, or immunoglobulin levels. Because many women wanting implants have had negative experiences with other contraceptives, it is important that the differences between this method and previous methods be explained.

Disadvantages

There are some disadvantages associated with the use of the implant systems. Implants cause disruption of bleeding patterns, especially during the first year of use, and some women or their partners find these changes unacceptable.[28] Endogenous estrogen is nearly normal, and unlike the estrogen-progestin contraceptives, progestin is not regularly withdrawn to allow endometrial sloughing. Consequently, the endometrium sheds at unpredictable intervals.

The implants must be inserted and removed in a surgical procedure performed by trained personnel. Women cannot initiate or discontinue the method without the assistance of a clinician. The incidence of complicated removals is approximately 5% for Norplant and lower for Implanon, an incidence that can be best minimized by good training and careful insertion.[29, 30] The implants can be visible under the skin. This sign of the use of contraception may be unacceptable for some women and for some partners.[28]

Implants do not provide protection against sexually transmitted infections (STIs) such as herpes, human papillomavirus, HIV, gonorrhea, or chlamydia. Although users may be less likely to use a second method because of the high contraceptive efficacy,[31] users at risk for STIs must use condoms as a second method to prevent infection.

Because the insertion and removal of implants require minor surgical procedures, initiation and discontinuation costs are higher than with oral contraceptives or barrier methods. The cost of implants plus fees for insertion total an amount that may seem high to patients unless they compare it with the total cost of using other methods for up to 5 years.[32] Nevertheless, short-term use is expensive compared with the relatively low initial costs of other reversible methods, and most women cannot be expected to use long-acting methods for their full duration of action.

Cultural factors can influence the acceptability of menstrual changes. Some cultures restrict a woman from participating in religious activity, household activities, or sexual intercourse while menstruating. All users must be aware of the possible menstrual changes. It is important to stress that all of the menstrual changes are expected, that they do not cause or represent illness, and that most women revert back to a more normal pattern with increasing duration of use.

Insertion and removal of implants is a new experience for most women. As with any new experience, women approach it with varying degrees of apprehension and anxiety. In reality, most patients are able to watch in comfort as implants are inserted or removed. Women should be told that the incisions used for the procedures are very small and heal quickly, leaving small scars that are usually difficult to see because of their location and size.

We encourage prospective users to see and touch implants. Women can be reassured that the implants are not damaged or move if the skin above them is accidentally injured. Normal activity cannot damage or displace the implants. Most women become unaware of their presence. A few women report sensing the implants if they are touched or manipulated for a prolonged period of time or after vigorous exercise. The implants are more visible in slender women with good muscle tone. Darker-skinned users may notice further darkening of the skin directly over the implants; this resolves after removal.

Efficacy

Contraceptive implants provide highly effective birth control. In a 3-year study of 635 women using Implanon, no pregnancies occurred.[33] In studies of Norplant conducted in 11 countries, totaling 12,133 woman-years of use, the pregnancy rate was 0.2 pregnancies per 100 woman-years of use.[8, 24] All but one of the pregnancies that occurred during this evaluation were present at the time of implant insertion. If these luteal phase insertions are excluded from analysis, the first-year pregnancy rate was 0.01 per 100 woman-years. In adolescents, Norplant implants provide better protection against unwanted pregnancy, compared with oral contraceptives, and an important factor is the better continuation rate with Norplant.[31, 34, 35] The contraceptive efficacy is maintained through 7 years of use in women who are not obese.

173

Failure Rates During the First Year of Use, United States [36,37]

Method	Percent of Women with Pregnancy	
	Lowest Expected	Typical
No method	85.0%	85.0%
Combination Pill	0.1%	7.6%
Progestin only	0.5%	3.0%
IUDs		
Levonorgestrel IUD	0.1%	0.1%
Copper T 380A	0.6%	0.8%
Implants		
Six levonorgestrel capsules (Norplant)	0.05%	0.2%
Two levonorgestrel rods (Jadelle)	0.06%	?
One etonogestrel rod (Implanon)	0.01%	?
Injectable	0.3%	0.3%
Female sterilization	0.2%	0.4%
Male sterilization	0.1%	0.15%

There are no weight restrictions for Norplant users, but heavier women (more than 70 kg) may experience slightly higher pregnancy rates in the later years of use compared with lighter women. Even in the later years, however, pregnancy rates for heavier women using Norplant are lower than with oral contraception. The differences in pregnancy rates by weight are probably due to the dilutional effect of larger body size on the low, sustained serum levels of levonorgestrel. Heavier women should not rely on Norplant beyond the 5-year limit. For slender women the duration of Norplant's efficacy may extend well past the fifth year of use. In some extended trials, no pregnancies have occurred into the seventh year.

The contraceptive efficacy of Implanon surpasses that of Norplant and sterilization.[16] Only a rare pregnancy occurs, resulting in a Pearl Index of about 0.01.[17, 38] In over 70,000 cycles, no pregnancies were recorded because of total inhibition of ovulation until ovulations were observed in the last 6 months of the 3-year period.[17, 33] Postmarketing surveillance of pregnancies in Australia, where nearly one-quarter of contraceptors relied on Implanon in 2004, revealed that of 173 pregnancies, only 13 could possibly have been failures of the method.[9] In Australia and the Netherlands, pregnancies commonly were the consequence of poor insertion technique, especially allowing the implant to fall unnoticed to the floor. Data are not available regarding the effect of body weight on the efficacy of Implanon, but unlike Norplant, progestin levels are not significantly lower in heavier women.

Implants have an immediate contraceptive effect when inserted within the first 7 days of a menstrual cycle, but when insertion is after day 7, a backup method of contraception is necessary for at least 3 days.[39]

Ectopic Pregnancy

The ectopic pregnancy rate during Norplant use is 0.28 per 1,000 woman-years.[8] *Although the risk of developing an ectopic pregnancy during use of Norplant is low, when pregnancy does occur, ectopic pregnancy should be suspected because approximately 30% of Norplant pregnancies are ectopic.* Because Implanon is more effective in inhibiting ovulation, we would expect the risk of ectopic pregnancy to be considerably less than that associated with Norplant.

Ectopic Pregnancy Rates per 1,000 Woman-Years[8, 40, 41,]

Non-contraceptive users, all ages	3.0–4.5
Copper T-380 IUD	0.20
Norplant	0.28

Menstrual Effects

Menstrual bleeding patterns are highly variable among users of implant contraception. With levonorgestrel implants, some alteration of menstrual patterns occur during the first year of use in approximately 80% of users, later decreasing to about 40%, and by the fifth year, to about 33%.[42, 43] The changes include alterations in the interval between bleeding, the duration and volume of menstrual flow, and spotting. Oligomenorrhea and amenorrhea also occur but are less common, less than 10% after the first year and diminishing thereafter. Irregular and prolonged bleeding usually occurs during the first year. Although bleeding problems occur much less frequently after the second year, they can occur at any time.[43, 44] Studies of the endometrium in Norplant users experiencing abnormal bleeding indicate the presence of enlarged venous sinusoids (fragile vessels) and a reduction in the expression of a protein factor (perivascular stromal cell tissue factor) involved in the initiation of hemostasis.[45] Within weeks after insertion, the density of endometrial small blood vessels increases and the endometrium regresses to an atrophic state.[46] It is believed that bleeding is a consequence of rapid endometrial regression and that the apparent increase in the number of blood vessels may reflect increased tortuosity accompanying the atrophic regression.

Implanon alters menstrual patterns, but amenorrhea occurs more often (21% of users in the first year, 30–40% after 1 year) than with Norplant.[4, 6] A single Implanon rod completely suppresses ovulation for 2.5 years, and, therefore, menses do not become more regular after the first 2 years as with Norplant. After 2 years, ovulation occurs in about half of the menstrual cycles. Bleeding is lighter and less frequent among Implanon users because more profound ovarian suppression results in less follicular estrogen production and less endometrial stimulation, nevertheless irregular bleeding continues to be a major reason for discontinuation.[6, 47]

Vaginal Bleeding Patterns[6]

	Implanon	Norplant	Statistically Different
Amenorrhea	22%	5%	Yes
Infrequent bleeding	27%	21%	Yes
Frequent bleeding	6%	3%	No
Prolonged bleeding	12%	9%	No

Despite an increase in the number of spotting and bleeding days over preinsertion menstrual patterns, hemoglobin concentrations rise in Norplant users because of a decrease in the average amount of menstrual blood loss.[48-51] Implanon likewise does not cause anemia.[4]

Implant users who can no longer tolerate prolonged bleeding benefit from a short course of oral estrogen: conjugated estrogens, 1.25 mg, or estradiol, 2 mg, administered daily for 7 days. A therapeutic dose of one of the prostaglandin inhibitors given during the bleeding helps to diminish flow, but estrogen is the most effective treatment.[52, 53] Another approach is to administer an estrogen-progestin oral contraceptive for 1–3 months.[54]

Although implants are very effective, pregnancy must be considered in women reporting amenorrhea who had been ovulating previously, as evidenced by regular menses prior to an episode of amenorrhea. A sensitive urine pregnancy test should be obtained. Women who remain amenorrheic throughout their use of implants are unlikely to become pregnant.[43] It is important to explain to patients the mechanism of the amenorrhea: the local progestational effect causing decidualization and atrophy.

Metabolic Effects

Exposure to the sustained, low doses of progestin delivered by the implants is not associated with significant metabolic changes. Studies of liver function,[3, 55, 56] blood coagulation,[3, 57-59] immunoglobulin levels,[60, 61] serum cortisol levels,[62] and blood chemistries[56, 60] have failed to detect changes outside of normal ranges in Norplant users.

No major impact on the lipoprotein profile can be demonstrated with Norplant.[55, 63, 64] Minor changes are transient, and, with prolonged duration of use, lipoproteins return to preinsertion levels. Long-term exposure to the low dose of levonorgestrel released by Norplant is unlikely to affect users' risk of atherogenesis, just as prolonged exposure to combined oral contraception has not (see Chapter 2). There are no clinically important effects on carbohydrate metabolism.[60, 65, 66] No effect on insulin sensitivity can be detected.[67] In a cohort study of 5 years' duration, no increase was observed in diabetes mellitus, depression, lupus erythematosus, cardiovascular diseases—in fact there was no increase in serious morbidity.[68]

There are no significant metabolic differences comparing Implanon and Norplant.[69] Neither implant system has important clinical effects on the lipoprotein profile, carbohydrate metabolism, thyroid and adrenal function, liver function tests, or the clotting mechanism.[3, 70-74] Implant contraception is a good choice for a woman at risk for estrogen-associated thromboembolism. Because of the lower androgenic characteristic of etonogestrel, Implanon does not cause a decrease in the levels of sex hormone-binding globulin.[71]

Measurements of bone density in young women reveal that Implanon and Norplant do not affect the teenage gain in bone; similar gains in bone were recorded in implant users and control subjects.[75, 76] In older women, an increase in forearm, spine, and femur bone density has been documented after 6 and 12 months of Norplant use.[77, 78] An international cross-section study reported a small loss in bone density with Norplant that was rapidly regained after discontinuation.[79]

A slight increase in gallbladder disease has been noted in Norplant users.[16, 80] This is at best just a word of caution because the association is weak and may reflect preexisting disease, and there is no apparent biologic mechanism.

Effects on Future Fertility

Circulating levels of progestin become too low to measure within 48 hours after removal of implants. Most women resume normal ovulatory cycles during the first month after removal. The pregnancy rates during the first year after removal are comparable with those of women not using contraceptive methods and trying to become pregnant. There are no long-term effects on future fertility nor are there any effects on sex ratios, rates of ectopic pregnancy, spontaneous miscarriage, stillbirth, or congenital malformations.[8, 24] The return of fertility after implant removal is prompt, and pregnancy outcomes are within normal limits. The rate and outcome of subsequent pregnancies are not influenced by duration of use.

For women who are spacing their pregnancies, the difference between implants and depot-medroxyprogesterone acetate in the timing of the return to fertility can be critical. Implants allow precise timing of pregnancy because the return of ovulation after removal is prompt. Etonogestrel serum levels are undetectable within one week after removal of Implanon, and ovulation can be expected in the first month after discontinuation.[2] Depot-medroxyprogesterone acetate, on the other hand, can cause up to 18 months' delay in return to fertility. By that time, 90% of users of either method have ovulated, but in the first several months, the difference is dramatic. By 3 months after removal, half of implant users have ovulated, but 10 months must elapse before half of depot-medroxyprogesterone acetate users are ovulatory.

Side Effects

The occurrence of serious side effects is very rare, no different in incidence than that observed in the general population. In addition to the menstrual changes, levonorgestrel implant users have reported the following side effects: headache, acne, weight change, mastalgia, hyperpigmentation over the implants, hirsutism, depression, mood changes, anxiety, nervousness, ovarian cyst formation, and galactorrhea.[8, 24, 42, 44, 81]

It is difficult, of course, to be certain which of these effects were actually caused by the levonorgestrel. For example, careful study fails to reveal a relationship between Norplant use and depressive symptoms.[82] Although most of these side effects are minor in nature, they can cause patients to discontinue the method. Patients often find common side effects tolerable after assurance that they do not represent a health hazard.[28] Many complaints respond to reassurance; others can be treated with simple therapies. The most common side effect experienced by users is headache; approximately 20% of women who discontinue use do so because of headache.[28, 81]

Stroke, thrombotic thrombocytopenic purpura, thrombocytopenia, and pseudotumor cerebri have been reported with Norplant.[83] However, it is by no means established that the incidence of these problems is increased, and there is little reason to suspect a cause-and-effect relationship. In the follow-up study conducted by the World Health Organization in 8 countries, no significant excess of cardiovascular events or malignant disease has been observed.[84]

Weight Change

Women using levonorgestrel implants more frequently complain of weight gain than of weight loss, but findings are variable.[80] In the Dominican Republic, 75% of those who changed weight lost weight, whereas in San Francisco, two-thirds gained weight. Assessment of weight change in Norplant users is confounded by changes in exercise, diet, and aging. Although an increase in appetite can be attributed to the androgenic activity of levonorgestrel, it is unlikely that the low levels with Norplant have any clinical impact. Counseling for weight changes focuses best on dietary review and dietary changes. Indeed, a 5-year follow-up of 75 women with Norplant implants could document no increase in the body mass index (nor was there a correlation between irregular bleeding and body weight).[85] A similar experience has been documented with Implanon.[5]

Mastalgia

Bilateral mastalgia, often occurring premenstrually, is usually associated with complaints of fluid retention. After pregnancy has been ruled out, reassurance and therapy aimed at symptomatic relief are indicated. This symptom decreases with increasing duration of implant use, and occurs at a lower rate comparing Implanon with Norplant.[5] Most implant users respond to treatment and do not elect to remove the implants. Careful assessments of the relationship between methylxanthines and mastalgia have failed to demonstrate a link. The most effective treatments for mastalgia are the following: danazol (200 mg/day), vitamin E (600 units/day), bromocriptine (2.5 mg/day), or tamoxifen (20 mg/day), but there are no studies of these treatments in implant users.

Galactorrhea

Galactorrhea is more common among women who have had insertion of the implants on discontinuation of lactation. Pregnancy and other possible causes should be ruled out by performing a pregnancy test and a thorough breast examination. Patients can be reassured that this is a common occurrence among implant and oral contraceptive users. Decreasing the amount of breast and nipple stimulation during sexual relations might alleviate the symptom, but if amenorrhea accompanies persistent galactorrhea, a prolactin level should be obtained.

Acne

Acne, with or without an increase in oil production, is the most common skin complaint among levonorgestrel implant users. The acne is caused by the androgenic activity of the levonorgestrel that produces a direct impact and causes a decrease in SHBG levels leading to an increase in free steroid levels (both levonorgestrel and testosterone).[14] This is in contrast to combined oral contraceptives that contain levonorgestrel, in which the estrogen effect on SHBG (an increase) produces a decrease in unbound, free androgens. Etonogestrel implants are less commonly associated with acne because this progestin is less androgenic than levonorgestrel.[5] Common therapies for complaints of acne include dietary change, practice of good skin hygiene with the use of soaps or skin cleansers, and application of topical antibiotics (e.g., 1% clindamycin solution or gel or topical erythromycin).

Ovarian Cysts

Unlike oral contraception, the low serum progestin levels maintained by implants do not suppress follicle-stimulating hormone (FSH), which continues to stimulate ovarian follicle growth in most users. The LH peak during the first 2 years of use, on the other hand, is usually abolished so that these follicles do not ovulate.[15] However, some continue to grow and cause pain or they are palpated at the time of pelvic examination.[86] Adnexal masses are approximately 8 times more frequent in Norplant users compared with normally cycling women. Because these are simple cysts (and most regress spontaneously within 1 month of detection), they need not be sonographically or laparoscopically evaluated.[30] Further evaluation is indicated if they became large and painful or fail to regress. Regular ovulators are

179

less likely to form cysts so the situation is likely to improve after 2 years of implant use. Etonogestrel implants suppress follicular development more profoundly; thus, ovarian cysts are less likely than with levonorgestrel implants.

Cancer

We can speculate on possible effects of implants based on our experience with oral contraceptives and depot-medroxyprogesterone acetate. The risk of endometrial cancer ought to be reduced. A study of the endometrial effects of Norplant failed to find any evidence of hyperplasia, even when levonorgestrel levels were low and endogenous estradiol production was normal.[87] The risk of ovarian cancer is also probably reduced, and we would expect a greater effect with Implanon because it more effectively suppresses ovulation. Breast and cervical cancer effects are difficult to assess because of confounding variables as they are with oral contraception and depot-medroxyprogesterone acetate. The low progestin dose of implants, however, would be unlikely to have effects different from other hormonal contraceptives.

Post-marketing Surveillance Study

A large 5-year follow-up study in developing countries confirmed the low pregnancy rates associated with Norplant, 0.23 per 100 woman-years for intrauterine pregnancy and 0.03 per 100 woman-years for ectopic pregnancy.[84] When the women using Norplant were compared with women using nonhormonal methods of contraception and to the expected population rates, there was no excess of cancers, connective tissue diseases, or cardiovascular events. Importantly, the complaints of headache and mood disturbances (including anxiety and depression) were similar to those reported by women using oral contraceptives, although higher than for women using IUDs.

Insertion and Removal

The usual personal and family medical history and physical examination should concentrate on factors that might contraindicate use of the various contraceptive options. If a patient elects to use contraceptive implants, a detailed description of the method, including effectiveness, side effects, risks, benefits, as well as insertion and removal procedures, should be provided. Before insertion, the patient is asked to read and sign a written consent for the surgical placement of the implants. The consent reviews the potential complications of the procedure that include reaction to the local anesthetic, infection, expulsion of the implants, superficial phlebitis, bruising, and the possibility of a subsequent difficult removal.

Insertion can be performed at any time during the menstrual cycle as long as pregnancy can be ruled out. If the patient's last menstrual period was abnormal, if she has recently had sexual intercourse without contraception, or if there are reasons to suspect pregnancy, a sensitive urine pregnancy test is a wise precaution. Based on cervical mucus changes, a backup method need be used no more than 3 days after insertion.[12] Implants can be inserted immediately postpartum but certainly should be initiated no later than the third postpartum week in nonbreastfeeding women and the third postpartum month in breastfeeding women. Acne and headache are less common in women who receive Norplant immediately postpartum, and there is no difference in postpregnancy weight loss compared with women who receive it 4–6 weeks later.[88]

Patients should be questioned about allergies to local anesthetics, antiseptic solutions, and tape. A discussion about the technique of insertion and anticipated sensations is an important part of preparing the patient for the experience. All patients approach insertion with some degree of apprehension that can be decreased by detailed explanations and preparation.[89, 90]

Selection of the site for placement of implants is based on both functional and aesthetic factors. Various sites (the upper leg, forearm, and upper arm) have been used in clinical trials. The nondominant, upper, inner arm is the best site. This area is easily accessible to the clinician with minimal exposure of the patient. It is well protected during most normal activities. It is not highly visible, and migration of the implants from this site has not been documented. The site of placement does not affect circulating progestin levels. Careful implant insertion is the key to trouble-free removal.

Implanon offers important insertion advantages compared with Norplant.[91] Of course, only one rod simplifies and shortens both insertion and removal. In addition, a preloaded applicator is provided that facilitates placement. If necessary, Implanon can usually be visualized by ultrasonography.[92] However, if a nonpalpable rod is not visible on ultrasonography, definitive localization is best achieved with magnetic resonance imaging (MRI).[93] Removal of the Implanon rod uses the "fingers alone" technique with a 2 mm incision.[94] Insertion complications (mainly deep insertions) are rare, and removal complications (difficulty finding the implant or a broken implant) occur at a much lower frequency than with Norplant.[91, 95]

Insertion Technique

Insertion is carried out under local anesthesia in the office or clinic by someone, usually a physician or nurse practitioner, trained in the technique described here.[96] The procedure takes 5–10 minutes for a 6-implant system, and 2–3 minutes for a single implant.

Required Equipment for Implanon Insertion

2.5-mL syringe.
0.5-inch, 25-gauge needle for injecting the anesthetic.
1% chloroprocaine or lidocaine without epinephrine.
Antiseptic solution.
Adhesive strip for puncture closures.
Adhesive bandage.

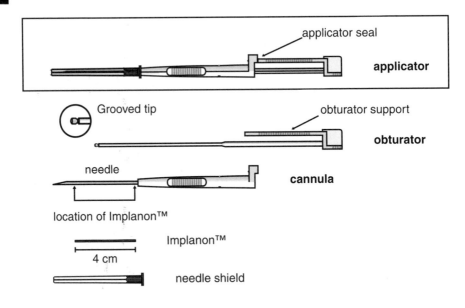

Positioning the Patient. The patient is placed in a supine position with the full length of her arm exposed. The upper inner arm is positioned by bending the elbow to 90 degrees and rotating the arm out, allowing full exposure of the insertion site at the junction of the biceps and triceps muscles. Adequate support under the arm should be provided to ensure comfort. To minimize the risk of infection, strict aseptic technique should be maintained throughout the procedure. An insertion site approximately

3–4 fingerbreadths (6–8 cm) superior and lateral to the medial epicondyle of the humerus is identified. A sterile drape is placed under the arm, and the insertion site on the arm is cleaned with an antiseptic such as povidone-iodine.

Anesthesia. Local anesthesia for the incision is obtained by raising a wheal of 1% chloroprocaine or lidocaine using a 25-gauge needle and injecting 1 mL under the skin along the track of the implant insertion needle.

Verify the presence of Implanon by looking carefully at the tip of the needle. If the implant is not visible, turn the applicator needle down and gently tap on a surface with the needle cover in place until the Implanon is seen, then tap the base of the applicator with the needle pointed up until the implant is no longer visible. Keep the applicator sterile.

183

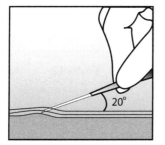
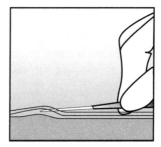

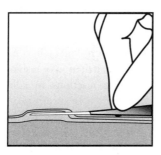

Incision and Placement. The insertion needle and its obturator can be pushed directly through the skin at no greater than a 20-degree angle without making an incision. The needle is advanced as superficially as possible under the skin by maintaining a slightly upward angle on the trocar. To minimize the chance of too deep an insertion, lift or tent the skin with the tip of the needle. If the skin dimples, the needle is too superficial; pull the needle back, and redirect.

Once the needle has been fully advanced, break the seal on the applicator by pressing the obturator support. Turn the obturator 90 degrees in either direction with respect to the cannula and fix the obturator with one hand. With the other hand, slowly pull the needle out of the arm, leaving the implant behind under the skin.

Immediately after insertion, palpate the implant to verify correct insertion. Look for the grooved tip of the obturator visible inside the needle. If the implant is not palpable and not within the needle, it must be located before contraception can be assured. If placement is in doubt, another contraceptive method must be used.

After the insertion, show the patient how to palpate the implant. Place an adhesive closure or bandage over the insertion site. Complete the patient chart label and the "User Card" that must be given to the patient.

Most women experience little pain during the insertion,[89] but, if it occurs, the discomfort can be relieved with aspirin, acetaminophen, or a non-steroidal-antiinflammatory agent. Infection or expulstion of the implants is rare (less than 1% with the Norplant system) and usually occurs when an implant is left pressing against the wound.[97]

The most commonly reported discomfort is a burning sensation during the injection of the local anesthetic. This effect of local anesthetic can be eliminated for most patients by adding 1 meq of sodium bicarbonate to each 10 mL of anesthetic (this shortens shelf life to 24 hours).[98] After the onset of anesthesia in 2–3 minutes, most women feel no more than a pressure sensation.

Complications of Insertion Potential complications include infection, hematoma formation, local irritation or rash over the implants, expulsion of the implant, and allergic reactions to adhesives of the dressing. The incidence of complications is minimized by clinician training and experience, and the use of strict aseptic technique. *Postinsertion pregnancies in Australia and the Netherlands were commonly due to a failure to insert the implant (allowing the implant to fall out prior to insertion). The clinician must make sure the implant is visualized in the trocar prior to insertion and after insertion is palpable under the skin.*

Infection The rate of infection varies among clinics and countries. The overall risk of infection after Norplant insertion is 0.8%.[97] Infections usually occur within the first week after insertion but can present as long as 4–5 months later. Infection can be treated either by the removal of the implant or the administration of oral antibiotics while the implant remains in place. One-third of insertion site infections treated with antibiotics are unresponsive to therapy and require removal.[97] There have been no reports of infections leading to serious injury. Rarely, a superficial phlebitis develops. If it resolves over 1–2 weeks with heat and elevation of the arm, the implants need not be removed.

Expulsion. Expulsion of one or more of the implants occurs in 0.4% of Norplant users, usually within the first few months.[97] The majority of expulsions are associated with concurrent infection at the insertion site. Another cause of expulsion is failure to advance the implants far enough from the incision, causing pressure on the incision by the distal tip of the implant.

Local Reactions. Although not common, hematomas can form. The use of a pressure dressing for 72 hours prevents enlargment. Application of an ice pack for 30 minutes immediately after insertion also helps. Local irritation, rash, pruritus, and pain occur in 4.7% of Norplant users, usually during the first month of use.[97] Allergies to skin closure strip adhesives or to latex gloves account for some reactions.[99] These problems resolve spontaneously, but itching can be relieved by topical corticoid steroids.

Removal Techniques Although implant removal is an office procedure requiring only a small amount of local anesthesia and a few simple instruments, instruction and practice are necessary.[98] Practicing on a model arm after viewing an instructional video makes first removals faster and less uncomfortable for both clinician and patient. A removal kit containing a model arm, a manual, and a compact disc illustrating basic technique is available at no charge from Organon Inc., by calling toll free (877) IMPLANON (467-5266). As for insertion, the patient should read and sign an informed consent to be filed in her medical record. We recommend that the patient be given a copy.

Proper positioning of the implant at the time of insertion is the most important factor influencing ease of removal. If the Norplant implants have been inserted with the distal tips (those away from the axilla) far apart or with implants crossing or touching one another, or too deeply, a larger incision and more time are required. Removal is easiest when the implants are just under the skin with their distal tips close together in a fan shape. The fibrous sheaths that form around implants can also make removal more difficult, especially if they are dense. The one and two implant systems can be removed faster and with less pain than the 6 Norplant capsules.[94]

Most removals are not painful (80% of our patients reported pain as "none" or "slight"), and systemic analgesia is not required.[100] Time for removal of 6 capsules ranges from 5 to 40 minutes, with an average of 20 minutes. For the single rod (Implanon), the average time is only 3 minutes. The most common cause of discomfort during the procedure is injection of the local anesthetic. This stinging sensation can be relieved if one meq sodium bicarbonate is added to each 10 mL of local anesthetic.[97] Patients may feel pressure or tugging from manipulation of the fibrous sheaths and the implants, but these sensations are not severe if the clinician waits a few minutes after injection of the local anesthetic. The sheaths that form around Implanon are less dense than those around Norplant capsules.

Removal with Instruments. This approach to removal is the one described in the Norplant package insert and has been used around the world for 15 years. The technique requires 3 small sterile drapes (one fenestrated), sterile gloves, antiseptic solution such as povidone-iodine, 25-gauge 1.5-inch needle with a 3-mL syringe, local anesthetic (1% lidocaine with 1:100,000 epinephrine, buffered with 1 meq sodium bicarbonate per 10 mL lidocaine), one curved and one straight mosquito clamp, 4 x 4 sterile gauze sponges, and a no. 11 blade scalpel. This method is more appropriate for removal of the 6-capsule Norplant system than for one or two rods, which can usually be removed using fingers alone.[94]

The patient is placed in a supine position with her arm flexed and externally rotated as for insertion. A thick book positioned under the patient's arm can make her more comfortable and provide a better operating field. A sterile towel is placed under the arm. The implants are best seen by stretching the skin above and below the implants. Palpate all 6 of the implants before starting; if some portion of every implant cannot be felt, it may be better to sonographically or radiographically image (see below) the impalpable ones before removal because when the palpable implants are gone, they are lost as landmarks.

The skin is cleaned with the antiseptic solution, preparing a wide area above and below the implants so that the incision won't be contaminated during manipulations for removal. Scrape the antiseptic solution from the skin lying over the implants (the sterile stick of a cotton tipped applicator can be used) and let the arm dry. This will leave an impression of the implants that helps find them for removal. Drape the arm with a fenestrated towel and use a third towel to create a sterile field for instruments on a Mayo stand or table.

Wearing sterile gloves, an incision site is selected by pressing down on the proximal ends of the capsules and palpating their distal tips with a finger.

Careful selection of the incision site is the most critical step for easy removal. The best incision site is right at the distal tips, midway between the most medial and lateral implants. This can be the same as the insertion site, but generally the removal incision is made a few millimeters higher up on the arm to ensure placing it as close as possible to the tips of all the implants.

A local anesthetic containing 1:100,000 epinephrine reduces bleeding and allows better visualization of the implants. The 25-gauge needle is used to raise a 1-cm wheal of local anesthetic just under the tips of the implants. About 2 mL are sufficient, although more may be required later. Injection of too much anesthetic over the implants can obscure the tips and make removal more difficult. A 3–5-mm incision is made with the no.11 scalpel right at the mid point of the cluster of implant tips. A larger incision is not usually required and can cause bleeding that can obscure the implants. Implants can be removed by the clinician either sitting or standing, but if sitting, a wheeled stool allows repositioning as needed.

The implant that is most superficial and closest to the incision is removed first. This implant is pushed gently toward the incision with the fingers until the tip is visible and can be grasped with a curved mosquito clamp. The fibrous sheath covering the implant is dissected away using a finger covered with an opened gauze sponge. If the sheath is too dense for the sponge, it can be cautiously dissected with the straight clamp, a needle tip, or, for really dense sheaths, with the scalpel, taking care not to cut open the implant. If the point of the scalpel blade is used to nick the sheath over the thick silastic plug at the tip of the implant, the implant itself will not be cut, but if the sheath is incised across the thin walls of the implant, the implant can be severed and require removal in two portions. If the sheath must be incised with the scalpel, the incision should be along, not across, the implant.

Once the sheath is opened and the white tip of the first implant is exposed, it is grasped with the straight clamp. The curved clamp is released and the implant is gently pulled out. This procedure is repeated with the remaining implants.

If the implant tips cannot be guided to the incision with digital pressure on the skin above the implants, the jaws of the straight mosquito are inserted into the incision and opened just beneath the skin to separate the tissue layers. The straight clamp is removed, and the curved clamp is inserted with the tips pointing upward toward the skin. The clamp is opened and the implant is guided down between the jaws with a forefinger on the skin above the implant. This downward pressure on the tips of the clamp is often the most painful part of the removal procedure. When the implant is pushed between the jaws of the clamp, the clamp is secured at the first or second ratchet. Too much pressure on the implant can fracture the silastic capsule, making removal more difficult. The implant should not be pulled out with the curved clamp. If the implant cannot be seen, after gentle traction, the clamp handle is flipped 180 degrees until it points in the opposite direction, toward the patient's head. A portion of the sheath is cleared with an opened sponge, or if necessary, the scalpel tip, incising longitudinally, not across the implant. The exposed portion is then grasped with the straight clamp, the curved clamp is released, and the implant is removed with gentle traction. The procedure is repeated until all the implants are removed.

At the completion of the procedure, the implants should be counted to ensure that all have been removed. If any of the implants have been broken, the pieces should be aligned and compared with an intact capsule to determine that all of the implant has been removed. An adhesive strip is used to close the incision while pinching the skin edges together. A pressure dressing is then applied as after insertion, and removed the next day. The fibrous sheaths can remain for months causing the patient to think that implants were left behind. For that reason, it is important to show the implants to the patient at the time of removal.

If removal of some of the implants is difficult, painful, or prolonged, the procedure should be interrupted and the patient should return in a few weeks to complete the removal. The remaining implants are easier to remove after bleeding and swelling subsides. A new incision can be made closer to the implants that are difficult to remove the first time. Even if some of the implants remain, the patient should immediately begin to use another method of contraception.

Removal with Fingers Alone. Implants can be removed with less pain and bleeding and through a smaller incision if the use of instruments is avoided. The amount of trauma and bruising in the surrounding tissues is decreased, the scar is less visible, and the risk of breaking the implants is reduced. The disadvantage of this approach is that it may not be successful for implants that are poorly aligned or too deeply inserted. This technique is especially appropriate for the one- and two-rod systems.[94]

After preparation of the patient, the distal tip of the implant is palpated. If the implant cannot be felt, removal should be postponed until it has been localized with ultrasonography or radiography. No more than 0.5 mL of buffered lidocaine with epinephrine is injected into the dermis immediately under the implant tip, raising a wheal of about 1 cm in diameter. Too much anesthetic makes it difficult to locate the implant tip under the skin. The area of the injection should be massaged to disperse the anesthetic. Pressure is applied with fingers on the proximal (axillary) end of the implant so that the distal tips presses up against the skin. A 2–3-mm longitudinal incision is made through the skin onto the tip of the implant until the rubbery sensation of the implant can be felt against the point of the scalpel blade. The fibrous sheath is incised by nicking the sheath with the tip of the scalpel blade against the implant tip. It may take several passes across the tip with the scalpel held in different directions to fully open the sheath.

As the sheath is opened, the end of the implant comes into view. With finger pressure on its other end, the implant can be pushed through the incision until it can be grasped with mosquito forceps or fingers and pulled out. The incision is closed with an adhesive strip and covered with a sterile gauze and a pressure bandage.

Holding the implant up against the incision with finger pressure is critical for success with this "pop out" technique. If pressure is released, the implant slips back to the position defined by the fibrous sheath around it. As the implant is manipulated using the fingers of both hands, the scalpel must be held so that it is immediately available to incise the sheath without releasing the implant. It is best to keep the scalpel in one hand with thumb and index finger while manipulating the implant, holding the implant with the rest of the fingers of both hands.

If the implant does not move toward the incision with finger pressure, it can be grasped with a hemostatic or vasectomy clamp, but the incision usually must be lengthened 2–3 mm to admit the clamp. The procedure followed is then as previously described for instrumental removals. It may be necessary to inject more local anesthetic, but not more than 1 mL at a time where the clamp is applied to the implant.

Difficult Removals. The incidence of difficult removals in the large post-marketing surveillance study of Norplant was 10.1 per 1,000 removals.[84] Removal is more difficult if the implants are broken during attempts to extract them. Once an implant is damaged, it can fracture repeatedly with further attempts to grasp it with clamps. To decrease this risk, the implants should be grasped at their ends whenever possible and as little traction as possible should be used for exposure and removal. If the scalpel is required to open the fibrous sheath around the implant, care should be taken to avoid slicing the capsule. If it has not been possible to grasp the end of implant, to open the fibrous sheath, incise along the length of the implant; cut longitudinally, not across, the implant. Rarely, removal of cut or broken implants requires an additional incision at the proximal end of the implant so that the remaining piece can be removed. Even more rarely, an implant can neither be palpated under the skin nor found through an incision. Such "lost" implants are most easily located with a high frequency

(7–10 megahertz), short focus ultrasound just prior to the removal procedure to help place the incision directly over the implant.[101] Use a transverse
orientation to identify the shadow (the implant itself is more difficult to
see), measure the depth, and draw lines representing the location on the
surface of the skin using a paper clip as a marker.

When an implant is not palpable, imaging techniques for localization are
required. Three techniques are particularly useful: mammography, sonography, and digital subtraction fluoroscopy.[102] Compression film screen
mammography is superior to standard plain film radiography.
Ultrasonography requires a linear array transducer (preferably 7 MHz)
applied to the upper arm with its long axis oriented perpendicular to the
long axis of the humerus. The transducer is slowly moved until the characteristic acoustic shadowing of the implant is visualized. To measure the
depth of each capsule, the transducer is repositioned along the axis of the
implant to identify the length and both ends. Depth is determined using
electronic calipers. Real-time sonography guidance can be useful during
the removal procedure. Digital subtraction fluoroscopy relies on ghost
images caused by motion during acquisition. Because it is readily available
and can be employed during removal, sonography is a first choice.

Another instrumental technique employs a modified vasectomy forceps
and is very useful for removing deeply or asymmetrically placed Norplant
implants. It requires a larger incision made in the center of the field of
implants. The vasectomy forceps is advanced under the skin toward the
mid portion of the implants. Those in the center are grasped first (in the
middle of each implant), pulled into the incision, and cleaned free of their
fibrous sheath as in the standard technique. The implant is then extracted,
bending it in the middle in a "U" shape. The implants furthest away from
the incision are removed last by advancing the forceps under the skin.[103]

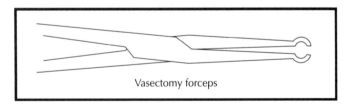

Vasectomy forceps

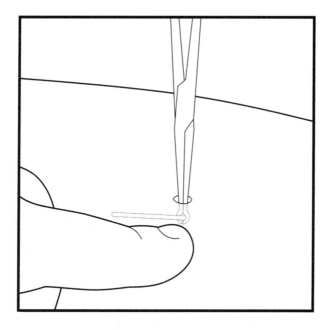

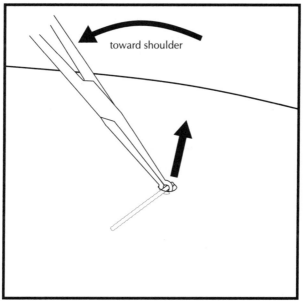

toward shoulder

We have found this approach to be especially useful for deeply placed, single capsules that are otherwise difficult to remove. The incision is made directly above the mid portion of the implant as determined by sonography or compression radiography. The scalpel blade (or a 25-gauge needle) is advanced to the depth of the implant as determined by imaging to feel for the capsule. The vasectomy forcep is advanced along the same track until the capsule can be grasped and elevated into the incision, freed from its fibrous sheath, and extracted.

Experienced clinicians agree that about half of difficult removals are due to improper placement.[29, 104] With one and two implant systems, removals are easier, but careful insertion remains the real secret to trouble-free removal.

Reasons for Termination

Although implants are long-term methods (2–7 years), only approximately 30% of women continue Norplant for 5 years (although in some cultures 5-year continuation rates reach 65–70%). Discontinuation occurs at a rate of 10–15% yearly, about the same as for intrauterine contraception but lower than for barrier or oral contraception.[8, 44, 89, 105] Bothersome side effects, such as menstrual changes, headache, or weight change, are the primary reasons for termination of implant use.[28, 81, 106, 107] Menstrual changes are the most common cause for discontinuation of implants in the first year of use. An unspoken concern for many patients and their partners is the fact that bleeding irregularity interferes with sexual interactions. Users who cannot tolerate these symptoms request removal in the first 2 years of use whereas women who want another pregnancy, the most common personal reason for removal, are more likely to terminate use in the third or fourth year. Headache has been observed at a lower rate with Implanon than with Norplant.[5]

User Acceptance of Contraceptive Implants

Overall, interview surveys throughout the world have indicated that women perceive sustained-release methods as highly acceptable methods of contraception.[90, 107–110] The most popular feature of implants is their ease of use. Approximately 20% of U.S. patients reported that friends and relatives notice their implants. This may be a greater problem in warmer climates with less encompassing clothing. Only 25% of the women who report that the implants were noticed were bothered by this attention.[28]

In the United States, the primary motivations for implant use have been problems with previous contraceptive methods and ease of implant use. Although fear of pain during implant insertion is a prominent source of anxiety for many women, the actual pain experienced does not match the expectations. The level of satisfaction has been high in self-motivated and well-informed users.[111] Teenagers provide an example of well-documented success. Their 1-year pregnancy rates are much lower and continuation rates much higher than that with oral contraceptives.[31, 112-115] However, teenage discontinuation of the method due to side effects (especially irregular bleeding and weight gain) is more common with Norplant.[34] The lower rate of irregular bleeding with Implanon contributes to higher patient acceptability, but irregular bleeding continues to be the major reason for discontinuation.[6, 26, 107]

Counseling Women

Frank information about negative factors such as irregular bleeding avoids surprise and disappointment and encourage women to continue use long enough to enjoy the positive attributes such as convenience, safety, and efficacy. Open discussion of side effects leads to public and media awareness of the disadvantages as well as the advantages of these methods. Helping women decide if they are good candidates for use of implants before they invest too much time and money in long-acting contraception is a very important objective of good counseling.

Common patient questions regarding contraceptive implants are

- Is it effective?
- How is it inserted and removed, how long do these procedures take, does it hurt, and will it leave scars?
- Will the implants be visible under the skin?
- Will the implants be uncomfortable or restrict movement of the arm?
- Will the implants move in the body?
- Will the implants be damaged if they are touched or bumped?
- Will this contraceptive change sexual drive and enjoyment?
- What are the short- and long-term side effects?
- Are there any effects on future fertility?
- What do the implants look and feel like?
- What happens if pregnancy occurs during use?
- How long will it take for the method to be effective after insertion?
- Can a partner tell if this method is being used?

LNG Rod — The Two Rod System

The two-implant system, Norplant-2 or Jadelle, uses levonorgestrel suspended in a silastic matrix and covered with a silastic membrane.[116] Bleeding, pregnancy, and continuation rates are like those of the 6-capsule system, but insertion and removal are easier.[24] Each rod measures 2.5 mm in diameter and 4.3 cm in length, contains 75 μg levonorgestrel, and releases the drug at the same dosage as Norplant.[116] Long-term clinical trials indicate that the performance and side effects are similar to Norplant, but removal is faster.[117, 118] This method is approved but not sold in the United States.

Another Single-Rod System

Uniplant. The newer progestins (desogestrel, gestodene, nestorone, nomegestrol, and norgestimate) are less androgenic than levonorgestrel and are useful in contraceptive implants. Uniplant (also Surplant) is a single-implant contraceptive, containing 55 mg nomegestrol acetate in a 4-cm silicone capsule with a 100 μg per day release rate. It provides contraception for 1 year.[119–121] A single silicone implant containing nestorone (Nestorone) is effective for 2 years; another version (Elcometrine) lasts 6 months.[16]

References

1. **Shastri PV,** Toxicology of polymers for implant contraceptives in women, Contraception 65:9, 2002.

2. **Huber J, Wenzl R,** Pharmacokinetics of Implanon. An integrated analysis, Contraception 58(Suppl):85S, 1998.

3. **Egberg N, van Beek A, Gunnervik C, Hulkko S, Hirvonen E, Larsson-Cohn U, Bennink HC,** Effects on the hemostatic sytem and liver function in relation to Implanon® and Norplant®, Contraception 58:93, 1998.

4. **Affandi B,** An integrated analysis of vaginal bleeding patterns in clinical trials of Implanon®, Contraception 58:99S, 1998.

5. **Urbancsek J,** An integrated analysis of nonmenstrual adverse events with Implanon®, Contraception 58(Suppl):109S, 1998.

6. **Zheng S-R, Zheng H-M, Qian S-Z, Sang G-W, Kaper RF,** A randomized multicenter study comparing the efficacy and bleeding pattern of a single-rod (Implanon®) and a six-capsule (Norplant®) hormonal contraceptive implant, Contraception 60:1, 1999.

7. **Haukkamaa M,** Contraception by Norplant subdermal capsules is not reliable in epileptic patients on anticonvulsant treatment, Contraception 33:559, 1986.

8. **Sivin I,** International experience with Norplant and Norplant-2 contraceptives, Stud Fam Plann 19:81, 1988.

9. **Woolrych MH, Hill R,** Unintended pregancies with the etonogestrel implant (Implanon): a case series from post-marketing experience in Australia, in press.

10. **Markarainen L, van Beek A, Tuomiyaara L, Asplund B, Bennink HC,** Ovarian function during the use of a single contraceptive implant (Implanon) compared with Norplant, Fertil Steril 69:714, 1998.

11. **Brache V, Faundes A, Johansson E, Alvarez F,** Anovulation, inadequate luteal phase, and poor sperm penetration in cervical mucus during prolonged use of Norplant implants, Contraception 31:261, 1985.

12. **Dunson TR, Blumenthal PD, Alvarez F, Brache V, Cochon L, Dalberth B, Glover L, Remsburg R, Vu K, Katz D,** Timing of onset of contraceptive effectiveness in Norplant implant users. Part I. Changes in cervical mucus, Fertil Steril 69:258, 1998.

13. **Brache V, Alvarez-Sanchez F, Faundes A, Tejada AS, Cochon L,** Ovarian endocrine function through five years of continuous treatment with Norplant subdermal contraceptive implants, Contraception 41:169, 1990.

14. **Affandi B, Cekan S, Boonkasemanti R, Samil RS, Diczfalusy E,** The interaction between sex hormone binding globulin and levonorgestrel released from Norplant, an implantable contraceptive, Contraception 35:135, 1987.

15. **Alvarez F, Brache V, Tejada AS, Faundes A,** Abnormal endocrine profile among women with confirmed or presumed ovulation during long-term Norplant use, Contraception 33:111, 1986.

16. **Meirik O, d'Arcangues C, for the WHO Consultation on Implantable Contraceptives for Women,** Implantable contraceptives for women, Hum Reprod Update 9:49, 2003.

17. **Croxatto HB, Mäkäräinen L,** The pharmacodynamics and efficacy of Implanon®, Contraception 58:91S, 1998.

18. **Makarainen L, van Beek A, Tuomivaara L, Asplund B, Coelingh Bennink H,** Ovarian function during the use of a single contraceptive implant: Implanon compared with Norplant, Fertil Steril 69:714, 1998.

19. **Croxatto HB, Diaz S, Salvatierra AM, Morales P, Ebensperger C, Brandeis A,** Treatment with Norplant subdermal implants inhibits sperm penetration through cervical mucus in vitro, Contraception 36:193, 1987.

20. **Segal SJ, Alvarez-Sanchez F, Brache V, Faundes A, Vilja P, Tuohimaa P,** Norplant implants: the mechanism of contraceptive action, Fertil Steril 56:273, 1991.

21. **Shaaban MM, Salem HT, Abdullah KA,** Influence of levonorgestrel contraceptive implants, Norplant, initiated early postpartum, upon lactation and infant growth, Contraception 32:623, 1985.

22. **Diaz S, Herreros C, Juez G, Casado ME, Salvatierra AM, Miranda P, Peralta O, Croxatto HB,** Fertility regulation in nursing women: influence of Norplant levonorgestrel implants upon lactation and infant growth, Contraception 32:53, 1985.

23. **Reinprayoon D, Taneepanichskul S, Bunyavejchevin S, Thaithumyanon P, Punnahitananda S, Tosukhowong P, Machielsen C, van Beek A,** Effects of the etonogestrel-releasing contraceptive implant (Implanon) on parameters of breastfeeding compared to those of an intrauterine device, Contraception 62:239, 2000.

24. **Sivin I, Stern J, Diaz S, Pavez M, Alvarez F, Brache V, Mishell Jr DR, Lacarra M, McCarthy T, Holma P, Darney P, Klaisle C, Olsson S-E, Odlind V,** Rates and outcomes of planned pregnancy after use of Norplant capsules, Norplant II rods, or levonorgestrel-releasing or copper TCu 380Ag intrauterine contraceptive devices, Am J Obstet Gynecol 166:1208, 1992.

25. **Diaz S, Pavez M, Cardenas H, Croxatto HB,** Recovery of fertility and outcome of planned pregnancies after the removal of Norplant subdermal implants or copper-T IUDs, Contraception 35:569, 1987.

26. **Croxatto HB,** Clinical profile of Implanon: a single-rod etonogestrel contraceptive implant, Eur J Contracept Reprod Health Care 5(Suppl 2):21, 2000.

27. **Kjos SL, Peters RK, Xiang A, Thomas D, Schaefer U, Buchanan TA,** Contraception and the risk of type 2 diabetes in Latino women with prior gestational diabetes, JAMA 280:533, 1998.

28. **Darney PD, Elizabeth A, Tanner S, MacPherson S, Hellerstein S, Alvardo A,** Acceptance and perceptions of Norplant among users in San Francisco, USA, Stud Fam Plann 21:152, 1990.

29. **Dunson TR, Amatya RN, Krueger SL,** Complications and risk factors associated with the removal of Norplant implants, Obstet Gynecol 85:543, 1995.

30. **Brache V, Faundes A, Alvarez F, Cochon L,** Non-menstrual adverse events during use of implantable contraceptives for women: data from clinical trials, Contraception 65:63, 2002.

31. **Darney PD, Callegari LS, Swift A, Atkinson ES, Robert AM,** Condom practices of urban teens using Norplant contraceptive implants, oral contraceptives, and condoms for contraception, Am J Obstet Gynecol 180:929, 1999.

32. **Trussell J, Leveque JA, Koenig JD, London R, Borden S, Henneberry J, LaGuardia KD, Stewart F, Wilson TG, Wysocki S, Strauss M,** The economic value of contraception: a comparison of 15 methods, Am J Public Health 85:494, 1995.

33. **Croxatto HB, Urbancsek J, Massai R, Coelingh Bennink H, van Beek A,** A multicentre efficacy and safety study of the single contraceptive implant Implanon. Implanon Study Group, Hum Reprod 14:976, 1999.

34. **Berenson AB, Wiemann CM, Rickerr VI, McCombs SL,** Contraceptive outcomes among adolescents prescribed Norplant implants versus oral contraceptives after one year of use, Am J Obstet Gynecol 176:586, 1997.

35. **Zibners A, Cromer BA, Hayes J,** Comparison of continuation rates for hormonal contraception among adolescents, J Pediatr Adolesc Gynecol 12:90, 1999.

36. **Trussell J, Vaughan B,** Contraceptive failure, method-related discontinuation and resumption of use: results from the 1995 National Survey of Family Growth, Fam Plann Perspect 31:64, 1999.

37. **Fu H, Darroch JE, Haas T, Ranjit N,** Contraceptive failure rates: new estimates from the 1995 National Survey of Family Growth, Fam Plann Perspect 31:58, 1999.

38. **Affandi B, Korver T, Geurts TB, Coelingh Bennink JH,** A pilot efficacy study with a single-rod contraceptive implant (Implanon) in 200 Indonesian women treated for < or = 4 years, Contraception 59:167, 1999.

39. **Brache V, Blumenthal PD, Alvarez F, Dunson TR, Cochon L, Faundes A,** Timing of onset of contraceptive effectiveness in Norplant® implant users. II. Effect on the ovarian function in the first cycle of use, Contraception 59:245, 1999.

40. **Centers for Disease Control and Prevention,** Ectopic pregnancy — United States, 1988–1989, MMWR 41:591, 1992.

41. **Franks AL, Beral V, Cates W, Jr., Hogue CJ,** Contraception and ectopic pregnancy risk, Am J Obstet Gynecol 163:1120, 1990.

42. **Sivin I, Alvarez-Sanchez F, Diaz S, Holma P, Coutinho E, McDonald O, Robertson DN, Stern J,** Three-year experience with Norplant subdermal contraception, Fertil Steril 39:799, 1983.

43. **Shoupe D, Mishell Jr DR, Bopp B, Fiedling M,** The significance of bleeding patterns in Norplant implant users, Obstet Gynecol 77:256, 1991.

44. **Sivin I, Diaz S, Holma P, Alvarez-Sanchez F, Robertson DN,** A four-year clinical study of Norplant implants, Stud Fam Plann 14:184, 1983.

45. **Runic R, Schatz F, Krey L, Demopoulos R, Thung S, Wan L, Lockwood CJ,** Alterations in endometrial stromal cell tissue factor protein and messenger ribonucleic acid expression in patients experiencing abnormal uterine bleeding while using Norplant-2 contraception, J Clin Endocrinol Metab 82:1983, 1997.

46. **Hickey M, Simbar M, Young L, Markham R, Russell P, Fraser IS,** A longitudinal study of changes in endometrial microvascular density in Norplant® implant users, Contraception 59:123, 1999.

47. **Mascarenhas L, van Beek A, Bennink H, Newton J,** A 2-year comparative study of endometrial histology and cervical cytology of contraceptive implant users in Birmingham, UK, Hum Reprod 13:3057, 1998.

48. **Nilsson C, Holma P,** Menstrual blood loss with contraceptive subdermal levonorgestrel implants, Fertil Steril 35:304, 1981.

49. **Fakeye O, Balogh S,** Effect of Norplant contraceptive use on hemoglobin, packed cell volume, and menstrual bleeding patterns, Contraception 39:265, 1989.

50. **Fraser IS, Weisberg E, Minehan E, Johansson ED,** A detailed analysis of menstrual blood loss in women using Norplant® and Nestorone® progestin-only contraceptive implants or vaginal rings, Contraception 61:241, 2000.

51. **International Collaborative Post-Marketing Surveillance of Norplant,** Post-marketing surveillance of Norplant® contraceptive implants: I. Contraceptive efficacy and reproductive health, Contraception 63:167, 2001.

52. **Diaz S, Croxatto HB, Pavez M, Belhadj H, Stern J, Sivin I,** Clinical assessment of treatments for prolonged bleeding in users of Norplant implants, Contraception 42:97, 1990.

53. **Kaewrudee S, Taneepanichskul S, Jaisamraun U, Reinprayoon D,** The effect of mefenamic acid on controlling irregular uterine bleeding secondary to Norplant® use, Contraception 60:25, 1999.

54. **Alvarez-Sanchez F, Brache V, Thevenin F, Cochon L, Faundes A,** Hormonal treatment for bleeding irregularities in Norplant implant users, Am J Obstet Gynecol 174:919, 1996.

55. **Shaaban MM, Elwan SI, El-Sharkawy MM, Farghaly AS,** Effect of subdermal lenonorgestrel contraceptive implants, Norplant, on liver functions, Contraception 30:407, 1984.

56. **Singh K, Viegas OAC, Liew D, Singh P, Ratnam SS,** Two-year follow-up of changes in clinical chemistry in Singaporean Norplant acceptors: metabolic changes, Contraception 39:129, 1989.

57. **Shaaban MM, Elwan SI, El-Kabsh MY, Farghaly SA, Thabet N,** Effect of levonorgestrel contraceptive implants, Norplant, on bleeding and coagulation, Contraception 30:421, 1984.

58. **Singh K, Viegas OAC, Koh SCL, Ratnam SS,** Effect of long-term use of Norplant implants on haemostatic function, Contraception 45:203, 1992.

59. **Viegas OAC, Koh SLC, Ratnam SS,** The effects of reformulated 2-rod Norplant implant on haemostasis after three years, Contraception 54:219, 1996.

60. **Croxatto HB, Diaz S, Robertson D, Pavez M,** Clinical chemistries in women treated with levonorgestrel implant (Norplant) or a TCu 200 IUD, Contraception 27:281, 1983.

61. **Abdulla K, Elwan SI, Salem HS, Shaaban MM,** Effect of early postpartum use of the contraceptive impants, Norplant, on the serum levels of immunoglobulin of the mothers and their breastfed infants, Contraception 32:261, 1985.

62. **Bayad M, Ibrahim I, Fayad M, Hassanein AA, Hafez ES, Abdalla MI,** Serum cortisol in women users of subdermal levonorgestrel implants, Contracept Delivery Syst 4:133, 1983.

63. **Roy S, Mishell Jr DR, Robertson D, Krauss RM, Lacarra M, Duda MJ,** Long-term reversible contraception with levonorgestrel-releasing Silastic rods, Am J Obstet Gynecol 148:1006, 1984.

64. **Otubu JAM, Towobola OA, Aisien AO, Ogunkeye OO,** Effects of Norplant contraceptive subdermal implants on serum lipids and lipoproteins, Contraception 47:149, 1993.

65. **Konje JC, Otolorin EO, Ladipo OA,** Changes in carbohydrate metabolism during 30 months on Norplant, Contraception 44:163, 1991.

66. **Koopersmith TB, Lobo RA,** Insulin sensitivity is unaltered by the use of the Norplant subdermal implant contraceptive, Contraception 51:197, 1995.

67. **Harper MA, Meis PJ, Steele L,** A prospective study of insulin sensitivity and glucose metabolism in women using a continuous subdermal levonorgestrel implant system, J Soc Gynecol Invest 4:86, 1997.

197

68. **Meirik O, Farley TMM, Sivin I, for the International Collaborative Post-Marketing Surveillance of Norplant,** Safety and efficacy of levonorgestrel implant, intrauterine device, and sterilization, Am J Obstet Gynecol 97:539, 2001.

69. **Suherman SK, Affandi B, Korver T,** The effects of Implanon on lipid metabolism in comparison with Norplant, Contraception 60:281, 1999.

70. **Mascarenhas L, van Beek A, Bennink H, Newton J,** Twenty-four month comparison of apolipoproteins A-1, A-II and B in contraceptive implant users (Norplant and Implanon) in Birmingham, United Kingdom, Contraception 58:215, 1998.

71. **Biswas A, Viegas OA, Bennink HJ, Korver T, Ratnam SS,** Effect of Implanon use on selected parameters of thyroid and adrenal function, Contraception 62:247, 2000.

72. **Biswas A, Viegas OA, Coeling Bennink JH, Korver T, Ratnam SS,** Implanon contraceptive implants: effects on carbohydrate metabolism, Contraception 63:137, 2001.

73. **Biswas A, Viegas OA, Roy AC,** Effect of Implanon and Norplant subdermal contraceptive implants on serum lipids—a randomized comparative study, Contraception 68:189, 2003.

74. **Dorflinger L,** Metabolic effects of implantable steroid contraceptives for women, Contraception 65:47, 2002.

75. **Cromer BA, Blair JM, Mahan JD, Zibners L, Naumovski Z,** A prospective comparison of bone density in adolescent girls receiving depot medroxyprogesterone acetate (Depo-Provera), levonorgestrel (Norplant), or oral contraceptives, J Pediatr 129:671, 1996.

76. **Beerthuizen R, van Beek A, Massai R, Makarainen L, Hout J, Bennink HJ,** Bone mineral density during long-term use of the progestagen contraceptive implant Implanon compared to a non-hormonal method of contraception, Hum Reprod 15:118, 2000.

77. **Naessen T, Olsson SE, Gudmundson J,** Differential effects on bone density of progestogen-only methods for contraception in premenopausal women, Contraception 52:35, 1995.

78. **Di X, Li Y, Zhang C, Jiang J, Gu S,** Effects of levonorgestrel-releasing subdermal contraceptive implants on bone density and bone metabolism, Contraception 60:161, 1999.

79. **Petitti DB, Piaggio G, Mehta S, Cravioto MC, Meirik O, for the WHO Study of Hormonal Contraception and Bone Health,** Steroid hormone contraception and bone mineral density: a cross-sectional study in an international population, Obstet Gynecol 95:736, 2000.

80. **International Collaborative Post-Marketing Surveillance of Norplant,** Post-marketing surveillance of Norplant® contraceptive implants: II. Non-reproductive health, Contraception 63:187, 2001.

81. **Gu S, Du M, Zhang L, Liu YL, Wang SH, Sivin I,** A 5-year evaluation of Norplant contraceptive implants in China, Obstet Gynecol 83:673, 1994.

82. **Westhoff C, Truman C, Kalmuss D, Cushman L, Rulin M, Heartwell S, Davidson A,** Depressive symptoms and Norplant® contraceptive implants, Contraception 57:241, 1998.

83. **Wysowski DK, Green L,** Serious adverse events in Norplant users reported to the Food and Drug Administration's MedWatch Spontaneous Reporting System, Obstet Gynecol 85:538, 1995.

84. **Fraser IS, Tiitinen A, Affandi B, Brache V, Croxatto HB, Diaz S, Ginsburg J, Gu S, Holma P, Johansson E, Meirik O, Mishell Jr DR, Nash HA, von Schoultz B, Sivin I,** Norplant® consensus statement and background review, Contraception 57:1, 1998.

85. **Pasquale SA, Knuppel RA, Owens AG, Bachmann GA,** Irregular bleeding, body mass index and coital frequency in Norplant contraceptive users, Contraception 50:109, 1994.

86. **Faundes A, Brache V, Tejada AS, Cochon L, Alvarez-Sanchez F,** Ovulatory dysfunction during continuous administration of low-dose levonorgestrel by subdermal implants, Fertil Steril 56:27, 1991.

87. **Darney PD, Taylor RN, Klaisle C, Bottles K, Zaloudek C,** Serum concentrations of estradiol, progesterone, and levonorgestrel are not determinants of endometrial histology or abnormal bleeding in long-term Norplant implant users, Contraception 53:97, 1996.

88. **Phemister DA, Lauarent S, Harrison Jr FNH,** Use of Norplant contraceptive implants in the immediate postpartum period: safety and tolerance, Am J Obstet Gynecol 172:175, 1995.

89. **Darney PD, Klaisle CM, Tanner S, Alvarado AM,** Sustained-release contraceptives, Curr Prob Obstet Gynecol Fertil 13:95, 1990.

198

90. **Zimmerman M, Haffey J, Crane E, Szumowski D, Alvarez F, Bhiromrut P, Brache V, Lubis F, Salah M, Shaaban MM, Shawly B, Sidiip S,** Assessing the acceptability of Norplant implants in four countries: findings from focus group research, Stud Fam Plann 21:92, 1990.

91. **Mascarenhas L,** Insertion and removal of Implanon: practical considerations, Eur J Contracept Reprod Health Care 5(Suppl 2):29, 2000.

92. **Lantz A, Nosher JL, Pasquale S, Siegel RL,** Ultrasound characteristics of subdermally implanted Implanon contraceptive rods, Contraception 56:323, 1997.

93. **Merki-Feld GS, Brekenfeld C, Migge B, Keller P,** Nonpalpable ultrasonographically not detectable Implanon rods can be localized by magnetic resonance imaging, Contraception 63:325, 2001.

94. **Zieman M, Klaisle C, Walker D, Bahisteri E, Darney P,** Fingers versus instruments for removing levonorgestrel contraceptive implants (Norplant), J Gynecol Tech 3:213, 1997.

95. **Edwards JE, Moore A,** Implanon: a review of clinical studies, Br J Fam Plann 24(Suppl):3, 1999.

96. **Bromham DR, Davey A, Gaffikin L, Ajello CA,** Materials, methods and results of the Norplant training program, Br J Fam Plann 10:256, 1995.

97. **Klavon SL, Grubb G,** Insertion site complications during the first year of Norplant use, Contraception 41:27, 1990.

98. **Nelson AL,** Neutralizing pH of lidocaine reduces pain during Norplant system insertion procedures, Contraception 51:299, 1995.

99. **Blain S, Oloto E, Meyrick I, Bromham D,** Skin reactions following Norplant® insertion and removal—possible causative factors, Br J Fam Plann 21:130, 1996.

100. **Darney PD, Klaisle CM, Walker DM,** The pop-out method of Norplant removal, Adv Contraception 8:188, 1992.

101. **Glauser SJ, Scharling ES, Stovall TG, Zagoria RJ,** Ultrasonography: usefulness in localization of the Norplant contraceptive implant system, J Ultrasound Med 14:411, 1995.

102. **Klaisle C, Zieman M, Allen J, Patel MD, Sickles EA, Darney PD,** Insertion, removal and imaging of subdermal contraceptive capsules, Am J Obstet Gynecol in press, 2000.

103. **Praptohardjo U, Wibowo S,** The "U" technique: a new method for Norplant implants removal, Contraception 48:526, 1993.

104. **Frank ML, Ditmore JR, Llegbodu AE, Bateman L, Poindexter III AN,** Characteristics and experiences of American women electing for early removal of contraceptive implants, Contraception 52:159, 1995.

105. **Smith A, Reuter S,** An assessment of the use of Implanon in three community services, J Fam Plann Reprod Health Care 28:193, 2002.

106. **Gu S, Sivin I, Du M, Zhang L, Ying-Lin L, Meng F, Wu S, Wang P, Gao Y, He X, Qi L, Chen C, Liu Y, Wang D,** Effectiveness of Norplant implants through seven years: a large-scale study in China, Contraception 52:99, 1995.

107. **Reuter S, Smith A,** Implanon: user views in the first year across three family planning services in the Trent Region, UK, Eur J Contracept Reprod Health Care 8:27, 2003.

108. **Salah M, Ahmed A, Abo-Eloyoun M, Shaaban MM,** Five-year experience with Norplant implants in Assiut, Egypt, Contraception 35:543, 1987.

109. **Bashayake S, Thapa S, Balogh A,** Evaluation of safety, efficacy, and acceptability of Norplant implants in Sri Lanka, Stud Fam Plann 19:39, 1988.

110. **Dugoff L, Jones III OW, Allen-Davis J, Hurst BS, Schlaff WD,** Assessing the acceptability of Norplant contraceptive in four patient populations, Contraception 52:45, 1995.

111. **Sivin I, Mishell Jr DR, Darney P, Wan L, Christ M,** Levonorgestrel capsule implants in the United States: a 5-year study, Obstet Gynecol 92:337, 1998.

112. **Cromer BA, Smith RD, Blair JM, Dwyer J, Brown RT,** A prospective study of adolescents who choose among levonorgesterone implant (Norplant), medroxyprogesterone acetate (Depo-Provera), or the combined oral contraceptive pill as contraception, Pediatrics 94:687, 1994.

113. **Cullins VE, Remsburg RE, Blumenthal PD, Huggins GR,** Comparison of adolescent and adult experience with Norplant levonorgestrel contraceptive implants, Obstet Gynecol 83:1026, 1994.

114. **Polaneczky M, Slap G, Forke C, Rappaport A, Sondheimer S,** The use of levonorgestrel implants (Norplant) for contraception in adolescent mothers, New Engl J Med 331:1201, 1994.

115. **Berenson AB, Wiemann CM,** Use of levonorgestrel implants versus oral contraceptives in adolescence: a case-control study, Am J Obstet Gynecol 172:1128, 1995.

116. **Sivin I, Lähteenmäki P, Ranta S, Darney P, Klaisle C, Wan L, Mishell Jr DR, Lacarra M, Viegas OAC, Bilhareus P, Koetsawang S, Piya-Anant M, Diaz S, Pavez M, Alvarez F, Brache V, LaGuardia K, Nash H, Stern J,** Levonorgestrel concentrations during use of levonorgestrel rod (LNG ROD) implants, Contraception 55:81, 1997.

117. **Sivin I, Alvarez F, Mishell Jr DR, Darney P, Wan L, Brache V, Lacarra M, Klaisle C, Stern J,** Contraception with two levonorgestrel rod implants. A 5-year study in the United States and Dominican Republic, Contraception 58:275, 1998.

118. **Wan LS, Stiber A, Lam LY,** The levonorgestrel two-rod implant for long-acting contraception: 10 years of clinical experience, Obstet Gynecol 102:24, 2003.

119. **Coutinho EM,** One year contraception with a single subdermal implant containing nomegestrel acetate (Uniplant), Contraception 47:94, 1993.

120. **Haukkamaa M, Laurikka-Routti M, Heikinheimo O, Moo-Young A,** Contraception with subdermal implants releasing the progestin ST-1435: a dose-finding study, Contraception 45:49, 1992.

121. **Diaz S, Schiappacasse V, Pavez M, Zepeda A, Moo-Young AJ, Brandeis A, Lahteenmaki P, Croxatto HB,** Clinical trial with Nestorone subdermal contraceptive implants, Contraception 51:33, 1995.

200

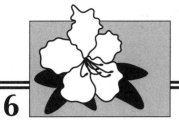

6

Injectable Contraception

D epot-medroxyprogesterone acetate is the most thoroughly studied progestin-only contraceptive. Although its approval for contraception in the United States is relatively recent (1992), it has been available in some countries since the mid-1960s. Much of our knowledge of the safety, efficacy, and acceptability of long-acting hormonal contraception comes from Indonesia, Sri Lanka, Thailand, and Mexico where depot-medroxyprogesterone acetate has been used and studied for decades. The long-delayed approval as a contraceptive in the United States was based on political and economic considerations not scientific ones.[1]

Depot-medroxyprogesterone acetate is formulated as microcrystals, suspended in an aqueous solution. The correct dose for contraceptive purposes is 150 mg intramuscularly (gluteal or deltoid) every 3 months. A comparative trial established that the 100-mg dose is significantly less effective.[2] The contraceptive level is maintained for at least 14 weeks, providing a safety margin for one of the most effective contraceptives available, about 1 pregnancy per 100 women after 5 years of consistent use.[2, 3] A newer formulation allows the self-administration of a subcutaneous dose of 104 mg every 3 months.[4-6]

Depot-medroxyprogesterone acetate is not a "sustained-release" system; it relies on higher peaks of progestin to inhibit ovulation and thicken cervical mucus. The difference between serum levels of progestins in a sustained-release system like Implanon and a depot system like depot-medroxyprogesterone acetate is illustrated in the diagram.

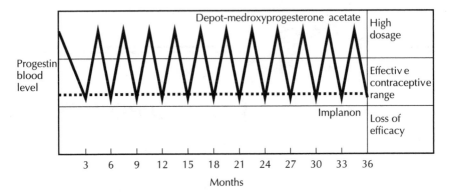

Other widely used injectables are norethindrone enanthate, 200 mg every 2 months, and the monthly injectables Lunelle (25 mg medroxyprogesterone acetate and 5 mg estradiol cypionate) and Mesigyna (50 mg norethindrone enanthate and 5 mg estradiol valerate).

Mechanism of Action

The mechanism of action of depot-medroxyprogesterone acetate is different from the other lower dose, progestin-only methods because, in addition to thickening of the cervical mucus and alteration of the endometrium, the circulating level of the progestin is high enough to effectively block the LH surge, and, therefore, ovulation does not occur.[7] Suppression of FSH is not as intense as with the combination oral contraceptive; therefore, follicular growth is maintained sufficiently to produce estrogen levels comparable to those in the early follicular phase of a normal menstrual cycle.[8] Symptoms of estrogen deficiency, such as vaginal atrophy or a decrease in breast size, do not occur.

Accidental pregnancies occurring at the time of the initial injection of depot-medroxyprogesterone acetate have been reported to be associated with higher neonatal and infant mortality rates, probably due to an increased risk of intrauterine growth restriction.[9, 10] The timing of the first injection is, therefore, very important. To ensure effective contraception, the first injection should be administered within the first 5 days of the menstrual cycle (before a dominant follicle emerges), or a backup method is necessary for 2 weeks.[5, 11–13] The duration of action can be shortened if attention is not paid to proper administration. The intramuscular injection must be given deeply by the Z-track technique and not massaged. It is prudent to avoid locations at risk for massage by daily activities.

Efficacy

The efficacy of this method (in both the intramuscular and subcutaneous formulations) is slightly better than that of sterilization and better than that of all the other temporary methods.[4-6, 14, 15] In a comparison of the intramuscular and subcutaneous methods, the blood levels of medroxyprogesterone acetate are approximately 30% lower with subcutaneous administration of the lower dose, but efficacy is not impaired.[5] Because serum concentrations are relatively high, efficacy is not influenced by weight (making this method a good choice for overweight women) or by the use of medications that stimulate hepatic enzymes.[5, 6] On the contrary, depot-medroxyprogesterone acetate is an excellent contraceptive choice for women taking antiepileptic drugs because the high progestin levels raise the seizure threshold.[16]

Failure Rates During the First Year of Use, United States[15, 17]

Method	Percent of Women with Pregnancy	
	Lowest Expected	Typical
No method	85.0%	85.0%
Combination pill	0.1	7.6
Progestin-only	0.5	3.0
IUDs		
Levonorgestrel IUD	0.1	0.1
Copper T 380A	0.6	0.8
Implant	0.05	0.2
Injectable	0.3	0.3

Indications

1. At least 1 year of birth spacing desired.
2. Highly effective long-acting contraception not linked to coitus.
3. Private, coitally independent method desired.
4. Estrogen-free contraception needed.
5. Breastfeeding.
6. Sickle cell disease.
7. Seizure disorder.

Absolute Contraindications

1. Pregnancy.
2. Unexplained genital bleeding.
3. Severe coagulation disorders.
4. Previous sex steroid-induced liver adenoma.

Relative Contraindications

1. Liver disease.
2. Severe cardiovascular disease.
3. Rapid return to fertility desired.
4. Difficulty with injections.
5. Severe depression.

Advantages

Like sustained-release forms of contraception, depot-medroxyprogesterone acetate is not associated with compliance problems and is not related to the coital event. Continuation rates are better and repeat pregnancy rates are reduced compared with oral contraceptive use in teenagers; however, continuation and repeat pregnancy rates are similar when adolescents begin these methods in the immediate postpartum period.[18, 19] Depot-medroxyprogesterone acetate is useful for women whose ability to remember contraceptive requirements is limited. It should be considered for women who lead disorganized lives or who are mentally retarded.

The freedom from the side effects of estrogen allows depot-medroxyprogesterone acetate to be considered for patients with congenital heart disease, sickle cell anemia, and a previous history of thromboembolism and for women over age 30 who smoke or have other risk factors such as hypertension or diabetes mellitus. The absolute safety in regard to thrombosis is mainly theoretical; it has not been proved in a controlled study. However, an increased risk of thrombosis has not been observed in epidemiologic evaluation of depot-medroxyprogesterone acetate users, and a World Health Organization (WHO) case-control study could find no evidence for increased risks of stroke, myocardial infarction, or venous thromboembolism.[3, 20]

Two case-control studies, one using data from the WHO Collaborative Study and one using the data from the U.K. general practice research database, assessed the risk of idiopathic venous thrombosis in users of progestins alone for therapeutic purposes, not for contraception, and concluded that therapeutic progestins alone may be associated with an increased risk of venous thromboembolism.[21, 22] These epidemiologic conclusions were based on extremely small numbers (only 3 cases in one report and 5 in the other) and had very wide confidence intervals. Patients who receive progestin only for therapeutic reasons are probably older and are more likely to have family histories of cardiovascular disease. In addition, a problem of preferential prescribing is present in that clinicians are more likely to promote the use of progestin only for women they perceive to be at greater risk of venous thromboembolism. Thus, it is likely that the case groups represented a higher risk group than the control groups in these reports. For these reasons, we do not believe progestins are associated with an increased risk of venous thromboembolism.

An important advantage exists for patients with sickle cell disease because evidence indicates an inhibition of in vivo sickling with hematologic improvement during treatment.[23] Both the frequency and the intensity of painful sickle cell crises are reduced.[24]

Another advantage is the finding that depot-medroxyprogesterone acetate increases the quantity of milk in nursing mothers, a direct contrast to the effect seen with combination oral contraception. The concentration of the drug in the breast milk is negligible, and no effects of the drug on infant growth and development have been observed.[25–27] In a careful study of male infants being breastfed by women treated with depot-medroxyprogesterone acetate, no metabolites of depot-medroxyprogesterone acetate could be detected in the infant's urine and no alterations could be observed in the infant levels of FSH, LH, testosterone, and cortisol.[28] Because of the slight positive impact on lactation, depot-medroxyprogesterone acetate can be administered immediately after delivery. A study to investigate the impact of early initiation found no adverse effects on breastfeeding.[29] In breast-feeding, overweight, Latina women with prior gestational diabetes, the progestin-only oral minipill was associated with a 3-fold increased risk of noninsulin dependent diabetes mellitus.[30] It is not known whether this might be a risk in all women who have experienced gestational diabetes or with all progestin-only methods; a prudent course would be to advise other methods for this special group of women.

As noted, depot-medroxyprogesterone acetate should be considered in patients with seizure disorders; an improvement in seizure control can be achieved probably because of the sedative properties of progestins.[16]

Other benefits associated with depot-medroxyprogesterone acetate use include a decreased risk of endometrial cancer comparable with that observed with oral contraceptives[31] and probably the same benefits associated with the progestin impact of oral contraceptives: reduced menstrual flow and anemia, less pelvic inflammatory disease (PID), less endometriosis, fewer uterine fibroids,[32] and fewer ectopic pregnancies. A failure to document a reduced risk of ovarian cancer by the World Health

Organization probably reflects the study's low statistical power and the high parity in the depot-medroxyprogesterone acetate users.[33]

Depot-medroxyprogesterone acetate, like oral contraception, may reduce the risk of pelvic inflammatory disease; however, the only study was hampered by small numbers.[34] Suppression of ovulation means that ectopic pregnancies are abolished and ovarian cysts are rare.

The greater the number of choices that women have, the more likely they are to find a contraceptive that works well for them. For some women the primary advantages of depot-medroxyprogesterone acetate are privacy and ease of use. No one but the user need know about the injection, and the 3-month schedule can be easy to maintain for women who do not mind injections. In some societies, injections are respected as efficacious, and depot-medroxyprogesterone acetate is the most popular contraceptive despite bleeding changes and other side effects.

Summary of Advantages

1. Easy to use, no daily or coital action required.
2. Safe, no serious health effects.
3. Very effective, as effective as sterilization, intrauterine contraception, and implant contraception.
4. Free from estrogen-related problems.
5. Private, use not detectable.
6. Lactation enhanced.
7. Noncontraceptive benefits.

Problems With Depot-Medroxyprogesterone Acetate

Major problems with depot-medroxyprogesterone acetate are irregular menstrual bleeding, breast tenderness, weight gain, and depression.[2, 3] By far, the most common problem is the change in menstrual bleeding. Up to 25% of patients discontinue in the first year because of irregular bleeding.[35] The bleeding is rarely heavy; in fact, hemoglobin values rise in depot-medroxyprogesterone acetate users. The incidence of irregular bleeding is 70% in the first year and 10% thereafter. Bleeding and spotting decrease progressively with each reinjection so that after 5 years, 80% of users are amenorrheic (compared with 10% of Norplant users).[36] With the subcutaneous preparation, the bleeding pattern is similar to that with the intramuscular product, and 55% achieve amenorrhea at the end of the first year of treatment.[4, 6] Irregular bleeding can be disturbing and annoying, and, for many patients, it inhibits sexuality; therefore, most users prefer the amenorrhea that comes with prolonged use.

If necessary, breakthrough bleeding can be treated with exogenous estrogen, 1.25 mg conjugated estrogens, or 2 mg estradiol, given daily for 7 days. A nonsteroidal antiinflammatory product given for a week is also effective, and another option is to administer an oral contraceptive for 1–3 months. Giving the depot-medroxyprogesterone acetate injection earlier (more frequently) does not change the bleeding pattern.[37] Most women can wait for amenorrhea without treatment if they know what to expect with time. Trying to regulate breakthrough bleeding with cyclic, repeated estradiol exposure has proved to be ineffective.[38]

About one-third of patients discontinue depot-medroxyprogesterone acetate by the end of 1 year, 50% by the end of 2 years, and about 80% by the end of 3 years.[39] The 1-year continuation rate in Texas public clinics was only 29%, much lower than reported elsewhere.[40] In a large international study, the most common medical reasons for discontinuing depot-medroxyprogesterone acetate during the first 2 years of use were the following:[3]

1. Headaches   —   2.3%
2. Weight gain   —   2.1%
3. Dizziness   —   1.2%
4. Abdominal pain   —   1.1%
5. Anxiety   —   0.7%

In Western societies, depression, fatigue, decreased libido, and hypertension are also encountered. Whether medroxyprogesterone acetate causes these side effects is difficult to know because they are very common complaints in nonusers as well.[41] When studied closely, no increase in depressive symptoms can be observed, even in women with significant complaints of depression prior to treatment.[42, 43]

Attempts to document a greater weight gain specifically associated with depot-medroxyprogesterone acetate have had mixed results, some finding no increase and others a small increase (e.g., about 4 kg over 5 years in one and 11 kg over 10 years in another).[44–47] In a placebo-controlled experiment, depot-medroxyprogesterone acetate had no effects on food intake, energy expenditure, or body weight.[48] With the subcutaneous method, an average weight gain of 1.5 kg was observed after one year.[4, 6] As with oral contraception, the weight gain may not be hormone-induced but reflect lifestyle and aging. On the other hand, specific individuals and certain ethnic groups may be more susceptible to weight gain; for example, significant weight gain was reported in Navajo women using depot-medroxyprogesterone acetate.[49]

Remember that if symptoms are truly due to the progestin, unlike pills and implants, depot-medroxyprogesterone acetate takes 6–8 months to be gone after the last injection.[5] Clearance is slower in heavier women. Approximately half of women who discontinue depot-medroxyprogesterone acetate can expect normal menses to return in 6 months after the last injection, but 25% wait a year before resumption of a normal pattern.[5, 36]

Several prospective studies have suggested that the use of depot-medroxyprogesterone acetate is associated with an increased risk of cervical infections, especially chlamydia.[50–52] This finding could very well be influenced by the inability to performed a randomized trial and reflect the difficulty in matching users and nonusers. The women who chose to use depot-medroxyprogesterone acetate in these cohort studies were notably different in their socioeconomic status, contraceptive practices, and sexual histories; thus, the results could reflect a higher rate of infection in the user group at baseline.

Anaphylaxis. As of 2004, there have been 3 case reports of anaphylactic shock within minutes after receiving intramuscular injections of depot-medroxyprogesterone aceate.[53–55] The reactions were most likely to one of the inert substances present in the injections: parabens, polyethylene glycols, and polysorbates. Depot-medroxyprogesterone acetate injections are best given by trained personnel in a clinic or office setting with resuscitation equipment and drugs available.

Breast Cancer

Medroxyprogesterone acetate, in large continuous doses, produced breast tumors in beagle dogs (perhaps because in dogs progestins stimulate growth hormone secretion, known to be a mammotrophic agent in dogs).[56] This is an effect unique with dogs and has not appeared in women after years of use. A very large, hospital-based, case-control WHO study conducted over 9 years in 3 developing countries indicated that exposure to depot-medroxyprogesterone acetate is associated with a very slightly increased risk in breast cancer in the first 4 years of use, but there was no evidence for an increase in risk with increasing duration of use.[57] The number of cases with recent use was not large, and the confidence intervals reflected this. A possible explanation for this finding is the combination of detection/surveillance bias and accelerated growth of an already present tumor, a situation similar to those described with oral contraceptives (Chapter 2) and postmenopausal hormone therapy.

Two earlier population-based, case-control studies indicated a possible association between breast cancer and depot-medroxyprogesterone acetate.

One, from Costa Rica, was based on only 19 cases.[58] The other, from New Zealand, did not find an increased relative risk in long-term users but did find an indication of increased risk shortly after initiating use at an early age, younger than age 25.[59] A pooled analysis of the WHO and New Zealand data indicated that the highest risk was in women who had received a single injection.[60] The risk, if real, is very slight, and it is equally possible that the suggestions of increased risk based on a small number of cases have not been free of confounding variables. A case-control study from Cape Town, South Africa, found no overall increase in the risk of breast cancer and no effect of increasing duration of use or recent use.[61] Because recent use may be the key factor, it is appropriate to emphasize that all of these studies did not find evidence for an overall increased risk of breast cancer, and the risk did not increase with duration of use. However, clinicians should consider informing patients that depot-medroxyprogesterone acetate might accelerate the growth of an already present occult cancer. We would expect such tumors to be detected at an earlier stage and grade of disease and to be associated with a better outcome.

Other Cancers

An increased risk of cervical dysplasia cannot be documented even with long-term use (4 or more years).[62] No increase in adenocarcinoma or adenosquamous carcinoma of the cervix could be detected in the WHO study.[63] The WHO study has not detected an increased risk of invasive squamous cell cancer of the cervix in depot-medroxyprogesterone acetate users; however, the risk of cervical carcinoma in situ was slightly elevated in the WHO case-control study, and it is not certain whether this is a real finding or a consequence of unrecognized biases, especially detection bias.[64, 65] In New Zealand, a modest increase in the risk of cervical dysplasia among users of depot-medroxyprogesterone acetate could be attributed to an increased prevalence of known risk factors for dysplasia among women who choose this method of contraception.[62] Nevertheless, it is prudent to insist on annual Pap smear surveillance in all users of contraception, no matter what method. Women at higher risk because of their sexual behavior (multiple partners, history of STIs) should have Pap smears every 6 months. An immature cellular pattern in Pap smears from long-term depot-medroxyprogesterone acetate users can suggest the presence of squamous intraepithelial premalignant lesions, but biopsies in these cases reveal epithelial atrophy.[66]

As noted, depot-medroxyprogesterone acetate is associated with a reduction in the risk of endometrial cancer, and there is probably a modest reduction in the risk of ovarian cancer. There is no evidence that liver cancer risk is changed by the use of depot-medroxyprogesterone acetate.[67]

Metabolic Effects

The impact of depot-medroxyprogesterone acetate on the lipoprotein profile is uncertain. Although some fail to detect an adverse impact and claim that this is due to the avoidance of a first-pass through effect in the liver, others have demonstrated a decrease in HDL-cholesterol and increases in total cholesterol and LDL-cholesterol.[68, 69] In a multicenter clinical trial by the World Health Organization, a transient adverse impact was present only in the few weeks after injection when blood levels were high.[70] The clinical impact of these changes, if any, have yet to be reported. It seems prudent to monitor the lipid profile annually in women using depot-medroxyprogesterone acetate for long durations. The emergence of significant adverse changes in LDL-cholesterol and HDL-cholesterol warrant reconsideration of contraceptive choice.

There are no clinically significant changes in carbohydrate metabolism or in coagulation factors.[71, 72] There are no studies available assessing the impact of depot-medroxyprogesterone acetate in women with diabetes mellitus or in women with previous gestational diabetes.

Effect on Bone Density. Clinicians are concerned that the contraceptive use of depot-medroxyprogesterone acetate is associated with the loss of bone. This is attributed to the fact that blood levels of estrogen with depot-medroxyprogesterone acetate are relatively lower over a period of time compared with a normal menstrual cycle, an idea that is supported by the demonstration that estrogen treatment prevents the bone loss.[73] Lumbar and hip bone loss has been documented in cross-sectional studies.[74, 75] The first of two studies in New Zealand was relatively small (30 women), but the second involved 200 women. This bone loss has also been observed in women receiving a high oral dose of medroxyprogesterone acetate, 50 mg daily, a dose that suppresses LH, resulting in low estrogen levels.[76] Another study documented decreased bone density, enhanced by lower body weight and duration of amenorrhea.[77] An American cross-sectional study indicated a greater bone loss with increasing duration of use, especially in younger women, 18–21 years old.[78]

The degree of bone loss in the previously mentioned studies is not as severe as that observed in the early postmenopausal years. Furthermore, this amount of bone loss is not so great that it cannot be regained. Bone density measurements in women who stopped using depot-medroxyprogesterone acetate indicated that the loss was regained in the lumbar spine but not in the femoral neck within 2 years even after long-term use, but in another cohort of past users, both spinal density and hip density were restored 30 months after discontinuation.[79, 80] Most importantly, cross-sectional studies of postmenopausal women in New Zealand and a large multicenter, worldwide population could not detect a difference in bone density comparing former users of depot-medroxyprogesterone acetate to never users, indicating that any loss of bone during use is regained.[81, 82]

A definitive response to this clinical concern is not possible because not all studies are in agreement. Cross-sectional studies and two studies making comparisons with IUD and Norplant users in Thailand found no bone loss in long-term (greater than 3 years) users of depot-medroxyprogesterone acetate.[83–87] And most importantly, longitudinal, prospective studies of bone fail to document bone loss in users of depot-medroxyprogesterone acetate. In Thailand, loss of forearm bone density could not be detected over 3 years of depot-medroxyprogesterone acetate use, suggesting that previous adverse findings could be explained by inadequate control of factors that affect bone, such as smoking and alcohol intake.[84] A small prospective study documented stable forearm bone density over a 6-month period of time, and a 2-year study could not detect any loss in cortical or trabecular bone in the radius.[88, 89] A cross-sectional study in England could not detect a decrease in the bone density of the lumbar spine or the femoral neck despite relatively low estradiol levels in amenorrheic women who had been receiving depot-medroxyprogesterone acetate for 1 to 16 years.[90]

Bone density increases rapidly and significantly during adolescence. Almost all of the bone mass in the hip and the vertebral bodies is accumulated in young women by age 18, and the years immediately following menarche are especially important.[91, 92] For this reason any drug that prevents this increase in bone density may increase the risk of osteoporosis later in life. Studies in adolescents have documented bone loss compared to normal controls and young women using oral contraceptives.[93, 94] Do adolescents who use depot-medroxyprogesterone acetate regain bone density after discontinuing this method of contraception, or are adolescents at greater risk for osteoporosis compared with women who use depot-medroxyprogesterone acetate later in life?

An example of bone loss that is regained is the bone loss associated with lactation. Secretion of calcium into the milk of lactating women approximately doubles the daily loss of calcium.[95] In women who breastfeed for 6 months or more, this is accompanied by significant bone loss even in the presence of a high calcium intake.[96] However, bone density rapidly returns to baseline levels in the 6 months after weaning.[97] The bone loss is due to increased bone resorption, probably secondary to the relatively low estrogen levels associated with lactation. Calcium supplementation has no effect on the calcium content of breast milk or on bone loss in lactating women who have normal diets.[98] Thus, studies indicate that any loss of calcium and bone associated with lactation is rapidly restored; therefore, there is no impact on the risk of postmenopausal osteoporosis.[99, 100]

In 2004, the U.S. Food and Drug Administration indicated a concern for the bone loss associated with depot-medroxyprogesterone acetate and warned that this method should not be used longer than 2 years unless it was the only option. We agree that concern is appropriate, but disagree with the warning. The mixed results, the degree of bone loss, some evidence that the bone loss is regained, and the similarity to the benign bone loss associated with lactation all argue that the use of depot-medroxyprogesterone acetate should not be limited by this concern and that supplemental estrogen treatment is not indicated (and would influence and complicate compliance). This concern requires ongoing surveillance of past users. However, at the present time, in our view, this should not be a reason to avoid this method of contraception, and there is no need to impose a time limit on duration of use. ***It is unlikely that bone loss occurs sufficiently to raise the risk of osteoporosis later in life.***

Galactorrhea. Galactorrhea is not associated with the use of depot-medroxyprogesterone acetate. Prolactin gene transcription is stimulated by estrogen and mediated by estrogen receptor binding to estrogen responsive elements. The increase in prolactin during pregnancy parallels the increase in estrogen beginning at 7–8 weeks gestation, and the mechanism for increasing prolactin secretion is believed to be estrogen suppression of the hypothalamic prolactin-inhibiting factor, dopamine, and direct stimulation of prolactin gene transcription in the pituitary.[101, 102] Although requiring estrogen for prolactin secretion, prolactin stimulation of breast milk production is prevented by progestational agents and pharmacologic amounts of estrogen. Only colostrum (composed of desquamated epithelial cells and transudate) is produced during gestation. Full lactation is inhibited by progesterone, which interferes with prolactin action at the alveolar cell prolactin receptor level. Both estrogen and progesterone are necessary for the expression of the lactogenic receptor, but progesterone antagonizes the positive action of prolactin on its own receptor while progesterone and pharmacologic amounts of androgens reduce prolactin binding.[103–105] In the mouse, inhibition of milk protein production is due to progesterone suppression of prolactin receptor expression.[106] The effective use of high doses of estrogen to suppress postpartum lactation indicates that pharmacologic amounts of estrogen also block prolactin action. For these reasons, exposure to high levels of progestational agents, such as depot medroxyprogesterone acetate, is not associated with the clinical problem of galactorrhea.

Effect on Future Fertility

The delay in becoming pregnant after ceasing use of depot-medroxyprogesterone acetate is a problem unique to injectable contraception; all the other temporary methods allow a more prompt return to fertility.[107] However, depot-medroxyprogesterone acetate does not permanently suppress ovarian function, and the concern that infertility with suppressed menstrual function may be caused by depot-medroxyprogesterone acetate has not been supported by epidemiologic data. The pregnancy rate in women discontinuing the injections because of a desire to become pregnant is normal.[108] By 18 months after the last injection, 90% of depot-medroxyprogesterone acetate users have become pregnant, the same proportion as for other methods.[109] The delay to conception is about 9 months after the last injection, and the delay does not increase with increasing duration of use. Because of this delay, women who want to conceive promptly after discontinuing their contraceptive should not use depot-medroxyprogesterone acetate. Suppressed menstrual function persisting beyond 18 months after the last injection is not due to the drug and deserves evaluation.

Short-Term Injectable Contraceptives

Monthly or every-other-month injectable combinations of estrogen and progestin are not new, having been developed over several decades.[110] This method of contraception is popular in China, Latin America, and Eastern Asia. A preparation widely used in China consists of 250 mg 17α-hydroxyprogesterone caproate and 5 mg estradiol valerate, known as Chinese Injectable No.1.

Lunelle (or Cyclofem)

Lunelle consists of 25 mg depot-medroxyprogesterone acetate and 5 mg estradiol cypionate and is administered every 28–30 days (not to exceed 33 days) as a deep intramuscular injection. This method is as effective as depot-medroxyprogesterone acetate but avoids the problems of menstrual irregularity and heavy bleeding, as well as amenorrhea.[111–116] In addition, the method is rapidly reversible; fertility rates after discontinuation are similar to oral contraceptives.[117] Besides the need for a monthly injection, another disadvantage is the likelihood that the combination of estrogen and progestin inhibits lactation. The requirement for a monthly injection can be made more convenient by the use of an automatic device for self-administration.[118] Approximately 80% of women who are amenorrheic on depot-medroxyprogesterone acetate develop vaginal bleeding if switched to Lunelle.[119] The same contraindications, concerns, problems, and probably benefits reported with oral contraception should apply to Lunelle.

213

Norethindrone Ethanthate

Norethindrone enanthate is given in a dose of 200 mg intramuscularly every 2 months. This progestin acts in the same way as depot-medroxy-progesterone acetate and has the same problems.[3] A combination (Mesigyna) of norethindrone enanthate (50 mg) with estradiol valerate (5 mg) given monthly provides effective contraception with good cycle control.[120] Compared with Lunelle, Mesigyna has less bleeding problems.[121] Fertility returns rapidly (by 1 month) after discontinuation.[117]

Dihydroxyprogesterone Acetophenide and Estradiol Enanthate

The combination of 150 mg dihydroxyprogesterone acetophenide with 10 mg estradiol enanthate (various brand names) is the most widely used injectable contraceptive in Latin America. As with Mesigyna and Lunelle, the monthly regimen allows regular, and even reduced, cyclic bleeding.[122] A lower dose (90 mg dihydroxyprogesterone acetophenide and 6 mg estradiol enanthate) provides the same effective contraception as the higher dose with similar bleeding patterns.[123]

References

1. **Rosenfield A, Maine D, Rochat R, Shelton J, Hatcher R,** The Food and Drug Administration and medroxyprogesterone acetate: what are the issues? JAMA 249:2922, 1983.

2. **WHO,** A multicentered phase III comparative clinical trial of depot-medroxyprogesterone acetate given three-monthly at doses of 100 mg or 150 mg: I. Contraceptive efficacy and side effects, Contraception 34:223, 1986.

3. **WHO,** Multinational comparative clinical evaluation of two long-acting injectable contraceptive steroids: norethisterone enanthate and medroxyprogesterone acetate. Final report, Contraception 28:1, 1983.

4. **Darney P, Jain J, Jakimiuk AJ,** Zero pregnancies with new low dose depot medroxyprogesterone acetate subcutaneous injection for contraception (abstract), Fertil Steril 82:S105, 2004.

5. **Jain J, Dutton C, Nicosia A, Wajszeczuk C, Bode FR, Mishell DR, Jr.,** Pharmacokinetics, ovulation suppression and return to ovulation following a lower dose subcutaneous formulation of Depo-Provera, Contraception 70:11, 2004.

6. **Jain J, Jakimiuk AJ, Bode FR, Ross D, Kaunitz AM,** Contraceptive efficacy and safety of DMPA-SC, Contraception 70:269, 2004.

7. **Mishell Jr DR,** Effect of 6 methyl-17-hydroxyprogesterone on urinary excretion of luteinizing hormone, Am J Obstet Gynecol 99:86, 1967.

8. **Fraser IS, Weisberg EA,** A comprehensive review of injectable contraception with special emphasis on depot medroxyprogesterone acetate, Med J Aust 1(Suppl):3, 1981.

9. **Pardthaisong T, Gray RH,** In utero exposure to steroid contraceptives and outcome of pregnancy, Am J Epidemiol 134:795, 1991.

10. **Gray RH, Pardthaisong T,** In utero exposure to steroid contraceptives and survival during infancy, Am J Epidemiol 134:804, 1991.

11. **Siriwongse T, Snidvonga W, Tantayaporn P, Leepipalboon S,** Effect of depot-medroxyprogesterone acetate on serum progesterone levels, when administered on various cycle days, Contraception 26:487, 1982.

12. **Petta C, Faúndes A, Dunson TR, Ramos M, DeLucio M, Faúndes D, Bahamondes L,** Timing of onset of contraceptive effectiveness in Depo-Provera users. I. Changes in cervical mucus, Fertil Steril 69:252, 1998.

13. **Petta CA, Faúndes A, Dunson TR, Ramos M, DeLucio M, Faúndes D, Bahamondes L,** Timing of onset of contraceptive effectiveness in Depo-Provera users. II. Effects on ovarian function, Fertil Steril 70:817, 1998.

14. **Harlap S, Kost K, Forrest JD,** Preventing Pregnancy, Protecting Health: A New Look at Birth Control Choices in the United States, The Alan Guttmacher Institute, New York, 1991.

15. **Fu H, Darroch JE, Haas T, Ranjit N,** Contraceptive failure rates: new estimates from the 1995 National Survey of Family Growth, Fam Plann Perspect 31:58, 1999.

16. **Mattson RH, Cramer JA, Caldwell BV, Siconolfi BC,** Treatment of seizures with medroxyprogesterone acetate: preliminary report, Neurology 34:1255, 1984.

17. **Trussell J, Vaughan B,** Contraceptive failure, method-related discontinuation and resumption of use: results from the 1995 National Survey of Family Growth, Fam Plann Perspect 31:64, 1999.

18. **O'Dell CM, Forke CM, Polaneczky MM, Sondheimer SJ, Slap GB,** Depot medroxyprogesterone acetate or oral contraception in postpartum adolescents, Obstet Gynecol 91:609, 1998.

19. **Polaneczky M, Guarnaccia M, Alon J, Wiley J,** Early experience with the contraceptive use of depo-medroxyprogesterone acetate in an inner-city population, Fam Plann Perspect 28:174, 1996.

20. **World Health Organization Collaborative Study of Cardiovascular Disease and Steroid Hormone Contraception,** Cardiovascular disease and use of oral and injectable progestogen-only contraceptives and combined injectable contraceptives. Results of an international, multicenter, case-control study, Contraception 57:315, 1998.

21. **Poulter NR, Chang CL, Farley TMM, Meirik O,** Risk of cardiovascular diseases associated with oral progestagen preparations with therapeutic indications, Lancet 354:1610, 1999.

22. **Vasilakis C, Jick H, del Mar Melero-Montes M,** Risk of idiopathic venous thromboembolism in users of progestagens alone, Lancet 354:1610, 1999.

23. **DeCeular K, Gruber C, Hayes R, Serjeant GR,** Medroxyprogesterone acetate and homozygous sickle-cell disease, Lancet ii:229, 1982.

24. **de Abood M, de Castillo Z, Guerrero F, Espino M, Austin KL,** Effect of Depo-Provera® or Microgynon® on the painful crises of sickle-cell anemia patients, Contraception 56:313, 1997.

25. **Jimenez J, Ochoa M, Soler MP, Portales P,** Long-term follow-up of children breast-fed by mothers receiving depot-medroxyprogesterone acetate, Contraception 30:523, 1984.

26. **Zacharias S, Aguilena J, Assanzo JR, Zanatu J,** Effects of hormonal and non-hormonal contracepters on lactation and incidence of pregnancy, Contraception 33:203, 1986.

27. **Pardthaisong T, Yenchit C, Gray R,** The long-term growth and development of children exposed to Depo-Provera during pregnancy or lactation, Contraception 45:313, 1992.

28. **Virutamasen P, Leepipatpaiboon S, Kriengsinyot R, Vichaidith P, Muia PN, Sekadde-Kigondu CB, Mati JKG, Forest MG, Dikkeschei LD, Wolthers BG, d'Arcangues C,** Pharmacodynamic effects of depot-medroxyprogesterone acetate (DMPA) administered to lactating women on their male infants, Contraception 54:153, 1996.

29. **Halderman LD, Nelson AL,** Impact of early postpartum administration of progestin-only hormonal contraceptives compared with nonhormonal contraceptives on short-term breast-feeding patterns, Am J Obstet Gynecol 186:1250, 2002.

30. **Kjos SL, Peters RK, Xiang A, Thomas D, Schaefer U, Buchanan TA,** Contraception and the risk of type 2 diabetes in Latino women with prior gestational diabetes, JAMA 280:533, 1998.

31. **WHO** Collaborative Study of Neoplasia and Steroid Contraceptives, Depot-medroxyprogesterone acetate (DMPA) and risk of endometrial cancer, Int J Cancer 49:186, 1991.

32. **Lumbiganon P, Rugpao S, Phandhu-fung S, Laopaiboon M, Vudhikamraksa N, Werawatkul Y,** Protective effect of depot-medroxyprogesterone acetate on surgically treated uterine leiomyomas: a multicentre case-control study, Br J Obstet Gynaecol 103:909, 1996.

33. **WHO** Collaborative Study of Neoplasia and Steroid Contraceptives, Depot-medroxyprogesterone acetate (DMPA) and risk of epithelial ovarian cancer, Int J Cancer 49:191, 1991.

34. **Gray RH,** Reduced risk of pelvic inflammatory disease with injectable contraceptives, Lancet i:1046, 1985.

35. **Cromer BA, Smith RD, Blair JM, Dwyer J, Brown RT,** A prospective study of adolescents who choose among levonorgestrel implant (Norplant), medroxyprogesterone acetate (Depo-Provera), or the combined oral contraceptive pill as contraception, Pediatrics 94:687, 1994.

36. **Gardner JM, Mishell DR, Jr.,** Analysis of bleeding patterns and resumption of fertility following discontinuation of a long-acting injectable contraceptive, Fertil Steril 21:286, 1970.

37. **Harel Z, Biro FM, Kollar LM,** Depo-Provera in adolescents: effects of early second injection or prior oral contraception, J Adolesc Health 16:379, 1995.

38. **Goldberg AB, Cardenas LH, Hubbard AE, Darney PD,** Post-abortion depot medroxyprogesterone acetate continuation rates: a randomized trial of cyclic estradiol, Contraception 66:215, 2002.

39. **Smith RD, Cromer BA, Hayes JR, et al.,** Medroxyprogesterone acetate (Depo-Provera) use in adolescents: uterine bleeding and blood pressure patterns, patient satisfaction, and continuation rates, Adolesc Pediatr Gynecol 8:24, 1995.

40. **Sangi-Haghpeykar M, Poindexter AN, Bateman L, Ditmore JR,** Experiences of injectable contraceptive users in an urban setting, Obstet Gynecol 88:227, 1996.

41. **Westhoff C, Wieland D, Tiezzi L,** Depression in users of depo-medroxyprogesterone acetate, Contraception 51:351, 1995.

42. **Westhoff C, Truman C, Kalmuss D, Cushman L, Davidson A, Rulin M, Heartwell S,** Depressive symptoms and Depo-Provera, Contraception 57:237, 1998.

43. **Gupta N, O'Brien R, Jacobsen LJ, Davis A, Zuckerman A, Supran S, Kulig J,** Mood changes in adolescents using depot-medroxyprogesterone acetate for contraception: a prospective study, J Pediatr Adolesc Gynecol 14:71, 2001.

44. **Moore LL, Valuck R, McDougall C, Fink W,** A comparative study of one-year weight gain among users of medroxyprogesterone acetate, levonorgestrel implants, and oral contraceptives, Contraception 52:215, 1995.

45. **Mainwaring R, Hales HA, Stevenson K, Hatasaka HH, Poulson AM, Jones KP, Peterson CM,** Metabolic parameters, bleeding, and weight changes in U.S. women using progestin only contraceptives, Contraception 51:149, 1995.

46. **Taneepanichskul S, Reinprayoon D, Khaosaad P**, Comparative study of weight change between long-term DMPA and IUD acceptors, Contraception 58:149, 1998.

47. **Bahamondes L, Del Castillo S, Tabares G, Arce XE, Perrotti M, Petta C**, Comparison of weight increase in users of depot medroxyprogesterone acetate and copper IUD up to 5 years, Contraception 64:223, 2001.

48. **Pelkman CL, Chow M, Heinbach RA, Rolls BJ**, Short-term effects of a progestational contraceptive drug on food intake, resting energy expenditure, and body weight in young women, Am J Clin Nutr 73:19, 2001.

49. **Espey E, Steinhart J, Ogburn T, Qualls C**, Depo-provera associated with weight gain in Navajo women, Contraception 62:55, 2000.

50. **Jacobson DL, Peralta L, Farmer M, Graham NM, Gaydos C, Zenilman J**, Relationship of hormonal contraception and cervical ectopy as measured by computerized planimetry to chlamydial infection in adolescents, Sex Transm Dis 27:313, 2000.

51. **Baeten JM, Nyange PM, Richardson BA, Lavreys L, Chohan B, Martin HL, Mandaliya K, Nidinya-Achola JO, Bwayo JJ, Kreiss JK,** Hormonal contraception and risk of sexually transmitted disease acquisition: results form a prospective study, Am J Obstet Gynecol 185:380, 2001.

52. **Morrison CS, Bright P, Wong EL, Kwok C, Yacobson I, Gaydos CA, Tucker HT, Blumenthal PD,** Hormonal contraceptive use, cervical ectopy, and the acquisition of cervical infections, Sex Transm Dis 31:561, 2004.

53. **Brooks G,** Anaphylactoid shock with medroxyprogesterone acetate: a case report, J La State Med Soc 126:397, 1974.

54. **Rajapaksa DS,** Anaphylaxis to Depo-Provera? Ceylon Med J 38:158, 1993.

55. **Selo-Ojeme DO, Tillisi A, Welch CC,** Anaphylaxis from medroxyprogesterone acetate, Obstet Gynecol 103:1045, 2004.

56. **Jordan A,** Toxicology of depot medroxyprogesterone acetate, Contraception 49:18901, 1994.

57. **WHO** Collaborative Study of Neoplasia and Steroid Contraceptives, Breast cancer and depot-medroxyprogesterone acetate: a multinational study, Lancet 338:833, 1991.

58. **Lee NC, Rosero-Bixby L, Oberle MW, Grimaldo C, Whatley AS, Rovira EZ,** A case-control study of breast cancer and hormonal contraception in Costa Rica, J Natl Cancer Inst 79:1247, 1987.

59. **Paul C, Skegg DCG, Spears GFS,** Depot medroxyprogesterone (Depo-Provera) and risk of breast cancer, Br Med J 299:7591, 1989.

60. **Skegg DCG, Noonan EA, Paul C, Spears GFS, Meirik O, Thomas DB,** Depot-medroxyprogesterone acetate and breast cancer: a pooled analysis of the World Health Organization and the New Zealand studies, JAMA 273:799, 1995.

61. **Shapiro S, Rosenberg L, Hoffman M, Truter H, Cooper D, Rao S, Dent D, Gudgeon A, van Zyl J, Katzenellenbogen J, Bailie R,** Risk of breast cancer in relation to the use of injectable progestogen contraceptives and combined estrogen/progestogen contraceptives, Am J Epidemiol 151:396, 2000.

62. **The New Zealand Contraception and Health Study Group,** History of long-term use of depot-medroxyprogesterone acetate in patients with cervical dysplasia; case-control analysis nested in a cohort study, Contraception 50:443, 1994.

63. **Thomas DB, Ray RM, and the WHO Collaborative Study of Neoplasia and Steroid Contraceptives,** Depot-medroxyprogesterone acetate (DMPA) and risk of invasive adenocarcinomas and adenosquamous carcinomas of the uterine cervix, Contraception 52:307, 1995.

64. **WHO Collaborative Study of Neoplasia and Steroid Contraception,** Depot-medroxyprogesterone acetate (DMPA) and risk of invasive squamous cell cervical cancer, Contraception 45:299, 1992.

65. **Thomas DB, Ye Z, Ray RM, and the WHO Collaborative Study of Neoplasia and Steroid Contraception,** Cervical carcinoma in situ and use of depot-medroxyprogesterone acetate (DMPA), Contraception 51:25, 1995.

66. **Valente PT, Schantz HD, Trabal JF,** Cytologic changes in cervical smears associated with prolonged use of depot-medroxyprogesterone acetate, Cancer 84:328, 1998.

67. **WHO,** Depo-medroxyprogesterone acetate (DMPA) and cancer; memorandum from a WHO meeting, Bull World Health Organization 64:375, 1986.

68. **Garza-Fores J, De la Cruz DL, Valles de Bourges V, Sanchez-Nuncio R, Martinez M, Fuziwara JL, Perez-Palacios G,** Long-term effects of depot-medroxyprogesterone acetate on lipoprotein metabolism, Contraception 44:61, 1991.

69. **Enk L, Landgren BM, Lindberg U-B, Silverstolpe G, Crona N,** A prospective, one-year study on the effects of two long acting injectable contraceptives (depot-medroxyprogesterone acetate and norethisterone enanthate) on serum and lipoprotein lipids, Horm Metab Res 24:85, 1992.

70. **WHO,** A multicentre comparative study of serum lipids and apolipoproteins in long-term users of DMPA and a control group of IUD users, Contraception 47:177, 1993.

71. **Fahmy K, Khairy M, Allam G, Gobran F, Allush M,** Effect of depo-medroxyprogesterone acetate on coagulation factors and serum lipids in Egyptian women, Contraception 44:431, 1991.

72. **Fahmy K, Abdel-Razik M, Shaaraway M, Al-Kholy G, Saad S, Wagdi A, Al-Azzony M,** Effect of long-acting progestagen-only injectable contraceptives on carbohydrate metabolism and its hormonal profile, Contraception 44:419, 1991.

73. **Cundy T, Ames R, Horne A, Clearwater J, Roberts H, Gamble G, Reid IR,** A randomized controlled trial of estrogen replacement therapy in long-term users of depot-medroxyprogesterone acetate, J Clin Endocrinol Metab 88:78, 2003.

74. **Cundy T, Evans M, Roberts H, Wattie D, Ames R, Reid IR,** Bone density in women receiving depot-medroxyprogesterone acetate for contraception, Br Med J 303:13, 1991.

75. **Cundy T, Cornish J, Roberts H, Elder H, Reid IR,** Spinal bone density in women using depot-medroxyprogesterone contraception, Obstet Gynecol 92:569, 1998.

76. **Cundy T, Farquhar CM, Cornish J, Reid IR,** Short-term effects of high dose oral medroxyprogesterone acetate on bone density in premenopausal women, J Clin Endocrinol Metab 81:1014, 1996.

77. **Paiva LC, Pinto-Neto AM, Faúndes A,** Bone density among long-term users of medroxyprogesterone acetate as a contraceptive, Contraception 58:351, 1998.

78. **Scholes D, Lacroix AZ, Ott SM, Ichikawa LE, Barlow WE,** Bone mineral density in women using depot-medroxyprogesterone acetate for contraception, Obstet Gynecol 93:233, 1999.

79. **Cundy T, Cornish J, Evans MC, Roberts H, Reid IR,** Recovery of bone density in women who stop using medroxyprogesterone acetate, Br Med J 308:247, 1994.

80. **Scholes D, LaCroix AZ, Ichikawa LE, Barlow WE, Ott SM,** Injectable hormone contraception and bone density: results from a prospective study, Epidemiology 13:581, 2002.

81. **Orr-Walker BJ, Evans MC, Ames RW, Clearwater JM, Cundy T, Reid IR,** The effect of past use of the injectable contraceptive depot-medroxyprogesterone acetate on bone mineral density in normal post-menopausal women, Clin Endocrinol 49:615, 1998.

82. **Petitti DB, Piaggio G, Mehta S, Cravioto MC, Meirik O, for the WHO Study of Hormonal Contraception and Bone Health,** Steroid hormone contraception and bone mineral density: a cross-sectional study in an international population, Obstet Gynecol 95:736, 2000.

83. **Virutamasen P, Wangsuphachart S, Reinprayoon D, Kriengsinyot R, Leepipatpaiboon S, Gua C,** Trabecular bone in long-term depot-medroxyprogesterone acetate users, Asia Oceania J Obstet Gynaecol 20:269, 1994.

84. **Taneepanichskul S, Intaraprasert S, Theppisai U, Chaturachinda K,** Bone mineral density in long-term depot-medro-xyprogesterone acetate acceptors, Contraception 56:1, 1997.

85. **Taneepanichskul S, Intaraprasert S, Theppisai U, Chaturachinda K,** Bone mineral density during long-term treatment with Norplant implants and depot-medroxyprogesterone acetate, Contraception 56:153, 1997.

86. **Tharnprisarn W, Taneepanichskul S,** Bone mineral density in adolescent and young Thai girls receiving oral contraceptives compared with depot-medroxyprogsterone acetate: a cross-sectional study in young Thai women, Contraception 66:101, 2002.

87. **Perrotti M, Bahamondes L, Petta C, Castro S,** Forearm bone density in long-term users of oral combined contraceptives and depot-medroxyprogesteone acetate, Fertil Steril 76:469, 2001.

88. **Naessen T, Olsson SE, Gudmundson J,** Differential effects on bone density of progestogen-only methods for contraception in premenopausal women, Contraception 52:35, 1995.

218

89. **Merki-Feld GS, Neff M, Keller PJ,** A 2-year prospective study on the effects of depot-medroxyprogesterone acetate on bone mass—response to estrogen and calcium therapy in individual users, Contraception 67:79, 2003.

90. **Gbolade B, Ellis S, Murby B, Randall S, Kirkman R,** Bone density in long term users of depot-medroxyprogesterone acetate, Br J Obstet Gynaecol 105:790, 1998.

91. **Theitz G, Buch B, Rizzoli R, Slosman D, Clavien H, Sizonko PC, Bonjour JPH,** Longitudinal monitoring of bone mass accumulation in healthy adolescents: evidence for a marked reduction after 16 years of age at the levels of lumbar spine and femoral neck in female subjects, J Clin Endocrinol Metab 75:1060, 1992.

92. **Matkovic V, Jelic T, Wardlaw GM, Ilich J, Goel PK, Wright JK, Andon MB, Smith KT, Heaney RP,** Timing of peak bone mass in caucasian females and its implication for the prevention of osteoporosis: inference from a cross-sectional model, J Clin Invest 93:799, 1994.

93. **Cromer BA, Blair JM, Mahan JD, Zibners L, Naumovski Z,** A prospective comparison of bone density in adolescent girls receiving depot-medroxyprogesterone acetate (Depo-Provera), levonorgestrel (Norplant), or oral contraceptives, J Pediatr 129:671, 1996.

94. **Lara-Torre E, Edwards CP, Perlaman S, Hertweck SP,** Bone mineral density in adolescent females using depot medroxyprogesterone acetate, J Pediatr Adolesc Gynecol 17:17, 2004.

95. **Kumar R, Cohen WR, Epstein FH,** Vitamin D and calcium hormones in pregnancy, New Engl J Med 302:1143, 1980.

96. **Sowers M, Corton G, Shapiro B, Jannausch ML, Crutchfield M, Smith ML, Randolph JF, Hollis B,** Changes in bone density with lactation, JAMA 269:3130, 1993.

97. **Kalkwarf HJ, Specker BL,** Bone mineral loss during lactation and recovery after weaning, Obstet Gynecol 86:26, 1995.

98. **Kalkwarf HJ, Specker BL, Bianchi DC, Ranz J, Ho M,** The effect of calcium supplementation on bone density during lactation and after weaning, New Engl J Med 337:523, 1997.

99. **Laskey MA, Prentice A, Hanratty LA, Jarjou LM, Dibba B, Beavan SR, Cole TJ,** Bone changes after 3 mo of lactation: influence of calcium intake, breast-milk output, and vitamin D-receptor genotype, Am J Clin Nutr 67:685, 1998.

100. **Ritchie LD, Fung EB, Halloran BP, Turnlund JR, Van Loan MD, Cann CE, King JC,** A longitudinal study of calcium homeostasis during human pregnancy and lactation and after resumption of menses, Am J Clin Nutr 67:693, 1998.

101. **Tyson JE, Friesen HG,** Factors influencing the secretion of human prolactin and growth hormone in menstrual and gestational women, Am J Obstet Gynecol 116:377, 1973.

102. **Barberia JM, Abu-Fadil S, Kletzky OA, Nakamura RM, Mishell Jr DR,** Serum prolactin patterns in early human gestation, Am J Obstet Gynecol 121:1107, 1975.

103. **Murphy LJ, Murphy LC, Stead B, Sutherland RL, Lazarus L,** Modulation of lactogenic receptors by progestins in cultured human breast cancer cells, J Clin Endocrinol Metab 62:280, 1986.

104. **Simon WE, Pahnke VG, Holzel F,** In vitro modulation of prolactin binding to human mammary carcinoma cells by steroid hormones and prolactin, J Clin Endocrinol Metab 60:1243, 1985.

105. **Kelly PA, Kjiane J, Postel-Vinay M-C, Edery M,** The prolactin/growth hormone receptor family, Endocr Rev 12:235, 1991.

106. **Haslam SZ, Shyamala G,** Progesterone receptors in normal mammary gland: receptor modulations in relation to differentiation, J Cell Biol 86:730, 1980.

107. **Garza-Flores J, Cardenas S, Rodriguez V, Cravioto MC, Diaz-Sanchez V, Perez-Palacios G,** Return to ovulation following the use of long-acting injectable contraceptives: a comparative study, Contraception 31:361, 1985.

108. **Pardthaisong T,** Return of fertility after use of the injectable contraceptive Depo-Provera: updated analysis, J Biosoc Sci 16:23, 1984.

109. **Schwallie P, Assenze J,** The effect of depo-medroxyprogesterone acetate on pituitary and ovarian function, and the return of fertility following its discontinuation. A review, Contraception 10:181, 1974.

110. **Newton JR, d'Arcangues C, Hall PE,** A review of 'once-a-month' combined injectable contraceptives, J Obstet Gynaecol 14(Suppl 1):S1, 1994.

111. **WHO Special Programme of Research, Development and Research Training in Human Reproduction, Task Force on Long-Acting Systemic Agents for Fertility Regulation,** A multicentered phase III comparative study of two hormonal contraceptive preparations given once-a-month by intramuscular injection, Contraception 40:531, 1989.

219

112. **Cuong DT, Huong M,** Comparative phase III clinical trial of two injectable contraceptive preparations, depot-medroxyprogesterone acetate and Cyclofem in Vietnamese women, Contraception 54:169, 1996.

113. **Hall P, Bahamondes L, Diaz J, Petta C,** Introductory study of the once-a-month, injectable contraceptive Cyclofem® in Brazil, Chile, Columbia, and Peru, Contraception 56:353, 1997.

114. **Garza-Flores J, Morales del Olmo A, Fuziwara JL, Figueroa JG, Alonso A, Monroy J, Perez M, Urbina-Fuentes M, Guevara SJ, Cedeno E, Barrios R, Ferman JJ, Medina LM, Velezquez E, Perez-Palacios G,** Introduction of Cyclofem® once-a-month injectable contraceptive in Mexico, Contraception 58:7, 1998.

115. **Kaunitz AM, Garceau RJ, Cromie MA, and the Lunelle Study Group,** Comparative safety, efficacy, and cycle control of Lunelle™ monthly contraceptive injection (medroxy-progesterone acetate and estradiol cypionate injectable suspension) and Ortho-Novum® 7/7/7 oral contraceptive (Norethindrone/ethinyl estradiol triphasic), Contraception 60:179, 1999.

116. **Garceau RJ, Wajszczuk CJ, Kaunitz AM, for the Lunelle Study Group,** Bleeding patterns of women using Lunelle™ monthly contraceptive injections (medroxy-progesterone aceate and estradiol cypionate injectable suspension) compared with those of women using Ortho-Novum™ 7/7/7 (norethindrone/ethinyl estradiol triphasic) or other oral contraceptives, Contraception 62:289, 2000.

117. **Bahamondes L, Lavín P, Ojeda G, Petta C, Diaz J, Maradiegue E, Monteiro I,** Return of fertility after discontinuation of the once-a-month injectable contraceptive Cyclofem®, Contraception 55:307, 1997.

118. **Bahamondes L, Marchi NM, Nakagava HM, de Melo MLR, de Lourdes Cristofoletti M, Pellini E, Scozzafave RH, Petta C,** Self-administration with UniJect® of the once-a-month injectable contraceptive Cyclofem®, Contraception 56:301, 1997.

119. **Piya-Anant M, Koetsawang S, Patrasupapong N, Dinchuen P, d'Arcangues C, Piaggio G,** Pinol A, Effectiveness of Cyclofem® in the treatment of depot medroxyprogesterone acetate induced amenorrhea, Contraception 57:23, 1998.

120. **Kesseru EV, Aydinlik S, Etchepareborda JJ,** Multicentered, phase III clinical trial of norethisteone enanthate 50 mg plus estradiol valerate 5 mg as a monthly injectable contraceptive; final three-year report, Contraception 50:329, 1994.

121. **Sang GW, Shao QX, Ge RS, Chen JK, Song S, Fang KJ, He ML, Luo SY, Chen SF, Chen XB, Li MX, Wu SC, Sun GL, Zhou HE, Zhang SF, Zhu LL, Ye BL, Zhang JH, Ma FL, Jiang BY, Zhou ZQ, Dong QH, Shenm HC, Liu YX, Shao JY, Wang SX, Ming HD, Zhu ZR, Cheng HZ, Chen SH, Yu HY, Zhang ZY, Qing YN, Wang XY, Hall PE, d'Arcangues C, Snow RC,** A multicentred phase III comparative clinical trial of Mesigyna, Cyclofem, and injectable no. 1 given monthly by intramuscular injection to Chinese women. I. Contraceptive efficacy and side effects, Contraception 51:167, 1995.

122. **Martínez GH, Castañeda A, Correa JE,** Vaginal bleeding patterns in users of Perlutal®, a once-a-month injectable contraceptive consisting of 10 mg estradiol enanthate combined with 150 mg dihydroxyprogesterone acetophenide. A trial of 5462 woman-months, Contraception 58:21, 1998.

123. **Coutinho EM, Spinola P, Barbosa I, Gatto M, Tomaz G, Morais K, Yazlle ME, de Souza RN, Neto JSP, de Barros Leal W, Leal C, Hippolito SB, Abranches AD,** Multicenter, double-blind, comparative clinical study on the efficacy and acceptability of a monthly injectable contraceptive combination of 150 mg dihydroxyprogesterone acetophenide and 10 mg estradiol enanthate compared to a monthly injectable contraceptive combination of 90 mg dihydroxyprogesterone acetophenide and 6 mg estradiol enanthate, Contraception 55:175, 1997.

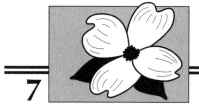

7

Intrauterine Contraception

Intrauterine contraceptives are used by over 100 million women world-wide, but only several hundred thousand of these are American. The growing need for reversible contraception in the United States would be well served by increasing utilization of intrauterine contraception with the intrauterine device (the IUD). The efficacy of modern IUDs in actual use is superior to that of oral contraception. Problems with IUD use can be minimized to a very low rate of minor side effects with careful screening and technique. We hope that American clinicians and patients "rediscover" this excellent method of contraception.

History

A frequently told, but not well-documented story, assigns the first use of intrauterine devices to caravan drivers who allegedly used intrauterine stones to prevent pregnancies in their camels during long journeys.

The forerunners of the modern IUD were small stem pessaries used in the 1800s, small button-like structures that covered the opening of the cervix and that were attached to stems extending into the cervical canal.[1] It is not certain whether these pessaries were used for contraception, but this seems to have been intended. In 1902, a pessary that extended into the uterus was developed by Hollweg in Germany and used for contraception. This pessary was sold for self-insertion, but the hazard of infection was great, earning the condemnation of the medical community.

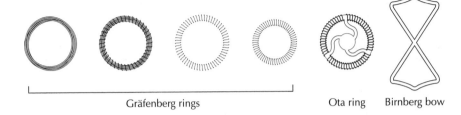

Gräfenberg rings   Ota ring   Birnberg bow

In 1909, Richter in Germany, reported success with a silkworm catgut ring that had a nickel and bronze wire protruding through the cervix.[2] Shortly after, Pust combined Richter's ring with the old button-type pessary and replaced the wire with a catgut thread.[3] This IUD was used during World War I in Germany, although the German literature was quick to report infections with its insertion and use. In the 1920s, Gräfenberg removed the tail and pessary because he believed this was the cause of infection. He reported his experience in 1930, using rings made of coiled silver and gold and then steel.[4]

The Gräfenberg ring was short-lived, falling victim to Nazi political philosophy that was bitterly opposed to contraception. The non-Aryan Gräfenberg was finally sent to jail, but he managed to flee Germany, dying in New York City in 1955. He never received the recognition that was his just due.

The Gräfenberg ring was associated with a high rate of expulsion. This was solved by Ota in Japan who added a supportive structure to the center of his gold- or silver-plated ring in 1934.[5] Ota also fell victim to World War II politics (he was sent into exile), but his ring continued to be used.

The Gräfenberg and Ota rings were essentially forgotten by the rest of the world throughout World War II. An awareness of the explosion in population and its impact began to grow in the first 2 decades after World War II. In 1959, reports from Japan and Israel by Ishihama and Oppenheimer, respectively, once again stirred interest in the rings.[6,7] The Oppenheimer report was in the American Journal of Obstetrics and Gynecology, and several American gynecologists were stimulated to use rings of silver or silk and others to develop their own devices.

In the 1960s and 1970s, the IUD thrived. Techniques were modified and a plethora of types were introduced. The various devices developed in the 1960s were made of plastic (polyethylene) impregnated with barium sulfate so that they would be visible on an x-ray. The Margulies Coil, developed by Lazer Margulies in 1960 at Mt. Sinai Hospital in New York City, was the first plastic device with a memory, which allowed the use of an inserter and reconfiguration of the shape when it was expelled into the uterus. The Coil was a large device (sure to cause cramping and bleeding), and its hard plastic tail proved risky for the male partner.

In 1962, the Population Council, at the suggestion of Alan Guttmacher, who that year became president of the Planned Parenthood Federation of America, organized the first international conference on IUDs in New York City. It was at this conference that Jack Lippes of Buffalo presented experience with his device, which fortunately as we will see, had a single filament thread as a tail. The Margulies Coil was rapidly replaced by the Lippes Loop, which quickly became the most widely prescribed IUD in the United States in the 1970s. A former World War II test pilot and engineer, Paul H. Bronnenkant, was making plastic parts for jukeboxes in his company, Hallmark Plastics, located next door to the Wurlitzer factory in Buffalo. Lippes' enlistment of Bronnenkant to develop his loop was so successful that Bronnenkant became an energetic advocate of the Lippes Loop; he carried heavy metal molds throughout the Far East to establish local production. A succeeding company, Finishing Enterprises, now directed by Bronnenkant's son, Lance Bronnenkant, is the original and continuing manufacturer of the TCu-380A. Beginning in 2004, an affiliate of Finishing Enterprises, FEI Women's Health, assumed responsibility for both the manufacturing and the marketing of the ParaGard TCu-380A IUD in the U.S.

The 1962 conference also led to the organization of a program established by the Population Council, under the direction of Christopher Tietze, to evaluate IUDs, the Cooperative Statistical Program. The Ninth Progress Report in 1970 was a landmark comparison of efficacy and problems with the various IUDs in use.[8]

Many other devices came along, but, with the exception of the four sizes of Lippes Loops and the two Saf-T-Coils, they had limited use. Stainless steel devices incorporating springs were designed to compress for easy insertion, but the movement of these devices allowed them to embed in the uterus, making them too difficult to remove. The Majzlin Spring is a memorable example.

The Dalkon Shield was introduced in 1970. Within 3 years, a high incidence of pelvic infection was recognized. There is no doubt that the problems with the Dalkon Shield were due to defective construction, pointed out as early as 1975 by Tatum.[9] The multifilamented tail (hundreds of fibers enclosed in a plastic sheath) of the Dalkon Shield provided a pathway for bacteria to ascend protected from the barrier of cervical mucus.

Although sales were discontinued in 1975, a call for removal of all Dalkon Shields was not issued until the early 1980s. The large number of women with pelvic infections led to many lawsuits against the pharmaceutical company, ultimately causing its bankruptcy. Unfortunately, the Dalkon Shield problem tainted all IUDs, and, ever since, media and the public in the United States have inappropriately regarded all IUDs in a single, generic fashion.

About the time of the introduction of the Dalkon Shield, the U.S. Senate conducted hearings on the safety of oral contraception. Young women who were discouraged from using oral contraceptives after these hearings turned to IUDs, principally the Dalkon Shield, which was promoted as suitable for nulliparous women. Changes in sexual behavior in the 1960s and 1970s, and failure to use protective contraception (condoms and oral contraceptives), led to an epidemic of sexually transmitted infections (STIs) and pelvic inflammatory disease (PID) for which IUDs were held partially responsible.[10]

The first epidemiologic studies of the relationship between IUDs and PID used women who depended on oral contraception or barrier methods as controls, and who were, therefore, at reduced risk of PID compared with noncontraceptors and IUD users.[11, 12] In addition, these first studies failed to control for the characteristics of sexual behavior that are now accepted as risk factors for PID (multiple partners, early age at first intercourse, and increased frequency of intercourse).[13] The Dalkon Shield magnified the risk attributed to IUDs because its high failure rate in young women who were already at risk of STIs led to septic spontaneous abortions and, in some cases, death.[14] Reports of these events led the American public to regard all IUDs as dangerous, including those that, unlike the Dalkon Shield, had undergone extensive clinical trials and postmarketing surveillance.

The 1980s saw the decline of IUD use in the United States as manufacturers discontinued marketing in response to the burden of litigation. Despite the fact that most of the lawsuits against the copper devices were won by the manufacturer, the cost of the defense combined with declining use affected the financial return. It should be emphasized that this action was the result of corporate business decisions related to concerns for profit and liability, not for medical or scientific reasons. It was not until 1988 that the IUD was returned to the U.S. market. The number of reproductive-aged women using the intrauterine device decreased by two-thirds from 1982 to 1988 and further decreased in 1995, from 7.1% to 2% to 0.8%, respectively.[15] Nevertheless, in the rest of the world, the IUD is the most widely used method of reversible contraception; currently, more than 100 million women use the IUD.

USE OF THE IUD IN THE U.S. AND THE WORLD[15, 16]

	U.S.A.	CHINA	WORLD
1981:	2.2 million women	42 million	60 million
1988:	0.7 million women	59 million	83 million
1995:	0.3 million women	75 million	106 million

The reason for the decline in the United States was the consumer fear of IUD-related pelvic infection. The final blow to the IUD in the United States came in 1985 with the publication of two reports indicating that the use of IUDs was associated with tubal infertility.[17, 18] Later, better controlled studies identified the Dalkon Shield as a high-risk device and failed to demonstrate an association between PID and other IUDs, except during the period shortly after insertion. Efforts to point out that the situation was different for the copper IUDs, and that, in fact, pelvic inflammatory disease was not increased in women with a single sexual partner,[19] failed to prevent the withdrawal of IUDs from the American market and the negative reaction to IUDs by the American public.

Ironically, the IUD declined in the country that developed the modern IUD. It is time for a revival!

225

The Modern IUD

The addition of copper to the IUD was suggested by Jaime Zipper of Chile, whose experiments with metals indicated that copper acted locally on the endometrium.[20] Howard Tatum combined Zipper's suggestion with the development of the T-shape to diminish the uterine reaction to the structural frame and produced the copper-T. The first copper IUD had copper wire wound around the straight shaft of the T, the TCu-200 (200 mm^2 of exposed copper wire), also known as the Tatum-T.[21] Tatum's reasoning was that the T-shape would conform to the shape of the uterus in contrast to the other IUDs that required the uterus to conform to their shape. Furthermore, the copper IUDs could be much smaller than those of simple, inert plastic devices and still provide effective contraception. Studies indicate that copper exerts its effect before implantation of a fertilized ovum; it may be spermicidal, or it may diminish sperm motility or fertilizing capacity. The addition of copper to the IUD and reduction in the size and structure of the frame improved tolerance, resulting in fewer removals for pain and bleeding.

The Cu-7 with a copper wound stem was developed in 1971 and quickly became the most popular device in the U.S. Both the Cu-7 and the Tatum-T were withdrawn from the United States market in 1986 by G. D. Searle and Company.

IUD development continued, however. More copper was added by Population Council investigators, leading to the TCu-380A (380 mm² of exposed copper surface area) with copper wound around the stem plus a copper sleeve on each horizontal arm.[22] The "A" in TCu-380A is for arms, indicating the importance of the copper sleeves. Making the copper solid and tubular increased effectiveness and the lifespan of the IUD. The TCu-380A has been in use in more than 30 countries since 1982, and, in 1988, it was marketed in the United States as the "ParaGard."

Efforts continue to develop IUDs that address the main problems of bleeding and cramping. The IUDs of the future will possibly be medicated and frameless.

Types of IUDs

Unmedicated IUDs

The Lippes Loop, made of plastic (polyethylene) impregnated with barium sulfate, is still used throughout the world (except in the United States). Flexible stainless steel rings are widely used in China but not elsewhere.[23]

Copper IUDs

The first copper IUDs were wound with 200 to 250 mm² of wire, and two of these are still available (except in the United States): the TCu-200 and the Multiload-250. The more modern copper IUDs contain more copper, and part of the copper is in the form of solid tubular sleeves, rather than wire, increasing efficacy and extending lifespan. This group of IUDs is represented in the United States by the TCu-380A (the ParaGard) and in the rest of the world by the TCu-220C, the Nova T, and the Multiload-375. The modern generation of IUDs in China includes a stainless steel ring with copper wire that also releases indomethacin (very effective with a low expulsion rate and less blood loss), a V-shaped copper IUD, and a copper IUD shaped like the uterine cavity.[23] The Sof-T is a copper IUD used only in Switzerland.

The TCu-380A is a T-shaped device with a polyethylene frame holding 380 mm² of exposed surface area of copper. The pure electrolytic copper wire wound around the 36-mm stem weighs 176 mg, and copper sleeves on the horizontal arms weigh 66.5 mg. A polyethylene monofilament is tied through the 3-mm ball on the stem, providing two white threads for detection and removal. The ball at the bottom of the stem helps reduce the risk of cervical perforation. The IUD frame contains barium sulfate, making it radiopaque. The TCu-380Ag is identical to the TCu-380A, but the copper wire on the stem has a silver core to prevent fragmentation and extend the lifespan of the copper. The TCu-380 Slimline has the copper sleeves flush at the ends of the horizontal arms to facilitate easier loading

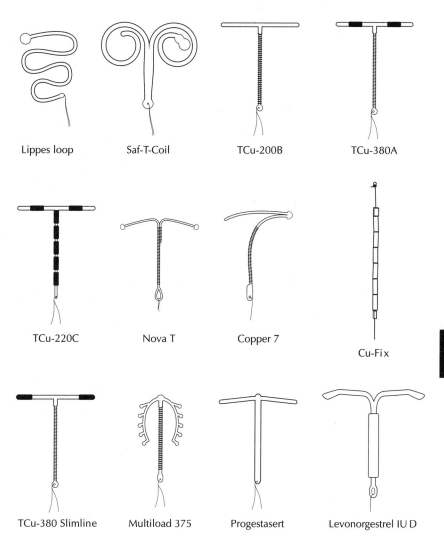

| Lippes loop | Saf-T-Coil | TCu-200B | TCu-380A |

| TCu-220C | Nova T | Copper 7 | Cu-Fix |

| TCu-380 Slimline | Multiload 375 | Progestasert | Levonorgestrel IU D |

and insertion. The performance of the TCu-380Ag and the TCu-380 Slimline is equal to that of the TCu-380A.[24, 25]

The Multiload-375 has 375 mm² of copper wire wound around its stem. The flexible arms were designed to minimize expulsions. This is a popular device in many parts of the world. The Multiload-375 and the TCu-380A are similar in their efficacy and performance.[26]

The Nova T is similar to the TCu-200, containing 200 mm² of copper; however, the Nova T has a silver core to the copper wire, flexible arms, and a large, flexible loop at the bottom to avoid injury to cervical tissue. There was some concern that the efficacy of the Nova T decreased after 3 years in World Health Organization (WHO) data; however, results from Finland and Scandinavia indicate low and stable pregnancy rates over 5 years of use.[26]

The CuSAFE-300 IUD has 300 mm² of copper in its vertical arm and a transverse arm with sharply bent ends that are adapted to the uterine cavity and help hold this IUD in the fundus. It is made from a more flexible plastic and is smaller than the world's two most popular IUDs, the TCu-380A and the Multiload-375. Pregnancy rates with the CuSAFE-300 are comparable to these two devices, but rates of removal for pain and bleeding are reported to be lower.[27]

The Hormone-Releasing IUD

The LNG-20 (Mirena), manufactured by Leiras-Schering A.G. in Finland, releases in vitro 20 μg of levonorgestrel per day.[28] This T-shaped device has a collar attached to the vertical arm, which contains 52 mg levonorgestrel dispersed in polydimethylsiloxane and released initially at a rate of 20 μg per day in vivo, progressively declining (reaching half of the initial rate after 5 years). The levonorgestrel IUD is approved for 5 years, but lasts up to 10 years, and reduces menstrual blood loss and pelvic infection rates.[29-31] Indeed, the levonorgestrel IUD is about as effective as endometrial ablation for the treatment of menorrhagia.[32] The local progestin effect directed to the endometrium can be utilized in patients on tamoxifen,[33] patients with dysmenorrhea,[34] and in postmenopausal women receiving estrogen therapy.[35, 36] Smaller devices releasing 5 μg or 10 μg levonorgestrel have been developed in Europe for use for at least 5 years in postmenopausal women.[36,37]

Future IUDs

The Ombrelle-250 and Ombrelle-380, designed to be more flexible in order to reduce expulsion and side effects, have been marketed in France. A frameless IUD, the FlexiGard (also known as the Cu-Fix or the GyneFIX), invented by Dirk Wildemeersch in 1983 in Belgium, consists of 6 copper sleeves (330 mm² of copper) strung on a surgical nylon (polypropylene) thread that is knotted at one end. The knot is pushed into the myometrium during insertion with a notched needle that works like a miniature harpoon. Because it is frameless, it has a low rate of removal for bleeding or pain, but a more difficult insertion may yield a higher expulsion rate.[38, 39] However, when inserted by experienced clinicians, the expulsion rate is very low, and the device is especially suited for nulligravid and nulliparous women.[40-42] This IUD is increasingly popular in Europe. A shorter system combined with a reservoir for the sustained release of levonorgestrel is being developed; a version (FibroPlant) that releases 14 μg levonorgestrel per day is being tested for perimenopausal and postmenopausal use.[43, 44]

Mechanism of Action

The contraceptive action of all IUDs is mainly in the uterine cavity. Ovulation is not affected, and the IUD is not an abortifacient.[45, 46] It is currently believed that the mechanism of action for IUDs is the production of an intrauterine environment that is spermicidal.

Nonmedicated IUDs depend for contraception on the general reaction of the uterus to a foreign body. It is believed that this reaction, a sterile inflammatory response, produces tissue injury of a minor degree but sufficient enough to be spermicidal. Very few, if any, sperm reach the ovum in the fallopian tube. Normally cleaving, fertilized ova cannot be obtained by tubal flushing in women with IUDs in contrast to noncontraceptors, indicating the failure of sperm to reach the ovum, and, thus, fertilization does not occur.[47] In women using copper IUDs, sensitive assays for human chorionic gonadotropin (hCG) do not find evidence of fertilization.[48, 49] This is consistent with the fact that the copper IUD protects against both intrauterine and ectopic pregnancies (see later).

The copper IUD releases free copper and copper salts that have both a biochemical and morphologic impact on the endometrium and produce alterations in cervical mucus and endometrial secretions. There is no measurable increase in the serum copper level. Copper has many specific actions, including the enhancement of prostaglandin production and the inhibition of various endometrial enzymes. The copper IUD is associated with an inflammatory response, marked by production in the endometrium of cytokine peptides known to be cytotoxic.[50] An additional spermicidal effect probably takes place in the cervical mucus.

The progestin-releasing IUD adds the endometrial action of the progestin to the foreign body reaction. The endometrium becomes decidualized with atrophy of the glands.[51] The progestin IUD probably has two mechanisms of action: inhibition of implantation and inhibition of sperm capacitation, penetration, and survival. The levonorgestrel IUD produces serum concentrations of the progestin about half those of Norplant so that ovarian follicular development and ovulation are also partially inhibited; after the first year, cycles are ovulatory in 50–75% of women, regardless of their bleeding patterns.[52] Finally, the progestin IUD thickens the cervical mucus, creating a barrier to sperm penetration. The progestin IUD decreases menstrual blood loss (about 40–50%) and dysmenorrhea; with the levonorgestrel IUD, bleeding can be reduced by 90% 1 year after insertion.[53] About 50% of women become amenorrheic 1 year after insertion of the levonorgestrel IUD.[54, 55] Average hemoglobin and iron levels increase over time compared with preinsertion values.[56]

Because of the favorable impact of locally released progestin on the endometrium, the levonorgestrel IUD is very effective for the treatment of menorrhagia, as effective as the administration of oral progestins (with less side effects), and compares favorably with surgical treatment (hysterectomy or endometrial ablation).[57-60] In addition, this IUD can be used to prevent and to treat endometrial hyperplasia. The levonorgestrel IUD may be associated with a slight increase in the formation of ovarian cysts, but they are asymptomatic and resolve spontaneously.[61]

Following removal of IUDs, the normal intrauterine environment is rapidly restored. *In large studies, there is no delay, regardless of duration of use, in achieving pregnancy at normal rates, which belies the assertion that IUD use is associated with infection leading to infertility.*[62-65] There has been no significant difference in cumulative pregnancy rates between parous and nulliparous or nulligravid women.[64, 65]

Efficacy of IUDs

Intrauterine Pregnancy

The TCu-380A is approved for use in the United States for 10 years. However, the TCu-380A has been demonstrated to maintain its efficacy over at least 12 years of use.[66] The TCu-200 is approved for 4 years and the Nova T for 5 years. The levonorgestrel IUD can be used for at least 7 years and probably 10 years.[26] The levonorgestrel device that releases 15–20 μg levonorgestrel per day is as effective as the new copper IUDs.[25, 29, 67, 68]

The nonmedicated IUDs never have to be replaced. The deposition of calcium salts on the IUD can produce a structure that is irritating to the endometrium. If bleeding increases after a nonmedicated IUD has been in place for some time, it is worth replacing it. Some clinicians (as do we) recommend replacing all older IUDs with the new, more effective copper IUDs.

First Year Clinical Trial Experience in Parous Women[69–71]

Device	Pregnancy Rate (%)	Expulsion Rate (%)	Removal Rate (%)
Lippes Loop	3	12–20	12–15
Cu-7	2–3	6	11
TCu-200	3	8	11
TCu-380A	0.5–0.8	5	14
Levonorgestrel IUD	0.2	6	17

Considering all IUDS together, the actual use failure rate in the first year is approximately 3%, with a 10% expulsion rate and a 15% rate of removal, mainly for bleeding and pain. With increasing duration of use and increasing age, the failure rate decreases, as do removals for pain and bleeding. The performance of the TCu-380A in recent years, however, has proved to be superior to previous IUDs.

231

Ten-Year Experience with ParaGard, TCu-380A
Rate per 100 users per year

	Year									
	1	2	3	4	5	6	7	8	9	10
Pregnancy	0.7	0.3	0.6	0.2	0.3	0.2	0.0	0.4	0.0	0.0
Expulsion	5.7	2.5	1.6	1.2	0.3	0.0	0.6	1.7	0.2	0.4
Bleeding/ Pain removal	11.9	9.8	7.0	3.5	3.7	2.7	3.0	2.5	2.2	3.7
Medical removals	2.5	2.1	1.6	1.7	0.1	0.3	1.0	0.4	0.7	0.3
Continuation	76.8	78.3	81.2	86.2	89.0	91.9	87.9	88.1	92.0	91.8
Number starting each year	4932	3149	2018	1121	872	621	563	483	423	325

Data from Population Council (*n* = 3536) and WHO (*n* = 1396) trials.

In careful studies, with attention to technique and participation by motivated patients, the failure rate with the TCu-380A and the other newer copper IUDs is less than one per 100 women per year.[26, 69, 72] The cumulative net pregnancy rate after 7 years of use is 1.5 per 100 woman-years, and after 12 years, only 1.9 per 100 women (not a single pregnancy was reported after 8 years of use).[66, 73] In developing countries, the failure rate with IUDs is less than that with oral contraception.[74] Failure rates are slightly higher in younger (less than age 25), more fertile women.

Women use IUDs longer than other reversible methods of contraception. The IUD continuation rate is higher than that with oral contraception, condoms, or diaphragms. This may reflect the circumstances surrounding the choice of an IUD (older, parous women).

Expulsion

Approximately 5% of patients spontaneously expel the TCu-380A within the first year. Women younger than age 20 have a higher expulsion rate than older women.[29, 75] This event can be associated with cramping, vaginal discharge, or uterine bleeding. However, in some cases, the only observable change is lengthening or absence of the IUD strings. Patients should be cautioned to request immediate attention if expulsion is suspected. A partially expelled IUD should be removed. If pregnancy or infection is not present, a new IUD can be inserted immediately (in this instance, antibiotic prophylaxis is recommended).

Ectopic Pregnancy

The previous use of an IUD does not increase the risk of a subsequent ectopic pregnancy.[65, 76, 77] The current use of an IUD offers some protection against ectopic pregnancy.[76–81] The largest study, a WHO multicenter study, concluded that IUD users were 50% less likely to have an ectopic pregnancy when compared with women using no contraception.[76] This protection is not as great as that achieved by inhibition of ovulation with oral contraception. Therefore, when an IUD user becomes pregnant, the pregnancy is more likely to be ectopic. However, the actual occurrence of an ectopic pregnancy in an IUD user is a rare event.

The lowest ectopic pregnancy rates are seen with the most effective IUDs, like the TCu-380A (90% less likely compared with noncontraceptors).[82] The rate is about one-tenth of the ectopic pregnancy rate associated with the Lippes Loop or with devices with less copper such as the TCu-200.[82] The progesterone-releasing IUD (that is no longer produced) had a higher rate, probably because its action was limited to a local effect on the endometrium,[79] but the reported rate was based on very small numbers and may have been inaccurate. Very few ectopic pregnancies have been reported with the levonorgestrel IUD, presumably because it is associated with a partial suppression of gonadotropins with subsequent disruption of normal follicular growth and development and, in a significant number of cycles, inhibition of ovulation.[25, 31, 68, 82, 83]

The risk of ectopic pregnancy does not increase with increasing duration of use with the TCu-380A or the levonorgestrel IUD.[25, 73] In a 7-year prospective study, not a single ectopic pregnancy was encountered with the levonorgestrel IUD, and in a 5-year study, only one.[25, 84] In 8,000 woman-years of experience in randomized multicenter trials, there has been only a single ectopic pregnancy reported with the TCu-380A (which is one-tenth the rate with the Lippes Loop or TCu-200).[25] Therefore, the risk of ectopic pregnancy during the use of the copper IUD or the levonorgestrel IUD is much lower compared with noncontraceptive users; however, if pregnancy occurs, the likelihood of an ectopic pregnancy is high.[85]

The protection against ectopic pregnancy provided by the TCu-380A and the levonorgestrel IUD makes these IUDs acceptable choices for contraception in women with previous ectopic pregnancies.

Ectopic Pregnancy Rates per 1,000 Woman-Years [82, 86]

Noncontraceptive users, all ages	3.00–4.50
Levonorgestrel IUD	0.20
TCu-380A IUD	0.20

Side Effects

With effective patient screening and good insertion technique, the copper and medicated IUDs are not associated with an increased risk of infertility after their removal. Even if IUDs are removed for problems, subsequent fertility rates are normal.[64, 65, 68]

The symptoms most often responsible for IUD discontinuation are increased uterine bleeding and increased menstrual pain. Within 1 year, 5–15% of women discontinue IUD use because of these problems. Smaller copper and progestin IUDs have reduced the incidence of pain and bleeding considerably, but a careful menstrual history is still important in helping a woman consider an IUD. Women with prolonged, heavy menstrual bleeding or significant dysmenorrhea may not be able to tolerate copper IUDs but may benefit from a progestin IUD.[53] Because bleeding and cramping are most severe in the first few months after IUD insertion, treatment with a nonsteroidal antiinflammatory drug (NSAID, an inhibitor of prostaglandin synthesis) during the first several menstrual periods can reduce bleeding and cramping and help a patient through this difficult time. Even persistent heavy menses can be effectively treated with NSAIDs.[87] NSAID treatment should begin at the onset of menses and be maintained for 3 days. A copper IUD is available in China that also releases a small amount of indomethacin; this device is associated with markedly less bleeding.[88]

It is not unusual to have a few days of intermenstrual spotting or light bleeding. Although aggravating, this does not cause significant blood loss. Such bleeding deserves the usual evaluation for cervical or endometrial pathology. These changes can be objectionable for women who are prevented from having intercourse while bleeding.

Following insertion of a modern copper IUD, menstrual blood loss increases by about 55%, and this level of bleeding continues for the duration of IUD use.[89] This is associated with a slight (1–2 day) prolongation of menstruation. Over a year's time, this amount of blood loss does not result in changes indicative of iron deficiency (e.g., serum ferritin). With longer use, however, ferritin levels are lower, suggesting a depletion of iron stores.[90] Assessment for iron depletion and anemia should be considered in long-term users and in women susceptible to iron deficiency anemia. In populations with a high prevalence of anemia, these changes occur more rapidly, and iron supplementation is recommended.[91]

Because of a decidualizing, atrophic impact on the endometrium, amenorrhea can develop over time with the progestin-containing IUD. With the levonorgestrel IUD, 70% of patients are oligomenorrheic and 30–40% are amenorrheic within 2 years.[55, 92] In a group of women who used the levonorgestrel IUD for more than 12 years, 60% were amenorrheic; 12% experienced infrequent, scanty bleeding; and 28% had regular but light bleeding.[56] For some women, the lack of periods is so disconcerting that they request removal. On the other hand, this effect on menstruation is manifested by an increase in blood hemoglobin levels.[25, 69] The levonorgestrel IUD is very effective when used to treat menorrhagia.[53, 93] This noncontraceptive benefit is of such a magnitude that this method of treatment achieves comparable results when compared to surgical methods such as endometrial ablation or hysterectomy.[32, 58, 59, 94] Bleeding is even reduced in the presence of leiomyomas, along with a reduction in myoma size.[95] The levonorgestrel IUD has been used successfully to treat endometriosis and especially dysmenorrhea associated with endometriosis.[96]

Sufficient progestin reaches the systemic circulation from the levonorgestrel-containing IUD so that androgenic side effects, such as acne and hirsutism, might occur; however, in one study no change could be detected in the circulating levels of sex hormone-binding globulin, and, therefore, clinical effects are unlikely.[97] More extensive clinical studies are needed to assess the impact of this IUD on the lipoprotein profile, but it is unlikely that the low dose of levonorgestrel has an important effect on cardiovascular risk.

Some women report an increased vaginal discharge while wearing an IUD. This complaint deserves examination for the presence of vaginal or cervical infection. Treatment can be provided with the IUD remaining in place.

Long-term use of the IUD is associated with impressive safety and lack of side effects. In a 7-year prospective study, the use of either the copper IUD or the levonorgestrel IUD beyond 5 years led to no increase in pelvic infection, no increase in ectopic pregnancy rates, no increase in anemia, and no increase in abnormal Pap smears.[25] Duration of use does not affect pregnancy rates or outcome.

The presence of copper may yield some benefits. There are epidemiologic data indicating that both the copper IUD and the inert IUD reduce the risks of endometrial cancer and invasive cervical cancer.[98–103] Presumably, this protective effect is due to induced biochemical alterations that affect cellular responses.

The copper IUD is not affected by magnetic resonance imaging, and, therefore, the copper IUD need not be removed before MRI, and neither patients nor workers need be excluded from MRIs or the MRI environment.[104, 105]

Infections

IUD-related bacterial infection is now believed to be due to contamination of the endometrial cavity at the time of insertion. Mishell's classic study indicated that the uterus is routinely contaminated by bacteria at insertion.[106] Infections that occur 3–4 months after insertion are believed to be due to acquired STIs not the direct result of the IUD. The early, insertion-related infections, therefore, are polymicrobial and are derived from the endogenous cervicovaginal flora, with a predominance of anaerobes.

A review of the WHO data base derived from all of the WHO IUD clinical trials concluded that the risk of pelvic inflammatory disease was 6 times higher during the 20 days after the insertion compared with later times during follow-up, but, most importantly, PID was extremely rare beyond the first 20 days after insertion.[107] In nearly 23,000 insertions, however, only 81 cases of PID were diagnosed, and a scarcity of PID was observed in those situations in which STIs are rare. There was no statistically significant difference comparing the copper IUD to the inert Lippes

Loop or progestin-containing IUD. These data confirm earlier studies that the risk of infection is highest immediately after insertion and that PID risk does not increase with long-term use.[14, 19] The problem of infection can be minimized with careful screening and the use of aseptic technique. Even women with insulin-dependent diabetes mellitus do not have an increased risk for infection.[108, 109]

Doxycycline (200 mg) or azithromycin (500 mg) administered orally 1 hour prior to insertion can provide protection against insertion-associated pelvic infection, but prophylactic antibiotics are probably of little benefit for women at low risk for STIs.

Compared with oral contraception, barrier methods, and hormonal IUDs, there is no reason to think that nonmedicated or copper IUDs can confer protection against STIs.[110] However, the levonorgestrel-releasing IUD has been reported to be associated with a protective effect against pelvic infection, and the copper IUD is associated with lower titers of anti-chlamydial antibody.[30, 111] In vitro, copper inhibits chlamydial growth in endometrial cells.[112] Thus, the association between IUD use and pelvic infection (and infertility) is now seriously questioned.[113] Women who use IUDs must be counseled to use condoms along with the IUD whenever they have intercourse with a partner who could be an STI carrier. Because sexual behavior is the most important modifier of the risk of infection, clinicians should ask prospective IUD users about numbers of partners, their partner's sexual practices, the frequency and age of onset of intercourse, and history of STIs.[114] Women at low risk are unlikely to have pelvic infections while using IUDs.[19]

It is not certain that the IUD is inappropriate for women who are at increased risk of bacterial endocarditis (previous endocarditis, rheumatic heart disease, or the presence of prosthetic heart valves). The bacteriologic contamination of the uterine cavity at insertion is short-lived.[106] Three studies have attempted to document bacteremia during IUD insertion or removal.[115-117] Only one of the three could find blood culture evidence of bacteremia, and it was present transiently in only a few patients.[117] In our view, the IUD is acceptable for patients at risk of bacterial endocarditis, *but antibiotic prophylaxis (amoxicillin 2 g) should be provided 1 hour before insertion or removal.*

Asymptomatic IUD users whose cervical cultures show gonorrheal or chlamydia infection should be treated with the recommended drugs without removal of the IUD. If, however, there is evidence that an infection has ascended to the endometrium or fallopian tubes, treatment must be instituted and the IUD removed promptly. Vaginal bacteriosis should be treated (metronidazole, 500 mg bid for 7 days), but the IUD need not be removed unless pelvic inflammation is present. There is no evidence that the prevalence of bacterial vaginosis is influenced by IUD use.[118]

For simple endometritis, in which uterine tenderness is the only physical finding, doxycycline (100 mg bid for 14 days) is adequate. If tubal infection is present, as evidenced by cervical motion tenderness, abdominal rebound tenderness, adnexal tenderness or masses, or elevated white blood count and sedimentation rate, parenteral treatment is indicated with removal of the IUD as soon as antibiotic serum levels are adequate. The previous presence of an IUD does not alter the treatment of PID. IUD-associated pelvic infection is more likely to be caused by non-STI organisms.[119]

Appropriate outpatient management of less severe infections:

> Cefoxitin (2 g intramuscularly) plus probenecid (1 g orally), or
> Ceftriaxone (250 mg IM) plus doxycycline (100 mg bid orally),
> for 14 days, or
> Levofloxacin (500 mg orally) once daily for 14 days, or
> Ofloxacin (400 mg orally) bid for 14 days.

Severe infections require hospitalization and treatment with:

> Cefoxitin (2 g intravenous qid), or
> Cefotetan (2 g intravenous bid)
> Plus doxycycline (100 mg bid orally or intravenous)
> Followed by 14 days of an oral regimen of antibiotics.

The following is an alternative regimen:

> Clindamycin (900 mg intravenously tid), plus
> Gentamicin (2 mg/kg intravenously or intramuscularly
> followed by 1.5 mg/kg tid), or
> Ofloxacin (400 mg intravenously bid) or,
> Levofloxacin (500 mg intravenously tid).

There is a suggestion (in cross-sectional studies) that the IUD use increases the risk of human immunodeficiency virus (HIV) transmission from man to woman, especially when the IUD is inserted or removed during exposure to the infected man.[120, 121] However, this is not a strong suggestion, because the risk with IUD use was ascertained compared with other contraceptive methods (which can protect against transmission), and the many and various influencing factors are difficult to adjust and control. In the only longitudinal study, no association was observed between IUD use and HIV acquisition by women.[122] In the only study reported, no evidence for female-to-male HIV transmission with IUD use was detected.[123] HIV-infected women who utilize IUDs for contraception do not have a greater incidence of complications (including pelvic inflammatory disease).[124]

Actinomyces

The significance of actinomycosis infection in IUD users is unclear. There are many reports of IUD users with unilateral pelvic abscesses containing gram-positive bacilli *Actinomyces*.[125–127] However, *Actinomyces,* part of the normal flora in the gastrointestinal tract, are found in Pap smears of up to 30% of plastic IUD wearers when cytologists take special care to look for the organisms. The rate is much lower (less than 1%) with copper devices and varies with duration of use.[125, 126, 128, 129] Furthermore, *Actinomyces* are commonly present in the normal vagina.[130] The clinician must decide whether to remove the IUD and treat the patient, treat with the IUD in place, or simply remove the IUD. These patients are almost always asymptomatic and without clinical signs of infection. If uterine tenderness or a pelvic mass is present, the IUD should always be removed after the initiation of treatment with oral penicillin G, 500 mg qid, for a month. Althernative antibiotic regimens include tetracycline 500 mg qid; doxycycline 100 mg bid; amoxicillin/clavulanate 500 mg bid If *Actinomyces* are present on the Pap smear of an asymptomatic well woman, in our view, it is not necessary to administer antibiotic treatment or to remove the IUD. Although it has been recommended that the IUD should be removed in this instance and replaced when a repeat Pap smear is negative, there is no evidence to support this recommendation. Another anaerobic, gram-positive rod, *Eubacterium nodatum,* resembles *Actinomyces* and has also been reported to be associated with colonization of an IUD.[131] *E. nodatum* can be mistaken for *Actinomyces* on Pap smears. Our recommendations can be applied to both *E. nodatum* and *Actinomyces.*

Pregnancy With an IUD In Situ
Spontaneous Miscarriage

Spontaneous miscarriage occurs more frequently among women who become pregnant with IUDs in place, a rate of approximately 40–50%. Because of this high rate of spontaneous miscarriage, IUDs should always be removed if pregnancy is diagnosed and the string is visible. Use of instruments inside the uterus should be avoided if the pregnancy is desired, unless sonographic guidance can help avoid rupture of the membranes.[132] After removal of an IUD with visible strings, the spontaneous miscarriage rate is approximately 30%.[133, 134] Combining ultrasonography guidance with carbon dioxide hysteroscopy, an IUD with a missing tail can be identified and removed during early pregnancy.[135] **If the IUD is easily removed** *without trauma or expelled during the first trimester, the risk of spontaneous miscarriage is not increased.*[136, 137]

Septic Abortion. In the past, if the IUD could not be easily removed from a pregnant uterus, the patient was offered induced abortion because it was believed that the risk of life-threatening septic, spontaneous miscarriage in the second trimester was increased 20-fold if the pregnancy continued with the IUD in utero. However, this belief was derived from experiences with the Dalkon Shield. There is no evidence that there is an increased risk of septic abortion if pregnancy occurs with an IUD in place other than the Shield.[137, 138] There have been no deaths in the United States since 1977 among women pregnant with an IUD.[139]

If a patient plans to terminate a pregnancy that has occurred with an IUD in place, the IUD should be removed immediately. If there is no evidence of infection, the IUD can safely be removed in a clinic or office.

If an IUD is in an infected, pregnant uterus, removal of the device should be undertaken only after antibiotic therapy has been initiated and if equipment for cardiovascular support and resuscitation is immediately available. These precautions are necessary because removal of an IUD from an infected, pregnant uterus can lead to septic shock.

Congenital Anomalies. There is no evidence that exposure of a fetus to medicated IUDs is harmful. The risk of congenital anomalies is not increased among infants born to women who become pregnant with an IUD in place.[137, 140] A case-control study did not find an increased incidence of IUD use in pregnancies resulting in limb-reduction deformities.[141]

Preterm Labor and Birth. The incidence of preterm labor and delivery is increased approximately 4-fold when an IUD is left in place during pregnancy.[137, 142–144]

Other Complications. Obstetrical complications at delivery (e.g., hemorrhage, stillbirth, and difficulties with placenta removal) have been reported only with the Dalkon Shield in situ.

IUD Insertion

Patient Selection

Patient selection for successful IUD use requires attention to menstrual history and the risk for STIs. Age and parity are not the critical factors in selection; the risk factors for STIs are the most important consideration. Women who have multiple sexual partners, whose partners have multiple partners, who are drug or alcohol dependent, and who are not in a stable sexual relationship are at greater risk of pelvic infection at the time of IUD insertion and at greater risk of acquiring an STI after IUD insertion.[17-19] It would be appropriate for these women to use condoms for STI protection and an IUD for effective contraception. Current, recent, or recurrent PID is a contraindication for IUD use. Hormonal and barrier methods are better choices for these women. Nulliparous and nulligravid women can safely use the IUD if both sexual partners are monogamous. In a national U.S. survey, only 13% of adults had more than one sexual partner in the previous year.[145] Most women are good candidates for the IUD. The levonorgestrel-releasing IUD (Mirena) performs as well as oral contraceptives when used by young nulliparous women.[146]

Patients with heavy menstrual periods should be cautioned regarding the increase in menstrual bleeding associated with the copper IUD. Women who are anticoagulated or have a bleeding disorder are obviously not good candidates for the copper IUD, but they might benefit from the progestin IUD.

There are other conditions that can compromise success. Women who have abnormalities of uterine anatomy (bicornuate uterus, submucous myoma, cervical stenosis) may not accommodate an IUD. The IUD is not a good choice when the uterine cavity is distorted by leiomyomas. According to conventional wisdom, the few individuals who have allergies to copper or have Wilson's disease (a prevalence of about 1 in 200,000) should not use copper IUDs; however, no cases of difficulty have ever been recorded and it is doubtful, considering the low exposure to copper, that there would be a problem. The amount of copper released into the circulation per day is less than that consumed in a normal diet.[147] Nevertheless, barrier methods or long-acting progestin-only methods are recommended for individuals with Wilson's disease.[148]

Immunosuppressed patients should not use IUDs. Patients at risk for endocarditis should be treated with prophylactic antibiotics at insertion and removal. In our view, cervical dysplasia does not preclude IUD insertion or continued use.

Because many older women have diabetes mellitus, it is worth emphasizing that no increase in adverse events has been observed with copper IUD use in women with either insulin-dependent or noninsulin-dependent diabetes.[108, 109, 149] Indeed, the IUD can be an ideal choice for a woman with diabetes, especially if vascular disease is present.

The IUD should not be dismissed just because the patient is an adolescent. Although the clinical performance of the IUD in a study of parous adolescents was not as good as in older women, it was still similar or slightly better than other reversible methods used by adolescents.[150] Given appropriate screening, counseling, and care, the IUD can provide long-term effective contraception for adolescents. There are no major differences in IUD efficacy and side effects comparing nulligravid women with parous women.[151] Nulligravid women who are past users of the IUD did not have an increased risk of tubal infertility in a case-control study, but long-term IUD users in a cohort study were reported to have reduced fertility compared with oral contraceptive users and short-term IUD users.[152, 153] The merits of the two studies can be debated (the cohort study had several confounding problems); by far most evidence indicates that IUD use does not impair fertility.[63–65, 68, 154, 155]

A careful speculum and bimanual examination is essential prior to IUD insertion. It is important to know the position of the uterus; undetected extreme posterior uterine position is the most common reason for perforation at the time of IUD insertion. However, perforation is rare; the incidence is estimated to be less than 1 per 3,000 insertions.[156] A very small or large uterus, determined by examination and sounding, can preclude insertion. For successful IUD use, the uterus should preferably not sound less than 6 cm or more than 9 cm.

Preferably, the absence of cervical or vaginal infection should be established before insertion. If this is not feasible, insertion should definitely be delayed if a mucopurulent discharge of the cervix or a significant vaginitis (including vaginal bacteriosis) is present.

Key Points in Patient Counseling

1. Protection against unwanted pregnancy begins immediately after insertion.
2. Menses can be longer and heavier (except with hormonal IUDs); tampons can be used.
3. There is a slightly increased risk of pelvic infection in the first few months after insertion.
4. Protection against infections transmitted through the vaginal mucosa requires the use of condoms.
5. Ectopic pregnancies can still occur.
6. The IUD can be spontaneously expelled; monthly palpation of the IUD strings is important to avoid unwanted pregnancies. If the strings are not felt or something hard is palpable (suggestive of the IUD frame), a clinician should be notified as soon as possible. Backup contraception should be provided until the patient can be examined.

Summary: IUD Use and Medical Conditions

1. A woman with a previous ectopic pregnancy can use a copper IUD or the levonorgestrel IUD.
2. Women with heavy menses and dysmenorrhea, including women who have a bleeding disorder or are anticoagulated, should consider the progestin-releasing IUD.
3. Women at risk for bacterial endocarditis should receive prophylactic antibiotics at insertion and removal.
4. Current, recent, or recurrent PID is a contraindication for IUD use.
5. Women with diabetes mellitus, either insulin-dependent or noninsulin-dependent, can use IUDs.
6. IUD insertion is relatively easier in breastfeeding women, and the rates of expulsion and uterine perforation are not increased.

Timing

An IUD can be safely inserted at any time after delivery, spontaneous miscarriage or induced abortion, or during the menstrual cycle. Expulsion rates were higher when the older, large plastic IUDs were inserted sooner than 8 weeks postpartum; however, studies indicate that the copper IUDs can be inserted between 4 and 8 weeks postpartum without an increase in pregnancy rates, expulsion, uterine perforation, or removals for bleeding and/or pain.[157, 158] Insertion can even occur immediately after a vaginal delivery; it is not associated with an increased risk of infection, uterine perforation, postpartum bleeding, or uterine subinvolution.[159] Postvaginal delivery insertion is not recommended if intrauterine infection is present, and a slightly higher expulsion rate is to be expected compared with insertion 4–8 weeks postpartum. The IUD can also be inserted at cesarean section; the expulsion rate is slightly lower than that with insertion immediately after vaginal delivery.[160]

Insertion of an IUD in breastfeeding women is relatively easier and is associated with a lower removal rate for bleeding or pain.[159] Reports disagree whether perforation is more common in lactating women.[159, 161, 162]

An IUD can be inserted immediately after a first-trimester abortion, but, after a second-trimester abortion, one should wait until uterine involution occurs.[163, 164]

Insertions can be more difficult if the cervix is closed between menses. The advantages of insertion during or shortly after a menstrual period include a more open cervical canal, the masking of insertion-related bleeding, and the knowledge that the patient is not pregnant. These relative advantages may be outweighed by the risk of unintended pregnancy if insertion is delayed to await menstrual bleeding. In addition, there is evidence that the expulsion rate and termination rates for pain, bleeding, and pregnancy are lower if insertions are performed after day 11 of the menstrual cycle, and the infection rate may be lower with insertions after the 17th cycle day.[165]

Technique for the TCu-380A

Inserting an IUD requires only a few minutes, has few complications, and is rarely painful, but preoperative examination, medication, and the right equipment ensures a good experience for your patient. After introducing a vaginal spectrum, the cervix is cleaned with chlorhexadine or povidone-iodine. Leave the antiseptic-soaked cotton-tipped applicator in the cervical canal during the procedures prior to insertion of the IUD. Place a paracervical block by injecting 1 mL of local anesthetic (1% chloroprocaine) into the cervical lip (anterior if the uterus is anterior in the pelvis and posterior if it lies posteriorly). Inclusion of atropine, 0.4 mg, in the anesthetic reduces the incidence of vasovagal reactions. After one minute, grasp the cervical lip with the tenaculum ratcheting it only to the first position in a slow, deliberate fashion. Use the tenaculum to move the cervix to the patient's right, revealing the left lateral vaginal fornix. Place the needle tip in the cervical mucosa at 3 o'clock, 1–2 cm lateral to the cervical os, advance it about 1.5 inches (4 cm) under the mucosa and inject about 4 mL of anesthetic, leaving an additional 1 mL behind under the mucosa as the needle is withdrawn. Now deflect the cervix to the patient's left and inject local anesthetic at 9 o'clock in similar fashion. Wait 2–3 minutes before proceeding. A very common mistake is to not allow sufficient time for anesthetic action.

Many women can tolerate IUD insertion, especially at the time of menses, without a paracervical block. For some women, however, insertion is less painful with local anesthetic and with administration of an NSAID 30–60 minutes prior to the procedure. If a paracervical block is not used, having the patient cough just as the tenaculum is applied reduces pain and the chance of a vasovagal reaction. An alternative approach for pain relief is to apply benzocaine 20% gel first at the tenaculum site then to leave a gel-soaked cotton-tipped applicator in the cervical canal for about 1 minute before inserting the IUD.[166]

Sound and measure the depth of the uterus (the insertion tube can be used for this purpose). The IUD is loaded into its insertion tube immediately prior to insertion. The arms of the TCu 380A must be folded manually, either with sterile gloves or through the sterile wrapper, and maneuvered into the end of the insertion tube, just enough to hold them in place during insertion. The insertion tube is advanced into the uterus to the

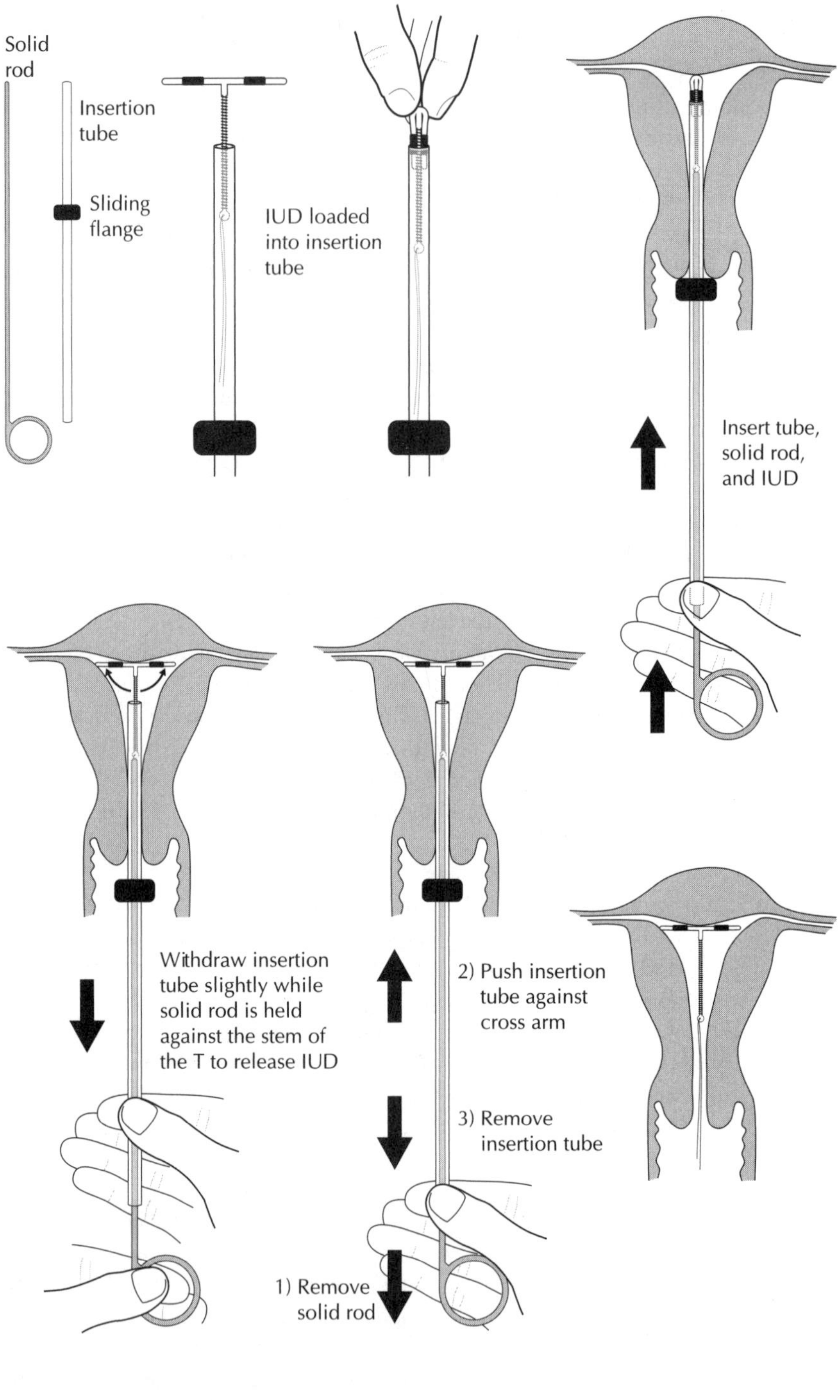

Solid
rod

Insertion
tube

Sliding
flange

IUD loaded
into insertion
tube

Insert tube,
solid rod,
and IUD

Withdraw insertion
tube slightly while
solid rod is held
against the stem of
the T to release IUD

2) Push insertion
tube against
cross arm

3) Remove
insertion tube

1) Remove
solid rod

244

correct depth as marked on the tube by a sliding plastic flange. The flange should be twisted to be in the same plane as the horizontal arms. When the insertion tube and IUD reach the fundus, withdraw a few millimeters. Check to make sure that the transverse arm of the IUD is in the horizontal plane so that the tips of the T rests in the cornual regions of the endometrial cavity. Placement in the vertical plane increases the risk of expulsion and pregnancy.[167] To release the TCu-380A, advance the solid rod until the resistance of the IUD is felt, fix the rod against the tenaculum, which is held in traction, and withdraw the insertion tube while the solid insertion rod is held against the stem of the T, releasing the transverse arms into high fundal position. Remove the solid rod and finally the inserter tube taking care not to pull on the strings. You can ensure that the TCu-380A is in a high fundal position if, after removing the solid rod, you push the inserter tube up against the cross arm of the T prior to withdrawing it completely from the cavity. Trim the strings to about 4 cm from the external os, and record their length in the chart. Shorter strings can cause unpleasant bristle-like sensations.

Patients with newly inserted IUDs should attempt to feel the strings before leaving the examining room. Giving them the cut ends of the strings as a sample of what to feel is helpful. Palpation should be performed monthly by the patient to verify continuing presence of the IUD after each menstrual flow. Caution the patient that the first 2 menses are typically heavier. As with all office procedures, patients should be provided a 24-hour phone number for urgent questions or concerns, and especially to report unusual pain, bleeding, or vaginal discharge.

A 1-month follow-up visit is recommended to identify problems amenable to counseling and treatment. Women experiencing heavier menstrual flow or irregular bleeding in the first month after insertion are at increased risk for removals because of bleeding and pain.[168] Intensified support along with treatment with an NSAID can maintain continuation of the method.

Technique for the Levonorgestrel IUD

Prepare for insertion as described above for the copper IUD. Open the sterile package, releasing the strings. Make sure that the slider is as far forward (toward the patient) as possible and that the arms of the IUD are horizontal. Holding the slider steady, pull on both strings to draw the IUD into the insertion tube until the knobs at the ends of the arms are closing the open end of the inserter. Fix the strings into the notch at the bottom of the inserter. Move the flange so that the forward surface is at the depth of the uterus as measured by the sound. Hold the slider firmly with a thumb or finger; move the inserter into the uterus until the flange is about 1.5–2.0 cm from the cervix (this allows space for the arms to open).

Holding the inserter steady, release the arms by pulling the slider back until it reaches the mark (the raised horizontal line); wait 10–30 seconds for the arms to completely open. Holding the slider in its new position, advance the inserter gently until the flange touches the cervix, placing the IUD high in the fundus. Release the IUD by pulling the slider down, making sure that the strings release from the notch. Remove the inserter and trim the strings.

Insertion against the anterior fundus is essential for maximal efficacy and low expulsion rates. Correct placement can be assessed with ultrasonography; this is especially useful when inserting IUDs in larger cavities (after a pregnancy or when myomas are present).

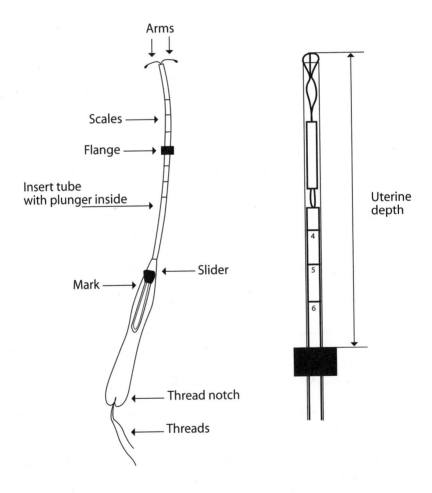

Prophylactic Antibiotics

Doxycycline (200 mg) administered orally 1 hour prior to insertion can provide protection against insertion-associated pelvic infection, but three double-blind randomized studies, two conducted in Africa and one in Turkey, found no significant advantage in the treated groups.[169–171] Azithromycin in a dose of 500 mg has also been used prophylactically, presumably offering more protection because of a longer half-life.[172] However, a randomized trial in low-risk women could find no effect on the subsequent rate of IUD removal or morbidity when 500 mg azithromycin was administered 1 hour before IUD insertion.[173] In women at low risk for STIs, the incidence of infection is so low that there is little benefit to be expected with prophylactic antibiotics.[174]

IUD Removal

Removal of an IUD can usually be accomplished by grasping the string with a ring forcep or uterine dressing forcep and exerting firm traction. If strings cannot be seen, they can often be extracted from the cervical canal by rotating two cotton-tipped applicators or a Pap smear cytobrush in the endocervical canal. If further maneuvers are required, a paracervical block should be administered. Oral administration of an NSAID beforehand reduces uterine cramping.

If IUD strings cannot be identified or extracted from the endocervical canal, a light plastic uterine sound should be passed into the endometrial cavity after administration of a paracervical block. A standard metal sound is too heavy and insensitive for this purpose. The IUD can frequently be felt with the sound and localized against the anterior or posterior wall of the uterus. The device can then be removed using a Facit polyp or alligator-type forcep directed to where the device was felt, taking care to open the forcep widely immediately on passing it through the internal cervical os so that the IUD can be caught between the jaws. If removal is not easily accomplished using this forcep, direct visualization of the IUD with sonography or hysteroscopy can facilitate removal. Sonography is less painful and more convenient and should be tried first.

Fertility returns promptly and pregnancies after removal of an IUD occur at a normal rate, sooner than after oral contraception.[62–65, 67, 68] Pregnancy outcome after IUD removal is assocated with a normal incidence of spontaneous miscarriage and ectopic pregnancy.[68]

If a patient wishes to continue use of an IUD, a new device can be placed immediately after removal of the old one. In this case, antibiotic prophylaxis is advised.

Embedded IUDs

If removal is not easily accomplished, direct visualization of the IUD with sonography or hysteroscopy can be helpful. Sonography is safer and less expensive.[132, 175] Transvaginal ultrasonography provides the best image to confirm the location of the IUD, but there is little room for the removal procedure. A better approach is to fill the bladder and use an abdominal sector transducer to image the uterine cavity as the forceps are introduced. One should open the forceps widely and see if the IUD moves when the forceps close on it. If it moves, one should close the forceps tightly and extract the IUD. If unsuccessful, the forceps is reintroduced in a different plane, keeping one jaw of the open forceps firmly against first the anterior and then the posterior uterine wall. If this approach is not successful, hysteroscopy is indicated.

Finding a Displaced IUD

When an IUD cannot be found, in addition to expulsion, one has to consider perforation of the uterus into the abdominal cavity (a very rare event) or embedment into the myometrium. All IUDs are radiopaque, but localizing them radiographically requires 2–3 views, is time-consuming and expensive, and does not allow intrauterine direction of instruments. A quick, real-time sonographic scan in the office is the best method to locate a lost IUD, whether or not removal is desired. If the IUD cannot be visualized with ultrasonography, abdominal x-rays are necessary because the IUD can be high and hidden.

If the IUD is identified perforating the myometrium or in the abdominal cavity, it should be removed using operative laparoscopy, usually under general anesthesia. If the IUD is in the uterine cavity, but cannot be grasped with a forceps under sonographic guidance, hysteroscopy is the best approach. Both routes may be helpful if an IUD is partially perforated.

Copper in the abdominal cavity can lead to adhesion formation, making laparoscopic removal difficult.[176] Although inert perforated devices without closed loops were previously allowed to remain in the abdominal cavity, current practice is to remove any perforated IUD. Because IUD perforations usually occur at the time of insertion, it is important to check for correct position by identifying the string within a few weeks after insertion. Uterine perforation itself is unlikely to cause more than transient pain and bleeding and can go undetected at the time of IUD insertion. If you believe perforation has occurred, prompt sonography is indicated so that the device can be removed before adhesion formation can occur.

This problem should be put into perspective. With the new generation of IUDs (copper and medicated), adhesion formation appears to be an immediate reaction that does not progress and rarely leads to serious complications.[177] In appropriate situations (in which the risk of surgery is considerable), clinician and patient may elect not to remove the translocated IUD in the absence of concerning symptoms.[178] However, a case has been reported of sigmoid perforation occurring 5 years after insertion, and the general consensus continues to favor removal of a perforated IUD immediately on diagnosis.[179]

IUD Myths

We hope the information in this chapter lays to rest 4 specific myths associated with IUDs. For emphasis, the following sentences provide the correct responses to what we believe are common misconceptions among clinicians:

1. IUDs are *NOT* abortifacients.
2. An increased risk of infection with the modern IUD is related *ONLY* to the insertion.
3. The modern IUD *HAS NOT* exposed clinicians to litigation.
4. IUDs *DO NOT* increase the risk of ectopic pregnancy.

References

1. **Huber SC, Piotrow PT, Orlans B, Dommer G,** Intrauterine devices, Pop Reports, Series B No. 2, 1975.

2. **Richter R,** Ein mittel zur verhutung der konzeption, Deutsche Med Wochenschrift 35:1525, 1909.

3. **Pust K,** Ein brauchbarer frauenschutz, Deutsche Med Wochenschrift 49:952, 1923.

4. **Gräfenberg E,** An intrauterine contraceptive method, In: Sanger M, Stone HM, eds. The Practice of Contraception: Proceedings of the 7th International Birth Control Conference, Zurich, Switzerland, Williams & Wilkins, Baltimore, 1930, pp 33–47.

5. **Ota T,** A study on birth control with an intra-uterine instrument, Jpn J Obstet Gynecol 17:210, 1934.

6. **Ishihama A,** Clinical studies on intrauterine rings, especially the present state of contraception in Japan and the experiences in the use of intra-uterine rings, Yokohama Med Bull 10:89, 1959.

7. **Oppenheimer W,** Prevention of pregnancy by the Graefenberg ring method: A re-evaluation after 28 years' experience, Am J Obstet Gynecol 78:446, 1959.

8. **Tietze C,** Evaluation of intrauterine devices. Ninth progress report of the cooperative statistical program, Stud Fam Plann 1:1, 1970.

9. **Tatum HJ, Schmidt FH, Phillips DM, McCarty M, O'Leary WM,** The Dalkon shield controversy, structural and bacteriologic studies of IUD tails, JAMA 231:711, 1975.

10. **Kessel E,** Pelvic inflammatory disease with intrauterine device use: A reassessment, Fertil Steril 51:1, 1989.

11. **Eschenbach DA, Harnisch JP, Holmes KK,** Pathogenesis of acute pelvic inflammatory disease: role of contraception and other risk factors, Am J Obstet Gynecol 128:838, 1977.

12. **Kaufman DW, Shapiro S, Rosenberg L, Monson RR, Miettinen OS, Stolley PD, Slone D,** Intrauterine contraceptive device use and pelvic inflammatory disease, Am J Obstet Gynecol 136:159, 1980.

13. **Kaufman DW, Watson J, Rosenberg L, Helmrich SP, Miller DR, Miettinen OS, Stolley PD, Shapiro S,** The effect of different types of intrauterine devices on the risk of pelvic inflammatory disease, JAMA 250:759, 1983.

14. **Lee NC, Rubin GL, Ory HW, Burkman RT,** Type of intrauterine device and the risk of pelvic inflammatory disease, Obstet Gynecol 62:1, 1983.

15. **Piccinino LJ, Mosher WD,** Trends in contraceptive use in the United States: 1982–1995, Fam Plann Perspect 30:4, 1998.

16. **Population Crisis Committee, Access to birth control:** A world assessment, Population Briefing Paper, Washington, DC, 1986.

17. **Daling JR, Weiss NS, Metch BJ, Chow WH, Soderstrom RM, Moore DE, Spadoni LR,** Stadel BV, Primary tubal infertility in relation to the use of an intrauterine device, New Engl J Med 312:937, 1985.

18. **Cramer DW, Schiff I, Schoenbaum SC, Gibson M, Belisle S, Albrecht B, Stillman RJ, Berger MJ, Wilson E, Stadel BV, Seible M,** Tubal infertility and the intrauterine device, New Engl J Med 312:941, 1985.

19. **Lee NC, Rubin GL, Borucki R,** The intrauterine device and pelvic inflammatory disease revisited: new results from the Womens' Health Study, Obstet Gynecol 72:1, 1988

20. **Zipper JA, Medel M, Prage R,** Suppression of fertility by intrauterine copper and zinc in rabbits: A new approach to intrauterine contraception, Am J Obstet Gynecol 105:529, 1969.

21. **Tatum HJ,** Milestones in intrauterine device development, Fertil Steril 39:141, 1983.

22. **Sivin I, Tatum HJ,** Four years of experience with the TCu 380A intrauterine contraceptive device, Fertil Steril 36:159, 1981.

23. **Sujuan G, Liuqu Z, Yuhao W, Feng L,** Chinese IUDs, In: Bardin CW, Mishell Jr DR, eds. Proceedings from the Fourth International Conference on IUDs, Butterworth-Heinemann, Boston, 1994, pp 308–318.

24. **Sivin I, Diaz S, Pavéz M, Alvarez F, Brache V, Diaz J, Odlind V, Olsson S-E, Stern J,** Two-year comparative trial of the gyne T 380 slimline and gyne T 380 intrauterine copper devices, Contraception 44:481, 1991.

25. **Sivin I, Stern J,** International Committee for Contraception Research, Health during prolonged use of levonorgestrel 20 mg/d and the copper TCu 380 Ag intrauterine contraceptive devices: a multicenter study, Fertil Steril 61:70, 1994.

250

26. **Chi I-c,** The TCu-380A (AG), MLCu375, and Nova-T IUDs and the IUD daily releasing 20 mg levonorgestrel — four pillars of IUD contraception for the nineties and beyond? Contraception 47:325, 1993.

27. **Kurz KM, Meier-Oehlke PA,** The Cu SAFE 300 IUD, a new concept in intrauterine contraception: first year results of a large study with follow-up of 1017 acceptors, Adv Contracept 7:291, 1991.

28. **Luukkainen T, Allonen H, Haukkamaa M, Lahteenmake P, Nilsson CG, Toivonen J,** Five years' experience with levonorgestrel-releasing IUDs, Contraception 33:139, 1986.

29. **Sivin I, Stern J, Coutinho E, Mattos CER, El Mahgoub S, Diaz S, Pavéz M, Alvarez F, Brache V, Thevinin F, Diaz J, Faundes A, Diaz MM, McCarthy T, Mishell Jr DR, Shoupe D,** Prolonged intrauterine contraception: a seven-year randomized study of the levonorgestrel 20 mcg/day (LNg 20) and the copper T380 Ag IUDs, Contraception 44:473, 1991.

30. **Toivonen J, Luukkainen T, Alloven H,** Protective effect of intrauterine release of levonorgestrel on pelvic infection: three years' comparative experience of levonorgestrel and copper-releasing intrauterine devices, Obstet Gynecol 77:261, 1991.

31. **Bilian X, Liying Z, Xuling Z, Mengchun J, Luukkainen T, Allonen H,** Pharmacokinetic and pharmacodynamic studies of levonorgestrel-releasing intrauterine device, Contraception 41:353, 1990.

32. **Crosignani PG, Vercellini P, Mosconi P, Oldani S, Cortesi I, De Giorgi O,** Levonorgestrel-releasing intrauterine device versus hysteroscopic endometrial resection in the treatment of dysfunctional uterine bleeding, Obstet Gynecol 90:257, 1997.

33. **Gardner FJE, Konje JC, Abrams KR, Brown LJR, Khanna S, Al-Azzawi F, Bell SC, Taylor DJ,** Endometrial protection from tamoxifen-stimulated changes by a levonorgestrel-releasing intrauterine system: a randomised controlled trial, Lancet 356:1711, 2000.

34. **Vercellini P, Aimi G, Panazza S, De Giorgi O, Pesole A, Crosignani PG,** A levonorgestrel-releasing intrauterine system for the treatment of dysmenorrhea associated with endometriosis: a pilot study, Fertil Steril 72:505, 1999.

35. **Varila E, Wahlstrom T, Rauramo I,** A 5-year follow-up study on the use of a levonorgestrel intrauterine system in women receiving hormone replacement therapy, Fertil Steril 76:969, 2001.

36. **Raudaskoski T, Tapanainen J, Tomas E, Luotola H, Pekonen F, Ronni-Sivula H, Timonen H, Riphagen F, Laatikainen T,** Intrauterine 10 microg and 20 microg levonorgestrel systems in postmenopausal women receiving oral oestrogen replacement therapy: clinical, endometrial and metabolic responses, Br J Obstet Gynaecol 109:136, 2002.

37. **Wollter-Svensson LO, Stadberg E, Andersson K, Mattsson LA, Odlind V, Persson I,** Intrauterine administration of levonorgestrel 5 and 10 microg/24 hours in perimenopausal hormone replacement therapy. A randomized clinical study during one year, Acta Obstet Gynecol Scand 76:449, 1997.

38. **UNDP, UNFPA, and WHO Special Programme of Research, Development and Research Training in Human Reproduction, World Bank: IUD Research Group,** The Tcu 380A IUD and the frameless IUD "the Flexigard:" interim three-year data from an International Multicenter Trial, Contraception 52:77, 1995.

39. **Rosenberg MJ, Foldesy R, Mishell Jr DR, Speroff L, Waugh MS, Burkman R,** Performance of the TCu380A and Cu-Fix IUDs in an international randomized trial, Contraception 53:197, 1996.

40. **Van Kets H, Van der Pas H, Thiery M, Wildemeersch D, Vrijens M, Van Trappen Y, Temmerman M, DePypere H, Delbarge W, Dhont M, Defoort P, Schacht EH, Bátárl I, Barri P, Martinez F, Iglesias Cortit LH, Creatsas G, Shangchun W, Xiaoming C, Zuan-chong F, Yu-ming W, Andrade A, Reinprayoon D, Pizarro E,** The GyneFix® implant system for interval, postabortal and postpartum contraception: a significant advance in long-term reversible contraception, Eur J Contraception Reprod Health Care 2:1, 1997.

41. **Wildemeersch D, Batar I, Webb A, Gbolade BA, Delbarge W, Temmerman M, Dhont M, Gillebaud J, GyneFIX.** The frameless intrauterine contraceptive implant—an update for interval, emergency and postabortal contraception, Br J Fam Plann 24:149, 1999.

42. **Wu S, Hu J, Wildemeersch D,** Performance of the frameless GyneFix and the TCu380A IUDs in a 3-year multicenter, randomized, comparative trial in parous women, Contraception 61:91, 2000.

43. **Wildemeersch D, Dhont M, Temmerman M, Delbarge W, Schacht E, Thiery M,** GyneFix-LNG: preliminary clinical experience with a copper and levonorgestrel-releasing intrauterine system, Eur J Contracept Reprod Health Care 4:15, 1999.

44. **Wildemeersch D, Schacht E, Wildemeersch P,** Performance and acceptability of intrauterine release of levonorgestrel with a miniature delivery system for hormonal substitution therapy, contraception and treatment in peri and postmenopausal women, Maturitas 44:237, 2003.

45. **Sivin I,** IUDs are contraceptives, not abortifacients: a comment on research and belief, Stud Fam Plann 20:355, 1989.

46. **Ortiz ME, Croxatto HB,** The mode of action of IUDs, Contraception 36:37, 1987.

47. **Alvarez F, Guiloff E, Brache V, Hess R, Fernandez E, Salvatierra AM, Guerrero B, Zacharias S,** New insights on the mode of action of intrauterine contraceptive devices in women, Fertil Steril 49:768, 1988.

48. **Segal SJ, Alvarez-Sanchez F, Adejuwon CA, Brache De Mejla V, Leon P, Faundes A,** Absence of chorionic gonadotropin in sera of women who use intrauterine devices, Fertil Steril 44:214, 1985.

49. **Wilcox AJ, Weinberg CR, Armstrong EG, Canfield RE,** Urinary human chorionic gonadotropin among intrauterine device users: Detection with a highly specific and sensitive assay, Fertil Steril 47:265, 1987.

50. **Ämmälä M, Nyman T, Strengell L, Rutanen E-M,** Effect of intrauterine contraceptive devices on cytokine messenger ribonucleic acid expression in the human endometrium, Fertil Steril 63:773, 1995.

51. **Critchley HO, Wang H, Jones RL, Kelly RW, Drudy TA, Gebbie AE, Buckley CH, McNeilly AS, Glasier AF,** Morphological and functional features of endometrial decidualization following long-term intrauterine levonorgestrel delivery, Hum Reprod 13:1218, 1998.

52. **Barbosa I, Olsson SE, Odlind V, Goncalves T, Coutinho E,** Ovarian function after seven years' use of levonorgestrel IUD, Adv Contraception 11:85, 1995.

53. **Andersson J, Rybo G,** Levonorgestrel-releasing intrauterine device in the treatment of menorrhagia, Br J Obstet Gynaecol 97:690, 1990.

54. **Baldszti E, Wimmer-Puchinger B, Loschke K,** Acceptability of the long-term contraceptive levonorgestrel-releasing intrauterine system (Mirena): a 3-year follow-up study, Contraception 67:87, 2003.

55. **Hidalgo M, Bahamondes L, Perrotti M, Diaz J, Dantas-Monteiro C, Petta C,** Bleeding patterns and clinical performance of the levonorgestrel-releasing intrauterine system (Mirena) up to two years, Contraception 65:129, 2002.

56. **Ronnerdag M, Odlind V,** Health effects of long-term use of the intrauterine levonorgestrel-releasing system. A follow-up study over 12 years of continuous use, Acta Obstet Gynecol Scand 78:716, 1999.

57. **Irvine GA, Campbell-Brown MB, Lumsden MA, Heikkila A, Walker JJ, Cameron IT,** Randomised comparative trial of the levonorgestrel intrauterine system and norethisterone for treatment of idiopathic menorrhagia, Br J Obstet Gynaecol 105:592, 1998.

58. **Istre O, Trolle B,** Treatment of menorrhagia with the levonorgestrel intrauterine system versus endometrial resection, Fertil Steril 76:304, 2001.

59. **Romer T,** Prospective comparison study of levonorgestrel IUD versus Roller-Ball endometrial ablation in the management of refractory recurrent hypermenorrhea, Eur J Obstet Gynecol Reprod Biol 90:27, 2000.

60. **Hurskainen R, Teperi J, Rissanen P, Aalto A-M, Grenman S, Kivelä A, Kujansuu E, Vuorma S, Yliskoski M, Paavonen J,** Clinical outcomes and costs with the levonorgestrel-releasing intrauterine system or hysterectomy for treatment of menorrhagia. Randomized trial 5-year follow-up, JAMA 291:1456, 2004.

61. **Inki P, Hurskainen R, Palo P, Ekholm E, Grenman S, Kivela A, Kujansuu E, Teperi J, Yliskoski M, Paavonen J,** Comparison of ovarian cyst formation in women using the levonorgestrel-releasing intrauterine system vs. hysterectomy, Ultrasound Obstet Gynecol 20:381, 2002.

62. **Vessey MP, Lawless M, McPherson K, Yeates D,** Fertility after stopping use of intrauterine contraceptive device, Br Med J 283:106, 1983.

63. **Belhadj H, Sivin I, Diaz S, Pavéz M, Tejada A-S, Brache V, Alvarez F, Shoupe D, Breaux H, Mishell Jr DR, McCarthy T, Yo V,** Recovery of fertility after use of the levonorgestrel 20 mcg/day or copper T 380Ag intrauterine device, Contraception 34:261, 1986.

252

64. **Skjeldestadt FE, Bratt H,** Fertility after complicated and non-complicated use of IUDs. A controlled prospective study, Adv Contracept 4:179, 1988.

65. **Wilson JC,** A prospective New Zealand study of fertility after removal of copper intrauterine devices for conception and because of complications: a four-year study, Am J Obstet Gynecol 160:391, 1989.

66. **United Nations Development Programme/United Nations Population Fund/World Health Organization/World Bank, Special Programme of Research, Development and Research Training in Human Reproduction,** Long-term reversible contraception. Twelve years of experience with the TCu380A and TCu220C, Contraception 56:341, 1997.

67. **Sivin I, Stern J, Diaz J, Diaz MM, Faundes A, Mahgoub SE, Diaz S, Pavéz M, Coutinho E, Mattos CER, McCarthy T, Mishell DR, Jr., Shoupe D, Alvarez F, Brache V, Jimenez E,** Two years of intrauterine contraception with levonorgestrel and with copper: a randomized comparison of the TCu 380Ag and levonorgestrel 20 mcg/day devices, Contraception 35:245, 1987.

68. **Sivin I, Stern J, Diaz S, Pavez M, Alvarez F, Brache V, Mishell Jr DR, Lacarra M, McCarthy T, Holma P, Darney P, Klaisle C, Olsson S-E, Odlind V,** Rates and outcomes of planned pregnancy after use of Norplant capsules, Norplant II rods, or levonorgestrel-releasing or copper TCu 380Ag intrauterine contraceptive devices, Am J Obstet Gynecol 166:1208, 1992.

69. **Sivin I, Schmidt F,** Effectiveness of IUDs: a review, Contraception 36:55, 1987.

70. **Sivin I, el Mahgoub S, McCarthy T, Mishell DR, Jr., Shoupe D, Alvarez F, Brache V, Jimenez E, Diaz J, Faundes A, et al.,** Long-term contraception with the levonorgestrel 20 mcg/day (LNg 20) and the copper T 380Ag intrauterine devices: a five-year randomized study, Contraception 42:361, 1990.

71. **Meirik O, Farley TMM, Sivin I, for the International Collaborative Post-Marketing Surveillance of Norplant,** Safety and efficacy of levonorgestrel implant, intrauterine device, and sterilization, Am J Obstet Gynecol 97:539, 2001.

72. **Petta CA, Amatya R, Farr G,** Clinical evaluation of the TCu 380A IUD at six Latin American centers, Contraception 50:17, 1994.

73. **WHO Special Programme of Research, Development and Research Training in Human Reproduction, Task Force on the Safety and Efficacy of Fertility Regulating Methods,** The TCu 380A, TCu 220C, Multiload 250, and Nova T IUDs at 3, 5, and 7 years of use, Contraception 42:141, 1990.

74. **Farr G, Amatya R,** Contraceptive efficacy of the copper T 380A and copper T 200 intrauterine devices: results from a comparative clinical trial in six developing countries, Contraception 49:231, 1994.

75. **Rivera R, Chen-Mok M, McMullen S,** Analysis of client characteristics that may affect early discontinuation of the TCu-380A IUD, Contraception 60:155, 1999.

76. **WHO Special Programme of Research, Development and Research Training in Human Reproduction, Task Force on Intrauterine Devices for Fertility Regulation,** A multinational case-control study of ectopic pregnancy, Clin Reprod Fertil 3:131, 1985.

77. **Marchbanks PA, Annegers JE, Coulam CB, Strathy JH, Kurland LT,** Risk factors for ectopic pregnancy. A population based study, JAMA 259:1823, 1988.

78. **Ory HW,** Ectopic pregnancy and intrauterine contraceptive devices: new perspectives, Obstet Gynecol 57:2, 1981.

79. **Edelman DA, Porter CW,** The intrauterine device and ectopic pregnancy, Contraception 36:85, 1987.

80. **Makinen JL, Erkkola RU, Laippala PJ,** Causes of the increase in incidence of ectopic pregnancy — a study on 1017 patients from 1966 to 1985 in Turku, Finland, Am J Obstet Gynecol 160:642, 1989.

81. **Skjeldestad FE,** How effectively do copper intrauterine devices prevent ectopic pregnancy? Acta Obstet Gynecol Scand 76:684, 1997.

82. **Sivin I,** Dose- and age-dependent ectopic pregnancy risks with intrauterine contraception, Obstet Gynecol 78:291, 1991.

83. **Barbosa I, Bakos O, Olsson S-E, Odlind V, Johansson EDB,** Ovarian function during use of a levonorgestrel-releasing IUD, Contraception 42:51, 1990.

84. **Andersson K, Odlind V, Rybo G,** Levonorgestrel-releasing and copper-releasing (Nova T) IUDs during five years of use: a randomized comparative trial, Contraception 49:56, 1994.

253

85. **Backman T, Rauramo I, Huhtala S, Koskenvuo M,** Pregnancy during the use of levonorgestrel intrauterine system, Am J Obstet Gynecol 190:50, 2004.

86. **Franks AL, Beral V, Cates W, Jr., Hogue CJ,** Contraception and ectopic pregnancy risk, Am J Obstet Gynecol 163:1120, 1990.

87. **Cameron IT, Haining R, Lumsden M-A, Thomas VR, Smith SK,** The effects of mefenamic acid and norethisterone on measured menstrual blood loss, Obstet Gynecol 76:85, 1990.

88. **Zhao G, Minshi L, Pengdi Z, Ruhua X, Jiedong W, Renqing X,** A preliminary morphometric study on the endometrium from patients treated with indomethacin-releasing copper intrauterine device, Hum Reprod 12:1563, 1997.

89. **Milsom I, Andersson K, Jonasson K, Lindstedt G, Rybo G,** The influence of the Gyne-T 380S IUD on menstrual blood loss and iron status, Contraception 52:175, 1995.

90. **Task Force for Epidemiological Research on Reproductive Health, United Nations Development Programme/United Nations Population Fund/World Health Organization/World Bank Special Programme of Research, Develpment and Research Training in Human Reproduction,** Effects of contraceptives on hemoglobin and ferritin, Contraception 58:261, 1998.

91. **Hassan EO, El-Husseini M, El-Nahal N,** The effect of 1-year use of the CuT 380A and oral contraceptive pills on hemoglobin and ferritin levels, Contraception 60:101, 1999.

92. **Backman T, Huhtala S, Blom T, Luoto R, Rauramo I, Markku K,** Length of use and symptoms associated with premature removal of the levonorgestrel intrauterine system: a nationwide study of 17,360 users, Br J Obstet Gynaecol 107:335, 2000.

93. **Tang GW, Lo SS,** Levonorgestrel intrauterine device in the treatment of menorrhagia in Chinese women: efficacy versus acceptability, Contraception 51:231, 1995.

94. **Crosignani PG, Vercellini P, Apolone G, De Giorgi O, Cortesi I, Meschia M,** Endometrial resection versus vaginal hysterectomy for menorrhagia: long-term clinical and quality-of-life outcomes, Am J Obstet Gynecol 177:95, 1997.

95. **Fong YF, Singh K,** Effect of the levonorgestrel-releasing intrauterine system on uterine myomas in a renal transplant patient, Contraception 60:51, 1999.

96. **Lockhat FB, Emembolu JO, Konje JC,** The evaluation of the effectiveness of an intrauterine-administered progestogen (levonorgestrel) in the symptomatic treatment of endometriosis and in the staging of the disease, Hum Reprod 19:179, 2004.

97. **Pakarinen P, Lahteenmaki P, Rutanen EM,** The effect of intrauterine and oral levonorgestrel administration on serum concentrations of sex hormone-binding globulin, insulin and insulin-like growth factor binding protein-1, Acta Obstet Gynecol Scand 78:423, 1999.

98. **Castellsague X, Thompson WD, Dubrow R,** Intra-uterine contraception and the risk of endometrial cancer, Int J Cancer 54:911, 1993.

99. **Lassise DL, Savitz DA, Hamman RF, Baron AE, Brinton LA, Levines RS,** Invasive cervical cancer and intrauterine device use, Int J Epidemiol 20:865, 1991.

100. **Parazzini F, La Vecchia C, Negri E,** Use of intrauterine device and risk of invasive cervical cancer, Int J Epidemiol 21:1030, 1992.

101. **Hill DA, Weiss NS, Voigt LF, Beresford SAA,** Endometrial cancer in relation to intrauterine device use, Int J Cancer 70:278, 1997.

102. **Sturgeon SR, Brinton LA, Berman ML, Mortel R, Twiggs LB, Barrett RJ, Wilbanks GD, Lurain JR,** Intrauterine device use and endometrial cancer risk, Int J Epidemiol 26:496, 1997.

103. **Benshushan A, Paltiel O, Rojansky N, Brzezinski A, Laufer N,** IUD use and the risk of endometrial cancer, Eur J Obstet Gynecol Reprod Biol 105:166, 2002.

104. **Mark AS, Hricak H,** Intrauterine contraceptive devices: MR imaging, Radiology 162:311, 1987.

105. **Pasquale SA, Russer TJ, Foldesy R, Mezrich RS,** Lack of interaction between magnetic resonance imaging and the copper-T380A IUD, Contraception 55:169, 1997.

106. **Mishell Jr DR, Bell JH, Good RG, Moyer DL,** The intrauterine device: a bacteriologic study of the endometrial cavity, Am J Obstet Gynecol 96:119, 1966.

107. **Farley MM, Rosenberg MJ, Rowe PJ, Chen J-H, Meirik O,** Intrauterine devices and pelvic inflammatory disease: an international perspective, Lancet 339:785, 1992.

108. **Skouby SO, Molsted-Pedersen L, Kosonen A,** Consequences of intrauterine contraception in diabetic women, Fertil Steril 42:568, 1984.

109. **Kimmerle R, Weiss R, Bergert M, Kurz K,** Effectiveness, safety, and acceptability of a copper intrauterine deivce (Cu Safe 300) in type I diabetic women, Diabetes Care 16:1227, 1993.

110. **Buchan H, Villard-Mackintosh L, Vessey M, Yeates D, McPherson K,** Epidemiology of pelvic inflammatory disease in parous women with special reference to intrauterine device use, Br J Obstet Gynaecol 97:780, 1990.

111. **Mehanna MTR, Rizk MA, Ramadan M, Schachter J,** Chlamydial serologic characteristics among intrauterine contraceptive device users: does copper inhibit chlamydial infection in the female genital tract? Am J Obstet Gynecol 171:691, 1994.

112. **Kleinman D, Insler V, Sarov I,** Inhibition of Chlamydia trachomatis growth in endometrial cells by copper: possible relevance for the use of copper IUDs, Contraception 39:665, 1989.

113. **Kronmal RA, Whitney CW, Mumford SD,** The intrauterine device and pelvic inflammatory disease: the Women's Health Study reanalyzed, J Clin Epidemiol 44:109, 1991.

114. **Lee NC, Rubin GL, Grimes DA,** Measures of sexual behavior and the risk of pelvic inflammatory disease, Obstet Gynecol 77:425, 1991.

115. **Everett ED, Reller LB, Droegemueller W, Greer BE,** Absence of bacteremia after insertion or removal of intrauterine device, Obstet Gynecol 47:207, 1976.

116. **Hall SM, Jamieson JR, Witcomb MA,** Bacteraemia after insertion of intrauterine devices, S Afr Med J 50:12321, 1976.

117. **Murray S, Hickey JB, Houang E,** Significant bacteremia associated with replacement of intrauterine contraceptive device, Am J Obstet Gynecol 156:698, 1987.

118. **Shoubnikova M, Hellberg D, Nilsson S, Mårdh P-A,** Contraceptive use in women with bacterial vaginosis, Contraception 55:355, 1997.

119. **Jossens MOR, Schachter J, Sweet RL,** Risk factors associated with pelvic inflammatory disease of differing microbial etiologies, Obstet Gynecol 83:989, 1994.

120. **European Study Group,** Risk factors for male to female transmission of HIV, Br Med J 298:411, 1989.

121. **Musicco M, Nicolosi A, Saracco A, Lazzarin A,** IUD use and man to woman sexual transmission of HIV-1, In: Bardin CW, Mishell Jr DR, eds. Proceedings from the Fourth International Conference on IUDs, Butterworth-Heinemann, Boston, 1994, pp 179–188.

122. **Kapiga SH, Lyamuya EF, Lwihula GK, Hunter DJ,** The incidence of HIV infection among women using family planning methods in Dar-es-Salaam, Tanzania, AIDS 12:75, 1998.

123. **European Study Group on Heterosexual Transmission of HIV,** Comparison of female to male and male to female transmission of HIV in 563 stable couples, Br Med J 304:809, 1992.

124. **Sinei SK, Morrison CS, Sekadde-Kigondu C, Allen M, Kokonya D,** Complications of use of intrauterine devices among HIV-1-infected women, Lancet 351:1238, 1998.

125. **Chapin DS, Sullinger JC,** A 43-year old woman with left buttock pain and a presacral mass, New Engl J Med 323:183, 1990.

126. **Keebler C, Chatwani A, Schwartz R,** Actinomycosis infection associated with intrauterine contraceptive devices, Am J Obstet Gynecol 145:596, 1983.

127. **Fiorino AS,** Intrauterine contraceptive device-associated actinomycotic abscess and *Actinomyces* detection on cervical smear, Obstet Gynecol 87:142, 1996.

128. **Duguid HLD,** Actinomycosis and IUDs, Int Plann Parenthood Fed Med Bull 17:3, 1983.

129. **Petitti DB, Yamamoto D, Morgenstern N,** Factors associated with actinomyces-like organisms on Papanicolaou smear in users of IUDs, Am J Obstet Gynecol 145:338, 1983.

130. **Persson E, Holmberg K, Dahlgren S, Nielsson L,** *Actinomyces israelii* in genital tract of women with and without intrauterine contraception devices, Acta Obstet Gynecol Scand 62:563, 1983.

131. **Hill GB,** Eubacterium nodatum mimics *Actinomyces* in intrauterine device-associated infections and other settings within the female genital tract, Obstet Gynecol 79:534, 1992.

132. **Stubblefield P, Fuller A, Foster S,** Ultrasound-guided intrauterine removal of intrauterine contraceptive devices in pregnancy, Obstet Gynecol 72:961, 1988.

133. **Lewit S,** Outcome of pregnancy with intrauterine device, Contraception 2:47, 1970.

134. **Alvior Jr GT,** Pregnancy outcome with removal of intrauterine device, Obstet Gynecol 41:894, 1973.

135. **Assaf A, Gohar M, Saad S, El-Nashar A, Abdel Aziz A,** Removal of intrauterine devices with missing tails during early pregnancy, Contraception 45:541, 1992.

136. **Foreman H, Stadel BV, Schlesselman S,** Intrauterine device usage and fetal loss, Obstet Gynecol 58:669, 1981.

137. **United Kingdom Family Planning Research Network,** Pregnancy outcome associated with the use of IUDs, Br J Fam Plann 15:7, 1989.

138. **Williams P, Johnson B, Vessey M,** Septic abortion in women using intrauterine devices, Br Med J iv:263, 1975.

139. **Atrash HK, Frye A, Hogue CJR,** Incidence of morbidity and mortality with IUD in situ in the 1980s and 1990s, In: Bardin CW, Mishell Jr DR, eds. Proceedings from the Fourth International Conference on IUDs, Butterworth-Heinemann, Boston, 1994, pp 76–87.

140. **Guillebaud J,** IUD and congenital malformation, Br Med J i:1016, 1975.

141. **Layde PM, Goldberg MF, Safra MJM, Oakley GP,** Failed intrauterine device contraception and limb reduction deformities: a case-control study, Fertil Steril 31:18, 1979.

142. **Tatum HJ, Schmidt FH, Jain AK,** Management and outcome of pregnancies associated with the copper-T intrauterine contraceptive device, Am J Obstet Gynecol 127:869, 1976.

143. **Vessey M, Doll R, Peto R, Johnson B, Wiggins P,** A long-term follow-up study of women using different methods of contraception — an interim report, J Biosoc Sci 8:373, 1976.

144. **Chaim W, Mazor M,** Pregnancy with an intrauterine device in situ and preterm delivery, Arch Gynecol Obstet 252:21, 1992.

145. **Leigh BC, Temple MT, Trocki KF,** The sexual behavior of US adults: results from a national survey, Am J Public Health 83:1400, 1993.

146. **Suhonen S, Haukkamaa M, Jakobsson T, Rauramo I,** Clinical performance of a levonorgestrel-releasing intrauterine system and oral contraceptives in young nulliparous women: a comparative study, Contraception 69:407, 2004.

147. **Newton J, Tacchi D,** Long-term use of copper intrauterine devices, Br J Fam Plann 16:116, 1990.

148. **Haimov-Kochman R, Ackerman Z, Anteby EY,** The contraceptive choice for a Wilson's disease patient with chronic liver disease, Contraception 56:241, 1997.

149. **Kjos SL, Ballagh SA, La Cour M, Xiang A, Mishell DR, Jr.,** The copper T380A intrauterine device in women with Type II diabetes mellitus, Obstet Gynecol 84:1006, 1994.

150. **Diaz J, Pinto-Neto AM, Bahamondes L, Diaz M, Arce XE, Castro S,** Performance of the copper T 200 in parous adolescents: are copper IUDs suitable for these women? Contraception 48:23, 1993.

151. **Duenas JL, Albert A, Carrasco F,** Intrauterine contraception in nulligravid vs parous women, Contraception 53:23, 1996.

152. **Hubacher D, Lara-Ricalde R, Taylor DJ, Guerra-Infante F, Guzman-Rodriguez R,** Use of copper intrauterine devices and the risk of tubal infertility among nulligravid women, New Engl J Med 345:561, 2001.

153. **Doll H, Vessey M, Painter R,** Return of fertility in nulliparous women after discontinuation of the intrauterine device: comparison with women discontinuing other methods of contraception, Br J Obstet Gynaecol 108:304, 2001.

154. **Andersson K, Batar I, Rybo G,** Return to fertility after removal of a levonorgestrel-releasing intra-uterine device and Nova T, Contraception 46:575, 1992.

155. **Bastianelli C, Farris M, Lippa A, Lucantoni V, Valente A,** Use of intrauterine device by nulliparous women. Prospective study and preliminary data], Minerva Ginecol 50:231, 1998.

156. **Edelman D, Van Os W,** Safety of intrauterine contraception, Adv Contracept 6:207, 1990.

157. **Mishell Jr DR, Roy S,** Copper intrauterine contraceptive device event rates following insertion 4 to 8 weeks post partum, Am J Obstet Gynecol 143:29, 1982.

158. **Zhuang L, Wang H, Yang P,** Observations of the clinical efficacies and side effects of six different timings of IUD insertions, Clin J Obstet Gynecol 22:350, 1987.

159. **Chi I-c, Farr G,** Postpartum IUD contraception—A review of an international experience, Adv Contracept 5:127, 1989.

160. **Zhou S, Chi I-C,** Immediate postpartum IUD insertions in a Chinese hospital—A two-year follow-up, Int J Gynaecol Obstet 35:157, 1991.

161. **Chi I-c, Potts M, Wilkens L, Champion C,** Performance of the TCu-380A device in breastfeeding and non-breastfeeding women, Contraception 39:603, 1989.

162. **Andersson K, Ryde-Blomqvist E, Lindell K, Odlind V, Milsom I,** Perforations with intrauterine devices. Report from a Swedish survey, Contraception 57:251, 1998.

163. **Nielsen NC, Nygren K-G, Allonen H,** Three years of experience after post-abortal insertion of Nova-T and Copper-T-200, Acta Obstet Gynecol Scand 63:261, 1984.

164. **Querido L, Ketting E, Haspels AA,** IUD insertion following induced abortion, Contraception 31:603, 1985.

165. **White MK, Ory HW, Rooks JB, Rochat RW,** Intrauterine device termination rates and the menstrual cycle day of insertion, Obstet Gynecol 55:220, 1980.

166. **Rabin JM, Spitzer M, Dwyer AT, Kaiser IM,** Topical anesthesia for gynecologic procedures, Obstet Gynecol 73:1040, 1984.

167. **Anteby E, Revel A, Ben-Chetrit A, Rosen B, Tadmor O, Yagel S,** Intrauterine device failure: relation to its location within the uterine cavity, Obstet Gynecol 81:112, 1993.

168. **Stanback J, Grimes D,** Can intrauterine device removals for bleeding or pain be predicted at a one-month follow-up visit? A multivariate analysis, Contraception 58:357, 1998.

169. **Sinei SKA, Schulz KF, Laptey PR, Grimes D, Arnsi J, Rosenthal S, Rosenberg M, Rivon G, Njage P, Bhullar V, Ogendo H,** Preventing IUCD-related pelvic infection: The efficacy of prophylactic doxycycline at insertion, Br J Obstet Gynaecol 97:412, 1990.

170. **Lapido OA, Farr G, Otolorin E, Konje JC, Sturgen K, Cox P, Champion CB,** Prevention of IUD-related pelvic infection: the efficacy of prophylactic doxycycline at IUD insertion, Adv Contracept 7:43, 1991.

171. **Zorlu CG, Aral K, Cobanoglu O, Gurler S, Gokmen O,** Pelvic inflammatory disease and intrauterine devices: prophylactic antibiotics to reduce febrile complications, Adv Contracept 9:299, 1993.

172. **Walsh TL, Bernstein GS, Grimes DA, Frezieres R, Bernstein L, Coulson AH, IUD Study Group,** Effect of prophylactic antibiotics on morbidity associated with IUD insertion: results of a pilot randomized controlled trial, Contraception 50:319, 1994.

173. **Walsh T, Grimes D, Frezieres R, Nelson A, Bernstein L, Coulson A, Bernstein G,** for the IUD Study Group, Randomised controlled trial of prophylactic antibiotics before insertion of intrauterine devices, Lancet 351:1005, 1998.

174. **Grimes DA, Schulz KF,** Antibiotic prophylaxis for intrauterine contraceptive device insertion, Cochrane Database Syst Rev:CD001327, 2000.

175. **Sachs BP, Gregory K, McArdle C, Pinshaw A,** Removal of retained intrauterine contraceptive devices in pregnancy, Am J Perinatol 9:139, 1992.

176. **Gorsline J, Osborne N,** Management of the missing intrauterine contraceptive device: Report of a case, Am J Obstet Gynecol 153:228, 1985.

177. **Adoni A, Chetrit AB,** The management of intrauterine devices following uterine perforation, Contraception 43:77, 1991.

178. **Markovitch O, Klein Z, Gidoni Y, Holzinger M, Beyth Y,** Extrauterine mislocated IUD: is surgical removal mandatory? Contraception 66:105, 2002.

179. **Gronlund B, Blaabjerg J,** Serious intestinal complication five years after insertion of a Nova-T, Contraception 44:517, 1991.

257

8

Barrier Methods of Contraception

Barrier methods of contraception have been the most widely used contraceptive techniques throughout recorded history. These methods, the oldest of methods, are now being thrust into the forefront as we respond to the personal and social impact of sexually transmitted diseases (STDs). A new need for sexual safety has brought modern respect and new developments to the condom, while the other barrier methods continue to serve well for appropriate couples.

History

The use of vaginal contraceptives is probably as ancient as *Homo sapiens.* References to sponges and plugs appear in the earliest of writings. Substances with either barrier or spermicidal properties (or both) have included honey, alum, spices, oils, tannic acids, lemon juice, and even crocodile dung. However, the diaphragm and the cervical cap were not invented until the late 1800s, the same time period that saw the beginning of investigations with spermicidal agents.

Intravaginal contraception was widespread in isolated cultures throughout the world. The Japanese used balls of bamboo paper, Islamic women used willow leaves, and the women in the Pacific Islands used seaweed. References can be found throughout ancient writings to sticky plugs, made of gumlike substances, to be placed in the vagina prior to intercourse. In preliterate societies, an effective method had to have been the result of trial and error, with some good luck thrown in.

How was contraceptive knowledge spread? Certainly, until modern times, individuals did not consult clinicians for contraception. Contraceptive knowledge was folklore, undoubtedly perpetuated by the oral tradition. The social and technical circumstances of ancient times conspired to make communication of information very difficult. But even when knowledge was lacking, the desire to prevent conception was not. Hence, the widespread use of potions, body movements, and amulets; all of which can be best described as magic.

Egyptian papyri dating from 1850 B.C. refer to plugs of honey, gum, acacia, and crocodile dung. The descriptions of contraceptive techniques by Soranus are viewed as the best in history until modern times.[1] Soranus of Ephesus lived from 98 to 138 and has often been referred to as the greatest gynecologist of antiquity. He studied in Alexandria and practiced in Rome. His great text was lost for centuries and was not published until 1838.

Soranus gave explicit directions regarding how to make concoctions that probably combined a barrier with spermicidal action. He favored making pulps from nuts and fruits (probably very acidic and spermicidal) and advocated the use of soft wool placed at the cervical os. He described up to 40 different combinations.

The earliest penis protectors were just that, intended to provide prophylaxis against infection. In 1564, Gabriello Fallopius, one of the early authorities on syphilis, described a linen condom that covered the glans penis. The linen condom of Fallopius was followed by full covering with animal skins and intestines, but use for contraception cannot be dated to earlier than the 1700s.

There are many versions accounting for the origin of the word *condom*. Most attribute the word to a Dr. Condom, a physician in England in the 1600s. The most famous story declares that Dr. Condom invented the sheath in response to the annoyance displayed by Charles II at the number of his illegitimate children. All attempts to trace this physician have failed. This origin of the word can neither be proved nor disproved. Condom may be derived from the Latin *condon* that means "receptacle."[1]

By 1800, condoms were available at brothels throughout Europe, but nobody wanted to claim responsibility. The French called the condom the English cape; the English called condoms French letters.

Vulcanization of rubber dates to 1844, and, by 1850, rubber condoms were available in the United States. The vulcanization of rubber revolutionized transportation and contraception. The introduction of liquid latex and automatic machinery ultimately made reliable condoms both plentiful and affordable.

Diaphragms first appeared in publications in Germany in the 1880s. A practicing German gynecologist C. Haase wrote extensively about his diaphragm, using the pseudonym Wilhelm P.J. Mensinga. The Mensinga diaphragm retained its original design with little change until modern times.

The cervical cap was available for use before the diaphragm. A New York gynecologist E.B. Foote wrote a pamphlet describing its use around 1860. By the 1930s, the cervical cap was the most widely prescribed method of contraception in Europe. Why was the cervical cap not accepted in the United States? The answer is not clear. Some blame the more prudish attitude toward sexuality as an explanation for why American women had difficulty learning self-insertion techniques.

Scientific experimentation with chemical inhibitors of sperm began in the 1800s. By the 1950s, more than 90 different spermicidal products were being marketed, and some of them were used in the first efforts to control fertility in India.[2] With the availability of the intrauterine device and the development of oral contraception, interest in spermicidal agents waned, and the number of products declined.

In the last decades of the 1800s, condoms, diaphragms, pessaries, and douching syringes were widely advertised; however, they were not widely used. It is only since 1900 that the knowledge and application of contraception have been democratized, encouraged, and promoted. And it is only since 1960 that contraception teaching and practice became part of the program in academic medicine but not without difficulty. In the 1960s, Duncan Reid, chair of obstetrics at Harvard Medical School, organized and cared for women in a clandestine clinic for contraception. In Dr. Reid's Clinic at the Boston Lying-In Hospital, women were able to receive contraceptives not available elsewhere in the city.

In 1961, C. Lee Buxton, chair of obstetrics and gynecology at Yale Medical School, and Estelle Griswold, the 61-year-old executive director of Connecticut Planned Parenthood, opened four Planned Parenthood clinics in New Haven, in a defiant move against the current Connecticut law. In an obvious test of the Connecticut law, Buxton and Griswold were arrested at the Orange Street clinic, in a prearranged scenario scripted by Buxton and Griswold at the invitation of the district attorney. They were found guilty and fined $100, but imprisonment was deferred because the obvious goal was a decision by the United States Supreme Court. Buxton was forever rankled by the trivial amount of the fine. On June 7, 1965, the Supreme Court voted 7–2 to overturn the Connecticut law on the basis of a constitutional right of privacy. It was not until 1972 and 1973 that the last state laws prohibiting the distribution of contraceptives were overthrown.

261

Failure Rates During the First Year of Use, United States [3, 4]

Method	Percent of Women with Pregnancy	
	Lowest Expected	Typical
No method	85.0	85.0
Combination pill	0.1	7.6
Progestin-only	0.5	3.0
IUDs		
Levonorgestrel IUD	0.1	0.1
Copper T 380A	0.6	0.8
Implant	0.2	0.2
Injectable	0.3	0.3
Female sterilization	0.2	0.4
Male sterilization	0.1	0.15
Spermicides	6.0	25.7
Periodic abstinence		20.5
Calendar	9.0	
Ovulation method	3.0	
Symptothermal	2.0	
Postovulation	1.0	
Withdrawal	4.0	23.6
Cervical cap		
Parous women	20.0	40.0
Nulliparous women	9.0	20.0
Sponge		
Parous women	20.0	40.0
Nulliparous women	9.0	20.0
Diaphragm and spermicides	6.0	12.1
Condom		
Male	3.0	13.9
Female	5.0	21.0

Risks and Benefits Common to All Barrier Methods

Barrier methods (condoms and diaphragms) provide protection (about a 50% reduction) against sexually transmitted infections (STIs) and pelvic inflammatory disease (PID).[5–9] This includes infections caused by *chlamydia, Neisseria gonorrhoeae, trichomonas,* herpes simplex, cytomegalovirus, and human immunodeficiency virus (HIV); however, only the condom has been proved to prevent HIV infection. STI protection has a beneficial impact on the risk of tubal infertility and ectopic pregnancy.[7, 10] There have been no significant clinical studies on STIs and cervical caps or the female condom, but these methods should be effective. Women who have never used barrier methods of contraception are almost twice as likely to develop cancer of the cervix.[10, 11] The risk of toxic shock syndrome is increased with female barrier methods, but the actual incidence is so rare that this is not a significant clinical consideration.[12] Women who have had toxic shock syndrome, however, should be advised to avoid barrier methods.

Barrier Methods and Preeclampsia. An initial case-control study indicated that methods of contraception that prevented exposure to sperm were associated with an increased risk of preeclampsia.[13] This was not confirmed in a careful analysis of two large prospective pregnancy studies.[14] This latter conclusion was more compelling in that it was derived from a large, prospective, cohort data base.

The Diaphragm

The first effective contraceptive method under a woman's control was the vaginal diaphragm. Distribution of diaphragms led to Margaret Sanger's arrest in New York City in 1918. This was still a contentious issue in 1965 when the Supreme Court's decision in *Griswold v. Connecticut* ended the ban on contraception in that state. By 1940, one-third of contracepting American couples were using the diaphragm. This decreased to 10% by 1965 after the introduction of oral contraceptives and intrauterine devices and fell to about 1.9% in 1995 (Chapter 1).

Efficacy

Failure rates for diaphragm users vary from as low as 2% per year of use to a high of 23%. The typical use failure rate after 1 year of use is 12%.[3, 4] Older, married women with longer use achieve the highest efficacy, but young women can use diaphragms very successfully if they are properly encouraged and counseled. There have been no adequate studies to determine whether efficacy is different with and without spermicides.[15]

Side Effects

The diaphragm is a safe method of contraception that rarely causes even minor side effects. Occasionally, women report vaginal irritation due to the latex rubber or the spermicidal jelly or cream used with the diaphragm. Less than 1% discontinue diaphragm use for these reasons. Urinary tract infections are 2–3-fold more common among diaphragm users than among women using oral contraception.[16, 17] Possibly, the rim of the diaphragm presses against the urethra and causes irritation that is perceived as infectious in origin, or true infection may result from touching the perineal area or from incomplete emptying of the bladder. It is more probable that spermicides used with the diaphragm can increase the risk of bacteriuria with *E. coli,* perhaps due to an alteration in the normal vaginal flora.[18] Clinical experience suggests that voiding after sexual intercourse is helpful, and, if necessary, a single postcoital dose of a prophylactic antibiotic can be recommended. Postcoital prophylaxis is effective, using trimethoprim-sulfamethoxazole (1 tablet postcoitus), nitrofurantoin (50 or 100 mg postcoitus), or cephalexin (250 mg postcoitus).

Improper fitting or prolonged retention (beyond 24 hours) can cause vaginal abrasion or mucosal irritation. There is no link between the normal use of diaphragms and the toxic shock syndrome.[19] It makes sense, however, to minimize the risk of toxic shock by removing the diaphragm after 24 hours and during menses.

Benefits

Diaphragm use reduces the incidence of cervical gonorrhea, trichomoniasis, and chlamydia,[20] pelvic inflammatory disease,[7, 21] and tubal infertility.[5, 10] There are no data, as of yet, regarding the effect of diaphragm use on the transmission of the acquired immunodeficiency syndropme (AIDS) virus HIV, but because the vagina remains exposed, the diaphragm is unlikely to protect against HIV. An important advantage of the diaphragm is low cost. Diaphragms are durable and with proper care can last for several years.

Choice and Use of the Diaphragm

There are three types of diaphragms, and most manufacturers produce them in sizes ranging from 50 to 105 mm in diameter, in increments of 2.5 to 5 mm. Most women use sizes between 65 and 80 mm.

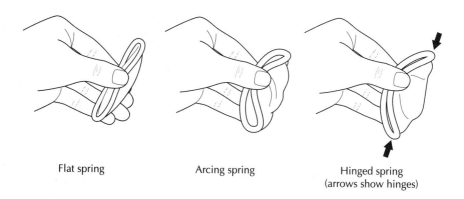

| Flat spring | Arcing spring | Hinged spring (arrows show hinges) |

The diaphragm made with a flat metal spring or a coil spring remains in a straight line when pinched at the edges. This type is suitable for women with good vaginal muscle tone and an adequate recess behind the pubic arch. However, many women find it difficult to place the posterior edge of these flat diaphragms into the posterior cul-de-sac and over the cervix.

Arcing diaphragms are easier to use for most women. They come in two types. The All-Flex type bends into an arc no matter where around the rim the edges are pinched together. The hinged type must be pinched between the hinges to form a symmetrical arc. The hinged type forms a narrower shape when pinched together and, thus, may be easier for some women to insert. The arcing diaphragms allow the posterior edge of the diaphragm to slip more easily past the cervix and into the posterior cul-de-sac. Women with poor vaginal muscle tone, cystocele, rectocele, a long cervix, or an anterior cervix of a retroverted uterus use arcing diaphragms more successfully.

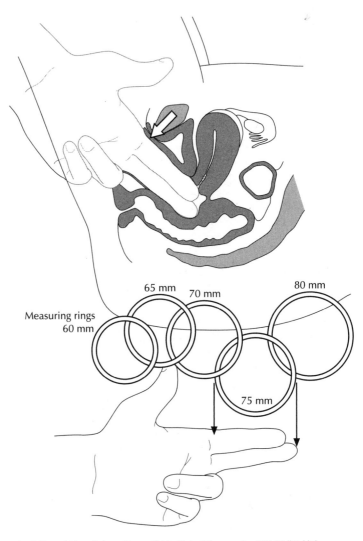

Measuring rings
60 mm
65 mm
70 mm
80 mm
75 mm

After S. Koperski from **Jackson, Berger, Keith,** *Vaginal Contraception*, G.K. Hall Publishers.

Fitting

Successful use of a diaphragm depends on proper fitting. The clinician must have available aseptic fitting rings or diaphragms themselves in all diameters. These devices should be scrupulously disinfected by soaking in a bleach solution. At the time of the pelvic examination, the middle finger is placed against the vaginal wall and the posterior cul-de-sac, while the hand is lifted anteriorly until the pubic symphysis abuts the index finger. This point is marked with the examiner's thumb to approximate the diameter of the diaphragm. The corresponding fitting ring or diaphragm is inserted, and the fit is assessed by both clinician and patient.

If the diaphragm is too tightly pressed against the pubic symphysis, a smaller size is selected. If the diaphragm is too loose (comes out with a cough or bearing down), the next larger size is selected. After a good fit is obtained, the diaphragm is removed by hooking the index finger under the rim behind the symphysis and pulling. It is important to instruct the patient in these procedures during and after the fitting. The patient should then insert the diaphragm, practice checking for proper placement, and attempt removal.

Timing

Diaphragm users need additional instruction about the timing of diaphragm use in relation to sexual intercourse and the use of spermicide. None of this advice has been rigorously assessed in clinical studies; therefore, these recommendations represent the consensus of clinical experience.

The diaphragm should be inserted no longer than 6 hours prior to sexual intercourse. About a tablespoonful of spermicidal cream or jelly should be placed in the dome of the diaphragm prior to insertion, and some of the spermicide should be spread around the rim with a finger. The diaphragm should be left in place for approximately 6 hours (but no more than 24 hours) after coitus. Additional spermicide should be placed in the vagina before each additional episode of sexual intercourse while the diaphragm is in place.

Reassessment

Weight loss, weight gain, vaginal delivery, and even sexual intercourse can change vaginal caliber. The fit of a diaphragm should be assessed every year at the time of the regular examination.

Care of the Diaphragm

After removal, the diaphragm should be washed with soap and water, rinsed, and dried. Powders of any sort need not and should not be applied to the diaphragm. It is wise to use water to periodically check for leaks. Diaphragms should be stored in a cool and dark location.

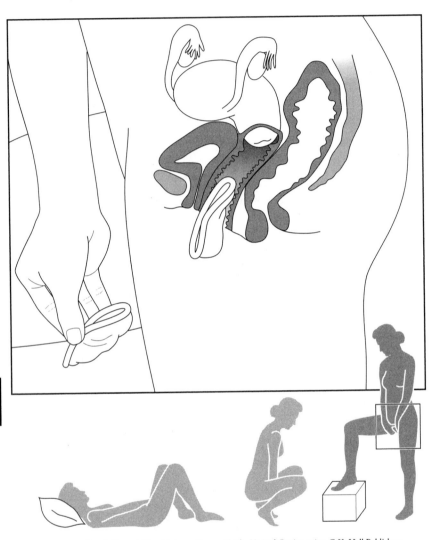

After S. Koperski from **Jackson, Berger, Keith**, *Vaginal Contraception*, G.K. Hall Publishers.

Diaphragm Insertion
Above: Compression of the diaphragm with the cavity
facing upward.
Below: Three commonly used positions for insertion.

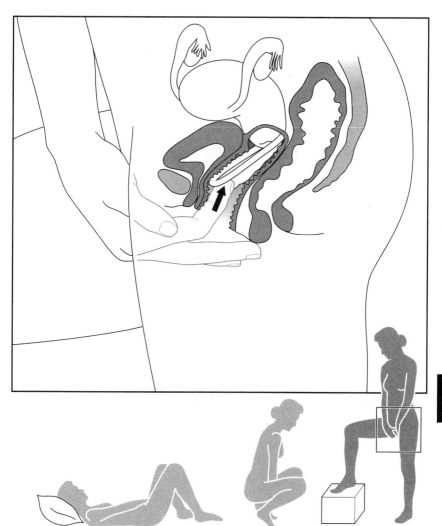

After S. Koperski from **Jackson, Berger, Keith**, *Vaginal Contraception*, G.K. Hall Publishers.

Diaphragm Insertion

The diaphragm is pushed into the vagina as far as it will go. The leading edge is behind the cervix. The front edge is behind the symphysis pubis.

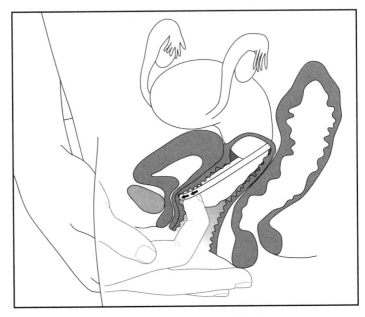

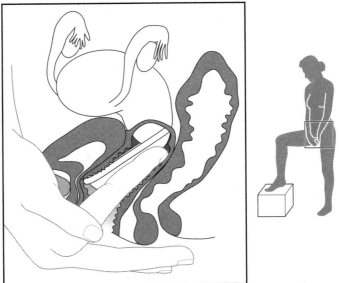

After S. Koperski from **Jackson, Berger, Keith**, *Vaginal Contraception*, G.K. Hall Publishers.

Checking Diaphragm Position

Above: Checking for forward movement; it should be snug.

Below: Feeling the cervix to make sure it is covered. Move the finger back and forth to feel the rim, then find the bulge in the middle.

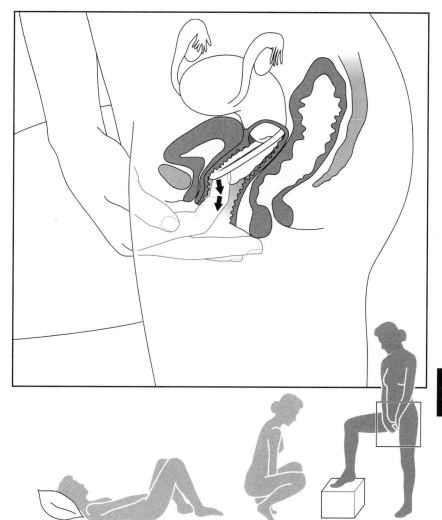

After S. Koperski from **Jackson, Berger, Keith**, *Vaginal Contraception*, G.K. Hall Publishers.

271

Diaphragm Removal

Insert the index finger under the front rim and pull downward and outward. An alternative method is to approach the diaphragm with the palm down and insert the finger between the outer edge and the vagina.

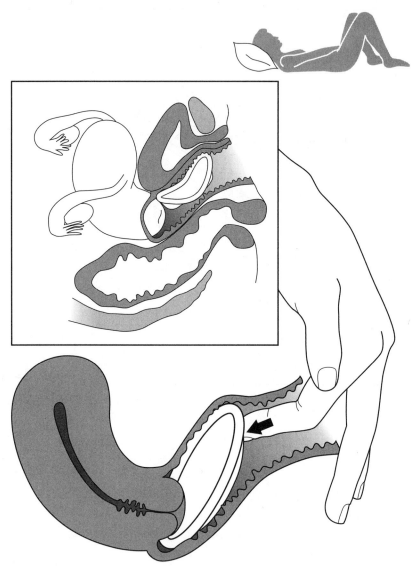

After S. Koperski from **Jackson, Berger, Keith**, *Vaginal Contraception*, G.K. Hall Publishers.

Incorrect Diaphragm Insertion

Above: The outer rim is correct, but the leading rim is in front of the cervix.

Below: Incorrect placement can be repositioned with a downward push on the outer edge.

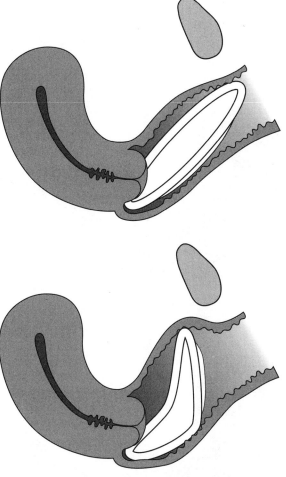

After S. Koperski from **Jackson, Berger, Keith**, *Vaginal Contraception*, G.K. Hall Publishers.

Incorrect Diaphragm Fit (Too Large)

Above: A diaphragm too large cannot fit behind the symphysis pubis.

Below: Forcing a diaphragm that is too large buckles the diaphragm and uncovers the cervix.

274

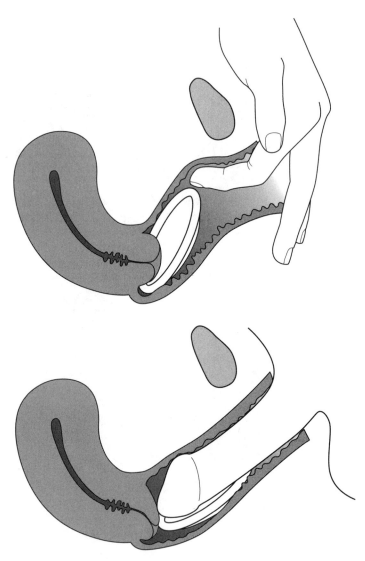

After S. Koperski from **Jackson, Berger, Keith**, *Vaginal Contraception*, G.K. Hall Publishers.

Incorrect Diaphragm Fit (Too Small)

Above: A diaphragm too small does not fit snugly behind the symphysis pubis.

Below: With a diaphragm too small, the penis displaces it and exposes the cervix.

The Cervical Cap

The cervical cap was popular in Europe long before its reintroduction into the United States. U.S. trials have demonstrated that the Prentif cervical cap is about as effective as the diaphragm but somewhat harder to fit (it comes in only 4 sizes) and more difficult to insert (it must be placed precisely over the cervix).[22, 23] Efficacy is significantly reduced in parous women.

The cervical latex Prentif cap has several advantages over the diaphragm. It can be left in place for a longer time (up to 48 hours), and it need not be used with a spermicide. However, a tablespoonful of spermicide placed in the cap before application is reported to increase efficacy (to a 6% failure rate in the first year) and to prolong wearing time by decreasing the incidence of foul-smelling discharge (a common complaint after 24 hours).[23]

The size of the cervix varies considerably from woman to woman, and the cervix changes in individual women in response to pregnancy or surgery. Proper fitting can be accomplished in about 80% of women. Women with a cervix that is too long or too short, or with a cervix that is far forward in the vagina, may not be suited for cap use. However, women with vaginal wall or pelvic relaxation, who cannot retain a diaphragm, may be able to use the cap.

Those women who can be fitted with one of the 4 sizes must first learn how to identify the cervix and then how to slide the cap into the vagina, up the posterior vaginal wall and onto the cervix. After insertion and after each act of sexual intercourse, the cervix should be checked to make sure that it is covered.

The cervical cap can be left in place for 2 days, but some women experience a foul-smelling discharge by 2 days. It must be left in place for at least 8 hours after sexual intercourse in order to ensure that no motile sperm are left in the vagina. To remove the cap (at least 8 hours after coitus), pressure must be exerted with a finger tip to break the seal. The finger is hooked over the cap rim to pull it out of the vagina. Bearing down or squatting or both can help to bring the cervix within reach of the finger.

The most common cause of failure is dislodgment of the cap from the cervix during sexual intercourse. There is no evidence that cervical caps cause toxic shock syndrome or dysplastic changes in the cervical mucosa.[24] It seems likely (although not yet documented) that cervical caps would provide the same protection from sexually transmitted infections as the diaphragm.

The FemCap, made of nonallergenic silicone rubber, is shaped like a sailor's hat, a design that allows a better fit over the cervix and in the vaginal fornices and provides a "brim" for easier removal.[25] This cap may be easier to fit and use. There are 3 sizes, one for nulliparous women and larger sizes for women who have had a vaginal delivery. In a randomized trial, the pregnancy rate with FemCap was nearly 2-fold higher compared with a diaphragm.[26]

Lea's Shield is a vaginal barrier contraceptive composed of silicone.[27, 28] This soft, pliable device comes in one size and fits over the cervix, held in place by the pressure of the vaginal wall around it. There is a collapsible valve that communicates with a 9-mm opening in the bowl that fits over the cervix. This valve allows equalization of air pressure during insertion and drainage of cervical secretions and discharge, permitting a snug fit over the cervix. A thick U-shaped loop attached to the anterior side of the bowl is used to stabilize the device during insertion and for removal. The thicker part of the device is shaped to fill the posterior fornix, thus contributing to its placement and stability over the cervix. The addition of a spermicide, placed in the bowl, is recommended. Lea's Shield is designed to remain in place for 48 hours after intercourse. Pregnancy rates are similar to other barrier methods, and no serious adverse effects have been reported.[29]

Ovés is a silastic cervical cap that is available in 3 sizes, with a loop for insertion and removal. Studies are limited to very small numbers of women, and there are no data on efficacy.[30]

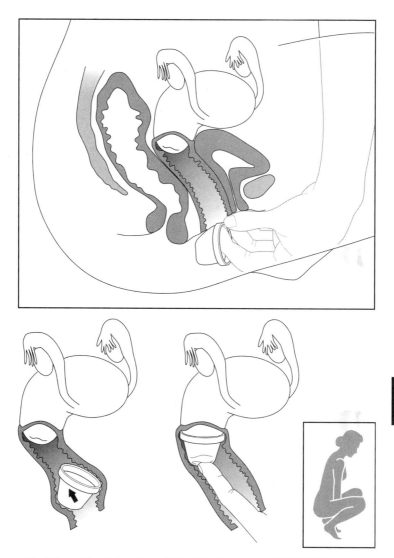

After S. Koperski from **Jackson, Berger, Keith**, *Vaginal Contraception*, G.K. Hall Publishers.

Insertion of the Cervical Cap

Above: The cap is pushed into the vagina with the index finger.
Below: The cap is pushed onto the cervix, and its position is checked by feeling the cervix through the cap.

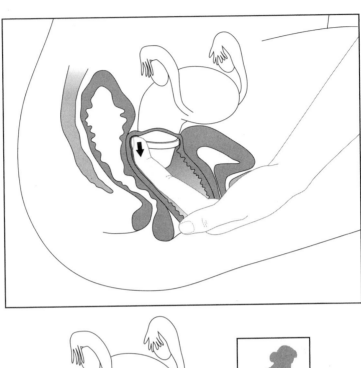

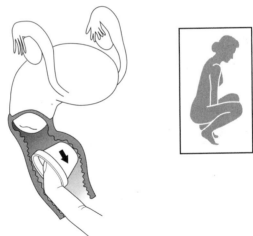

After S. Koperski from **Jackson, Berger, Keith**, *Vaginal Contraception*, G.K. Hall Publishers.

Removal of the Cervical Cap

Above: The index finger is placed behind the rim, and the cap
is dislodged with a downward motion.
Below: The cap is removed by inserting the finger into the cap.

The Contraceptive Sponge

The vaginal contraceptive sponge is a sustained-release system for a spermicide. The sponge also absorbs semen and blocks the entrance to the cervical canal. The Today sponge is a dimpled polyurethane disc impregnated with 1 g of nonoxynol-9. Approximately 20% of the nonoxynol-9 is released over the 24 hours that the sponge is left in the vagina. Production of the Today sponge in the United States ceased in 1995; it is available in Canada and can be purchased over the Internet. Protectaid is a polyurethane sponge available in Canada and Hong Kong (it also can be purchased over the Internet) that contains 3 spermicides and a dispersing gel.[31] The spermicidal agents are sodium cholate, nonoxynol-9, and benzalkonium chloride. This combination exerts antiviral actions in vitro.[32] The dispersing agent, polydimethysiloxane, forms a protective coating over the entire vagina, providing sustained protection.

To insert, the Today sponge is moistened with water (squeezing out the excess) and placed firmly against the cervix. There should always be a lapse of at least 6 hours after sexual intercourse before removal, even if the sponge has been in place for 24 hours before intercourse (maximal wear time, therefore, is 30 hours). It can be inserted immediately before sexual intercourse or up to 24 hours beforehand. It is removed by hooking a finger through the ribbon attached to the back of the sponge. The Protectaid sponge can be inserted up to 12 hours before intercourse, and it is easier to remove than the Today sponge. Obviously, the sponge is not a good choice for women with anatomic changes that make proper insertion and placement difficult.

In most studies, the effectiveness of the sponge exceeds that of foam, jellies, and tablets, but it is lower than that associated with diaphragm or condom use.[33-35] Some studies indicated higher failure rates (twice as high) in parous women, suggesting that one size may not fit all users.[36]

Discontinuation rates are generally higher among sponge users, compared with diaphragm and spermicide use. For some women, however, the sponge is preferred because it provides continuous protection for 24 hours regardless of the frequency of coitus. In addition, it is easier to use and less messy.

Side effects associated with the sponge include allergic reactions in about 4% of users. Another 8% complain of vaginal dryness, soreness, or itching. Some women find removal difficult. There is no risk of toxic shock syndrome, and, in fact, the nonoxynol-9 retards staphylococcal replication and toxin production. There has been some concern that the sponge may damage the vaginal mucosa and enhance HIV transmission.[37] Women using the sponge have lower rates of gonorrhea, trichomoniasis, and chlamydia.[7]

Spermicides

Jellies, creams, foams, melting suppositories, foaming tablets, foaming suppositories, and soluble films are used as vehicles for chemical agents that inactivate sperm in the vagina before they can move into the upper genital tract. Some are used together with diaphragms, caps, and condoms, but even used alone they can provide protection against pregnancy.

Various chemicals and a wide array of vehicles have been used vaginally as contraceptives for centuries. The first commercially available spermicidal pessaries were made in England in 1885 of cocoa butter and quinine sulfite. These or similar materials were used until the 1920s when effervescent tablets that released carbon dioxide and phenyl mercuric acetate were marketed. Modern spermicides, introduced in the 1950s, contain surface active agents that damage the sperm cell membranes. The agents currently used are nonoxynol-9, octoxynol-9, benzalkonium chloride, and menfegol. Most preparations contain 60–100 mg of these agents in each vaginal application, with concentrations ranging from 2–12.5%.

Representative Products

Vaginal Contraceptive Film
VCF (70 mg nonoxynol-9)

Foams
Delfen (nonoxynol-9, 12.5%)
Emko (nonoxynol-9, 8%)
Koromex (nonoxynol-9, 12.5%)

Jellies and Creams
Conceptrol (nonoxynol-9, 4%)
Delfen (nonoxynol-9, 12.5%)
Ortho Gynol (nonoxynol-9, 3%)
Ramses (nonoxynol-9, 5%)
Koromex Jelly (nonoxynol-9, 3%)

Suppositories
Encare (nonoxynol-9, 2.27%)
Koromex Inserts (nonoxynol-9, 125 mg)
Semicid (nonoxynol-9, 100 mg)

Advantage 24 is a contraceptive gel that adheres to the vaginal mucosa and provides longer availability of nonoxynol-9; it is intended to be effective for 24 hours. Although available without prescription, adequate clinical trial data are not available. Allendale-N9 is a vaginal contraceptive film

(VCF) that contains more nonoxynol-9 than VCF.[38] An Allendale film has also been developed that contains benzalkonium chloride instead of nonoxynol-9.[39] In addition to spermicidal activity, benzalkonium chloride is microbicidal and demonstrates activity against HIV.[40] Benzalkonium chloride is available for contraceptive use in the form of a suppository, in a sponge, or as a cream in several countries.

Although in vitro studies have demonstrated that spermicides kill or inactivate most STI pathogens, including HIV, it cannot be said that spermicides provide protection against sexually transmitted infections. Spermicides have been reported to prevent HIV seroconversion as well as to have no effect; therefore, spermicides by themselves cannot be counted on for protection against HIV.[41–45] In a controlled, clinical trial in female sex workers, nonoxynol-9 failed to protect against HIV transmission.[46] Clinical studies have indicated reductions in the risk of gonorrhea,[47–49] pelvic infections,[21] and chlamydial infection.[47, 49] However, these studies probably reflected condom use. In trials with a placebo, nonoxynol-9 provided no protection against gonorrhea or chlamydia.[46, 50, 51] Indeed, there is concern that frequent spermicide use may irritate the vagina and enhance HIV transmission.[42] Because of this concern, condom makers have discontinued the production of condoms lubricated with nonoxynol-9. There is little difference in the incidence of trichomoniasis, candidiasis, or bacterial vaginosis among spermicide users.[52] *The best evidence indicates that spermicides do not provide additional protection against STIs over that associated with condoms; therefore, spermicides should not be used without condoms if a primary objective is to prevent gonorrhea, chlamydia, or infection with HIV.*

Efficacy

Only periodic abstinence demonstrates as wide a range of efficacy in different studies as do the studies of spermicides. Efficacy seems to depend more on the population studied than the agent used. Efficacy ranges from less than 1% failure to nearly one-third in the first year of use. Failure rates of approximately 20–25% during a year's use are most typical.[4, 53] A randomized trial comparing VCF (72 mg nonoxynol-9) with Conceptrol foaming tablets (100 mg nonoxynol-9) recorded similar 6-month pregnancy rates (24.9% with the film and 28.0% with the tablet).[53] A randomized assessment of the various products concluded that a dose of 52.5 mg nonoxynol-9 was less effective (22% in 6 months) than those containing 100 mg or 150 mg (about 15% in 6 months; intermediate doses were not tested).[54] These are very high rates, amounting to approximately 30–40% for 1 year of use. *Although better than no method, spermicides alone should not be recommended for contraception unless method failure and pregnancy are acceptable.*

Spermicides require application 10–30 minutes prior to sexual intercourse. Jellies, creams, and foams remain effective for as long as 8 hours, but tablets and suppositories are good for less than 1 hour. If ejaculation does not occur within the period of effectiveness, the spermicide should be reapplied. Reapplication should definitely take place for each coital episode.

Vaginal postcoital douches are ineffective contraceptives even if they contain spermicidal agents. Postcoital douching is too late to prevent the rapid ascent of sperm (within seconds) to the fallopian tubes.

Advantages

Spermicides are relatively inexpensive and widely available in many retail outlets without prescription. This makes spermicides popular among adolescents and others who have infrequent or unpredictable sexual intercourse. In addition, spermicides are simple to use.

Side Effects

No serious side effects or safety problems have arisen in all the years that spermicides have been used. The only serious question raised was that of a possible association between spermicide use and congenital abnormalities or spontaneous miscarriages. Epidemiologic analysis, including a meta-analysis, concluded that there is insufficient evidence to support these associations.[55–57] Spermicides are not absorbed through the vaginal mucosa in concentrations high enough to have systemic effects.[58] Vaginal and cervical mucosal damage (de-epithelialization without inflammation) has been observed with nonoxynol-9, and the overall impact on HIV transmission, although unknown, is of concern.[59, 60]

The principal minor problem is allergy that occurs in 1–5% of users, related to either the vehicle or the spermicidal agent. Using a different product often solves the problem. Spermicide users also have an altered vaginal floral promoting the colonization of *E. coli*, leading to a greater susceptibility to urinary tract infections than with diaphragm/spermicide users.[17, 61]

The Search for Contraceptives to Prevent STIs

Research is underway to develop microbicides and contraceptives to prevent STIs. The ideal agent would be a topical microbicide that would prevent infection and be spermicidal. The road is long, extending from in vitro work to clinical application. An acceptable agent must avoid damage to vaginal epithelial cells and disruption of vaginal flora, and the delivery system must be user-friendly. However, it is unlikely that any new agent can match the latex condom, which is nearly 100% effective in blocking bacteria and viruses.

Condoms

Although awareness of condoms as an effective contraceptive method as well as protector against STIs has increased tremendously in recent years, a great deal remains to be accomplished to reach the appropriate level of condom use. Contraceptive efficacy and STI prevention must be linked together and publicly promoted. The male condom is the only contraceptive proved to prevent HIV infection.

There are three specific goals: correct use; consistent use; and affordable, easy availability. If these goals are met, the early 2000s will see the annual manufacture of 20 billion condoms per year.

Various types of condoms are available. Most are made of latex; polyurethane and silicone rubber condoms are also now manufactured. "Natural skin" (lamb's intestine) condoms are still obtainable (about 1% of sales). Latex condoms are 0.3–0.8 mm thick. Sperm that are 0.003 mm in diameter cannot penetrate condoms. The organisms that cause STIs and AIDS also do not penetrate latex condoms, but they can penetrate condoms made from intestine.[62, 63] Condom use (latex) is not believed to prevent transmission of human papillomavirus (HPV) because it is spread by skin contact. The use of spermicides or spermicide-coated condoms increases the incidence of *E. coli* bacteriuria and urinary tract infections due to either *E. coli* or *Staphylococcus saprophyticus* because of the spermicide-induced alteration in vaginal flora.[18, 64] Consistent use of condoms when one partner is HIV seropositive is highly effective in preventing HIV transmission; there was no seroconversion in 124 couples who used condoms consistently compared with 12.7% conversion after 24 months in couples with inconsistent use.[65, 66] Women who are partners of condom users are less likely to be HIV-positive.[67] An evaluation of the world's literature concluded that consistent use of condoms provides protection against HIV to a degree comparable to condom efficacy in preventing pregnancy (reflecting some inconsistent use and other routes of transmission).[66] In addition, condoms protect against transmission of the herpes simplex virus from infected men to women.[68]

Polyurethane condoms are expected to protect against STIs and HIV, based on in vitro efficacy as a barrier to bacteria and viruses. They are odorless, may have greater sensitivity, and are resistant to deterioration from storage and lubricants. Those individuals who have the infrequent problem of latex allergy can use polyurethane condoms. Breakage and slippage have been reported to be comparable with latex condoms.[69] However, in a randomized, well-designed study, the polyurethane condom had a 6-fold higher breakage rate, and another study comparing latex and polyurethane condoms found a higher pregnancy rate with the polyurethane condom.[70, 71]

Condoms can be straight or tapered, smooth or ribbed, colored or clear, lubricated or nonlubricated. These are all marketing ventures aimed at attracting individual notions of pleasure and enjoyment.[72] An often repeated concern is the alleged reduction in penile glans sensitivity that accompanies condom use.[72] This has never been objectively studied, and it is likely that this complaint is perception (or excuse) not based on reality. A clinician can overcome this objection by advocating the use of thinner (and more esoteric) condoms, knowing that any difference is also more of perception than reality.

As is true for most contraceptive methods, older, married couples experienced in using condoms and strongly motivated to avoid another pregnancy are much more effective users than young, unmarried couples with little contraceptive experience. This does not mean that condoms are not useful contraceptives for adolescents, who are likely to have sex unexpectedly or infrequently. The recent decline in the teen pregnancy rate partly reflects wider use of condoms by teens concerned about avoiding HIV infection.

Prospective users need instructions if they are to avoid pregnancy and STIs. A condom must be placed on the penis before it touches a partner. Uncircumcised men must pull the foreskin back. Prior to unrolling the condom to the base of the penis, air should be squeezed out of the reservoir tip with a thumb and forefinger. The tip of the condom should extend beyond the end of the penis to provide a reservoir to collect the ejaculate (a half-inch of pinched tip). If lubricants are used, they must be water based. Oil-based lubricants (such as Vaseline) weaken the latex. Couples should be concerned that any vaginal medication can compromise condom integrity. After intercourse, the condom should be held at the base as the still erect penis is withdrawn. Semen must not be allowed to spill or leak. The condom should be handled gently because fingernails and rings can penetrate the latex and cause leakage. If there is evidence of spill or leakage, a spermicidal agent should be quickly inserted into the vagina, and treatment should be initiated within 72 hours with an emergency contraception method.

Summary — Key Steps for Maximal Condom Efficacy

1. Use condoms for every act of coitus.
2. Place the condom before vaginal contact.
3. Create a reservoir at the tip.
4. Withdraw while the penis is still erect.
5. Hold the base of the condom during withdrawal.

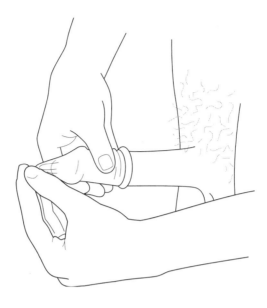

These instructions should be provided to new users of condoms who are likely to be reluctant to ask questions. Most condoms are acquired without medical supervision; therefore, clinicians should use every opportunity to inform patients about their proper use.

Inconsistent use explains most condom failures. Incorrect use accounts for additional failures; also, condoms sometimes break. Breakage rates range from 1–8 per 100 episodes of vaginal intercourse (and somewhat higher for anal intercourse), and slippage rates range from 1–5%.[73, 74] With experienced couples, condom failure due to breakage and slippage (sufficient to increase the risk of pregnancy or STIs) occurs at a rate of about 1%.[75] In a U.S. survey, one pregnancy resulted for every 3 condom breakages.[76] Concomitant use of spermicides lowers failure rates in case of breakage. In addition, even when there is slippage or breakage, the condom provides some protection against pregnancy and STIs because there is still a reduction in exposure to semen.[77]

Breakage is a greater problem for couples at risk for STIs. An infected man transmits gonorrhea to a susceptible woman approximately two-thirds of the time.[78] If the woman is infected, transmission to the man occurs one-third of the time.[79] The chances of HIV infection after a single sexual exposure ranges from 1 in 1,000 to 1 in 10.[80, 81]

Condom breakage rates depend on sexual behavior and practices, experience with condom use, the condition of the condoms, and manufacturing quality. Condoms remain in good condition for up to 5 years unless exposed to ultraviolet light, excessive heat or humidity, ozone, or oils. Condom manufacturers regularly check samples of their products to make sure they meet national standards. These procedures limit the proportion of defects to less than 0.1% of all condoms distributed. Contraceptive failure is more likely to be due to nonuse or incorrect use.

When a condom breaks, or if there is reason to believe spillage or leakage occurred, a woman should contact a clinician within 72 hours. Emergency contraception, as discussed in Chapter 3, should be provided. Couples who rely on condoms for contraception should be educated regarding emergency contraception, and an appropriate method should be kept available for self-medication (see Chapter 3).

For the immediate future, prevention of STIs and control of the AIDS epidemic requires a great increase in the use of condoms. We must all be involved in the effort to promote condom use. Condom use must be portrayed in the positive light of STI prevention. An important area of concentration is the teaching of the social skills required to ensure use by a reluctant partner. Using scare tactics about STIs to encourage condom use is not sufficient. A more positive approach can yield better compliance. It is useful to emphasize that prevention of STIs preserves future fertility. *For women not in a stable, monogamous relationship, a dual approach is recommended, combining the contraceptive efficacy and protection against PID offered by estrogen-progestin contraception with the use of a barrier method for prevention of viral STIs.*

The Female Condom

The female condom is a pouch made of polyurethane, which lines the vagina.[82] An internal ring in the closed end of the pouch covers the cervix and an external ring remains outside the vagina, partially covering the perineum. The female condom is prelubricated with silicone, and a spermicide need not be used. The female condom should be an effective barrier to STI infection. The female condom is impervious in vitro to cytomegalovirus and HIV;[83] however, high cost and acceptability are major problems. The integrity of the female condom is maintained with up to 8 multiple uses with washing, drying, and relubricating.[84] The devices are more cumbersome than condoms, and studies have indicated relatively high rates of problems such as slippage.[85] Women who have successfully used barrier methods and who are strongly motivated to avoid STIs are more likely to choose the female condom. With careful use, the efficacy rate should be similar to that of the diaphragm and the cervical cap.[86–88]

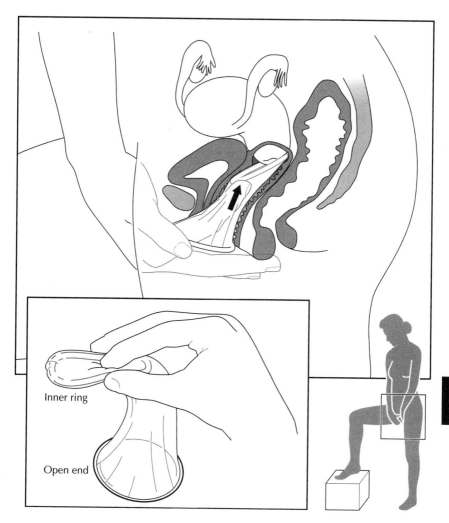

Inner ring

Open end

	Diaphragm	Cap	Sponge	Female Condom
Insertion before coitus, no longer than:	6 hrs	6 hrs	24 hrs	8 hrs
After coitus, should be left in place for:	6 hrs	8 hrs	6 hrs	6 hrs
Maximal wear time:	24 hrs	48 hrs	30 hrs	8 hrs

Future Developments

New barrier devices are being pursued, such as sponges incorporating several spermicides and cervical caps made of different materials. Chemical agents are being investigated that can combine spermicidal and antimicrobial actions, and vaginal spermicidal films of different materials and containing other spermicidal agents are being tested. Disposable diaphragms that release spermicide are in development. A one-size-fits-all diaphragm is being tested that can be obtained and used without a visit to a clinician.

References

1. **Himes NE,** Medical History of Contraception, Williams & Wilkins, Baltimore, 1936.

2. **Gamble CJ,** Spermicidal times as aids to the clinician's choice of contraceptive materials, Fertil Steril 8:174, 1957.

3. **Trussell J, Vaughan B,** Contraceptive failure, method-related discontinuation and resumption of use: results from the 1995 National Survey of Family Growth, Fam Plann Perspect 31:64, 1999.

4. **Fu H, Darroch JE, Haas T, Ranjit N,** Contraceptive failure rates: new estimates from the 1995 National Survey of Family Growth, Fam Plann Perspect 31:58, 1999.

5. **Grimes DA, Cates Jr W,** Family planning and sexually transmitted diseases, In: Holmes KK, Mardh P-A, Sparling PF, eds. Sexually Transmitted Diseases, 2nd ed, McGraw-Hill, New York, 1990, pp 1087–94.

6. **Cramer DW, Goldman MB, Schiff I, Belisla S, Albrecht B, Stadel B, Gibson M, Wilson E, Stillman R, Thompson I,** The relationship of tubal infertility to barrier method and oral contraceptive use, JAMA 257:2446, 1987.

7. **Rosenberg MJ, Davidson AJ, Chen J-H, Judson FN, Douglas JM,** Barrier contraceptives and sexually transmitted diseases in women: a comparison of female-dependent methods and condoms, Am J Pub Health 82:669, 1992.

8. **Rowe PJ,** You win some and you lose some — contraception and infections, Aust N Z Obstet Gynaecol 34:299, 1994.

9. **Cates Jr W, Stone K,** Family planning, sexually transmitted diseases and contraceptive choice: a literature update: part I, Fam Plann Perspect 24:75, 1992.

10. **Kost K, Forrest JD, Harlap S,** Comparing the health risks and benefits of contraceptive choices, Fam Plann Perspect 23:54, 1991.

11. **Coker AL, Hulka BS, McCann MF, Walton LA,** Barrier methods of contraception and cervical intraepithelial neoplasia, Contraception 45:1, 1992.

12. **Schwartz B, Gaventa S, Broome CV, Reingold AL, Hightower AW, Perlman JA, Wolf PH,** Nonmenstrual toxic shock syndrome associated with barrier contraceptives: report of a case-control study, Rev Infect Dis 11(Suppl):S43, 1989.

13. **Klonoff-Cohen HS, Savitz DA, Cefalo RC, McCann MF,** An epidemiologic study of contraception and preeclampsia, JAMA 262:3143, 1989.

14. **Mills JL, Klebanoff MA, Graubard BI, Carey JC, Berendes HW,** Barrier contraceptive methods and preeclampsia, JAMA 265:70, 1991.

15. **Cook L, Nanda K, Grimes D,** The diaphragm with and without spermicide for contraception: a Cochrane review, Hum Reprod 17:867, 2002.

16. **Fihn SD, Latham RH, Roberts P, Running K, Stamm WE,** Association between diaphragm use and urinary tract infection, JAMA 254:240, 1985.

17. **Hooton TM, Scholes D, Hughes JP, Winter C, Roberts PL, Stapleton AE, Stergachis A, Stamm WE,** A prospective study of risk factors for symptomatic urinary tract infection in young women, New Engl J Med 335:468, 1996.

18. **Hooton TM, Hillier S, Johnson C, Roberts P, Stamm WE,** *Escherichia coli* bacteriuria and contraceptive method, JAMA 265:64, 1991.

19. **Centers for Disease Control and Prevention,** Toxic shock syndrome, United States, 1970–1982, MMWR 31:201, 1982.

20. **Keith L, Berger G, Moss W,** Prevalence of gonorrhea among women using various methods of contraception, Br J Venereal Dis 51:307, 1975.

21. **Kelaghan J, Rubin GL, Ory HW, Layde PM,** Barrier method contraceptives and pelvic inflammatory disease, JAMA 248:184, 1982.

22. **Bernstein G, Kilzer LH, Coulson AH, Nakamara RM, Smith GC, Bernstein R, Frezieres R, Clark VA, Coan C,** Studies of cervical caps, Contraception 26:443, 1982.

23. **Richwald GA, Greenland S, Gerber MM, Potik R, Kersey L, Comas MA,** Effectiveness of the cavity-rim cervical cap: results of a large clinical study, Obstet Gynecol 74:143, 1989.

24. **Gollub EL, Sivin I,** The Prentif cervical cap and pap smear results: a critical appraisal, Contraception 40:343, 1989.

25. **Shihata AA,** The FemCap: a new contraceptive choice, Eur J Contracept Reprod Health Care 3:160, 1998.

26. **Mauck C, Callahan M, Weiner DH, Dominik R, and the FemCap® Investigators Group,** A comparative study of the safety and efficacy of FemCap®, a new vaginal barrier contraceptive, and the Ortho All-Flex® diaphragm, Contraception 60:71, 1999.

27. **Hunt WL, Gabbay L, Potts M,** Lea's Shield®, a new barrier contraceptive; preliminary clinical evaluations, three-day tolerance study, Contraception 50:551, 1994.

28. **Archer DF, Mauck CK, Viniegra-Sibal A, Anderson FD,** Lea's Shield®: a phase I postcoital study of a new contraceptive barrier device, Contraception 52:167, 1995.

29. **Mauck C, Glover LH, Miller E, Allen S, Archer DF, Blumenthal P, Rosenzweig BA, Dominik R, Sturgen K, Cooper J, Fingerhut F, Peacock L, Gabelnick HL,** Lea's Shield®: a study of the safety and efficacy of a new vaginal barrier contraceptive used with and without spermicide, Contraception 53:329, 1996.

30. **Roizen J, Richardson S, Tripp J, Hardwicke H, Lam TQ,** Oves contraceptive cap: short-term acceptability, aspects of use and user satisfaction, J Fam Plann Reprod Health Care 28:188, 2002.

31. **Courtot AM, Nikas G, Gravanis A, Psychoyos A,** Effects of cholic acid and "Protectaid" formulations on human sperm motility and ultrastructure, Hum Reprod 9:1999, 1994.

32. **Psychoyos A, Creatsas G, Hassan E,** Spermicidal and antiviral properties of cholic acid: contraceptive efficacy of a new vaginal sponge (Protectaid®) containing sodium cholate, Hum Reprod 8:866, 1993.

33. **Trussell J, Hatcher RA, Cates Jr W, Stewart FH, Kost K,** Contraceptive failure in the United States: an update, Stud Fam Plann 21:51, 1990.

34. **Edelman DA, McIntyre SL, Harper J,** A comparative trial of the Today contraceptive sponge and diaphragm: a preliminary report, Am J Obstet Gynecol 150:869, 1984.

35. **Creatsas G, Guerrero E, Guilbert E, Drouin J, Serfaty D, Lemieux L, Suissa S, Colin P,** A multinational evaluation of the efficacy, safety and acceptability of the Protectaid contraceptive sponge, Eur J Contracept Reprod Health Care 6:172, 2001.

36. **McIntyre SL, Higgins JE,** Parity and use-effectiveness with the contraceptive sponge, Am J Obstet Gynecol 155:796, 1986.

37. **Costello Daly C, Helling-Giese GE, Mati JK, Hunter DJ,** Contraceptive methods and the transmission of HIV: implications for family planning, Genitourin Med 70:110, 1994.

38. **Mauck CK, Baker JM, Barr SP, Johanson WM, Archer DF,** A phase I comparative study of three contraceptive films containing nonoxynol-9. Postcoital testing and coloposcopy, Contraception 56:97, 1997.

39. **Mauck CK, Baker JM, Barr SP, Abercrombie TJ, Archer DF,** A phase I comparative study of contraceptive films containing benzalkonium chloride and nonoxynol-9. Postcoital testing and coloposcopy, Contraception 56:89, 1997.

40. **Mendez F, Castro A,** Prevention of sexual transmission of AIDS/STD by a spermicide containing benzalkonium chloride, Arch AIDS Res 4:115, 1990.

41. **Hicks DR, Martin LS, Getchell JP, Health JL, Francis DP, McDougal JS, Curran JW, Voeller B,** Inactivation of HTLV-III/LAV-infected cultures of normal human lymphocytes by nonoxynol-9 in vitro, Lancet ii:1422, 1985.

42. **Kreiss J, Ngugi E, Holmes K, Ndinya-Achola J, Waiyaki P, Roberts PL, Ruminjo I, Sajabi R, Kimata J, Fleming TR, Anzala A, Holton D, Plummer F,** Efficacy of nonoxynol-9 contraceptive sponge use in preventing heterosexual acquisition of HIV in Nairobi prostitutes, JAMA 268:477, 1992.

43. **Zekeng L, Feldblum PJ, Oliver RM, Kaptue L,** Barrier contraceptive use and HIV infection among high risk women in Cameroon, AIDS 7:725, 1993.

44. **Wittkowski KM, Susser E, Kietz K,** The protective effect of condoms and nonoxynol-9 against HIV infection, Am J Public Health 88:590, 1998.

45. **Centers for Disease Control and Prevention,** Nonoxynol-9 spermicide contraception use—United States, 1999, MMWR 51:389, 2002.

46. **Van Damme L, Ramjee G, Alary M, Vuylsteke B, Chandeying V, Rees H, Sirivongrangson P, Mukenge-Tshibaka L, Ettiegne-Traore V, Uaheowitchai C, Karim SS, Masee B, Perriens J, Laga M, for the COL-1492 Study Group,** Effectiveness of COL-1492, a nonoxynol-9 vaginal gel, on HIV-1 transmission in female sex workers: a randomised controlled trial, Lancet 360:971, 2002.

47. **Louv WC, Austin H, Alexander WJ, Stagno S, Cheeks J,** A clinical trial of nonoxynol-9 as a prophylaxis for cervical *Neisseria gonorrhoeae* and *Chlamydia trachomatis* infections, J Infect Dis 158:518, 1988.

48. **Austin H, Louv WC, Alexander WJ,** A case-control study of spermicides and gonorrhea, JAMA 251:2822, 1984.

49. **Niruthisard S, Roddy RE, Chutivongse S,** Use of nonoxynol-9 and reduction in rate of gonococcal and chlamydial cervical infections, Lancet 339:1371, 1992.

50. **Roddy RE, Zekeng L, Ryan KA, Tamoufém U, Weir SS, Wong EL,** A controlled trial of nonoxynol 9 film to reduce male-to-female transmission of sexually transmitted diseases, New Engl J Med 339:504, 1998.

51. **Roddy RE, Zekeng L, Ryan KA, Tamoufe U, Tweedy KG,** Effect of nonoxynol-9 gel on urogenital gonorrhea and chlamydial infection: a randomized controlled trial, JAMA 287:1117, 2002.

52. **Barbone F, Austin H, Louv WC, Alexander WJ,** A follow-up study of methods of contra-ception, sexual activity, and rates of trichomoniasis, candidiasis, and bacterial vaginosis, Am J Obstet Gynecol 163:510, 1990.

53. **Raymond E, Dominik R, and The Spermicide Trial Group,** Contraceptive effectiveness of two spermicides: a randomized trial, Obstet Gynecol 93:896, 1999.

54. **Raymond EG, Chen PL, Luoto J, for the Spermicide Trial Group,** Contraceptive effectiveness and safety of five nonoxynol-9 spermicides: a randomized trial, Obstet Gynecol 103:430, 2004.

55. **Louik C, Mitchell AA, Werler MM, Hanson JW, Shapiro S,** Maternal exposure to spermicides in relation to certain birth defects, New Engl J Med 317:474, 1987.

56. **Bracken MB, Vita K,** Frequency of non-hormonal contraception around conception and association with congenital malformations in offspring, Am J Epidemiol 117:281, 1983.

57. **Einarson TR, Koren G, Mattice D, Schechter-Tsafiri O,** Maternal spermicide use and adverse reproductive outcome: a meta-analysis, Am J Obstet Gynecol 162:655, 1990.

58. **Malyk B,** Preliminary results: serum chemistry values before and after the intravaginal administration of 5% nonoxynol-9 cream, Fertil Steril 35:647, 1981.

59. **Niruthisard S, Roddy RE, Chutivonge S,** The effects of frequent nonoxynol-9 use on vaginal and cervical mucosa, Sex Transm Dis 268:521, 1991.

60. **Roddy RE, Cordero M, Cordero C, Fortney JA,** A dosing study of nonoxynol-9 and genital irritation, AIDS 4:165, 1993.

61. **Hooton TM, Fennell CL, Clark AM, Stamm WE,** Nonoxynol-9: differential antibacterial activity and enhancement of bacterial adherence to vaginal epithelial cells, J Infect Dis 164:1216, 1991.

62. **Stone KM, Grimes DA, Magder LS,** Primary prevention of sexually transmitted diseases. A primer for clinicians, JAMA 255:1763, 1986.

63. **Van de Perre P, Jacobs D, Sprecher-Goldberger S,** The latex condom, an efficient barrier against sexual transmission of AIDS-related viruses, AIDS 1:49, 1987.

64. **Fihn SD, Boyko EJ, Normand EH, Chen C-L, Grafton JR, Hunt M, Yarbro P, Scholes D, Stergachis A,** Association between use of spermicide-coated condoms and *Escherichia coli* urinary tract infection in young women, Am J Epidemiol 144:512, 1996.

65. **DeVincenzi I, for the European Study Group on Heterosexual Transmission of HIV,** A longitudinal study of human immunodeficiency virus transmission by heterosexual partners, New Engl J Med 331:341, 1994.

66. **Davis KR, Weller SC,** The effectiveness of condoms in reducing heterosexual transmission of HIV, Fam Plann Perspect 31:272, 1999.

67. **Diaz T, Schable B, Chu SY, and the Supplement to HIV and AIDS Surveillance Project Group,** Relationship between use of condoms and other forms of contraception among human immunodeficiency virus-infected women, Obstet Gynecol 86:277, 1995.

68. **Wald A, Langenberg AG, Link K, Izu AE, Ashley R, Warren T, Tyring S, Douglas JM, Jr., Corey L,** Effect of condoms on reducing the transmission of herpes simplex virus type 2 from men to women, JAMA 285:3100, 2001.

69. **Rosenberg MJ, Waugh MS, Solomon HM, Lyszkowski ADL,** The male polyurethane condom: a review of current knowledge, Contraception 53:141, 1996.

291

70. **Frezieres RG, Walsh TL, Nelson AL, Clark VA, Coulson AH,** Breakage and acceptability of a polyurethane condom: a randomized, controlled study, Fam Plann Perspect 30:73, 1998.

71. **Steiner MJ, Dominik R, Rountree RW, Nanda K, Dorflinger L,** Contraceptive effectiveness of a polyurethane condom and a latex condom: a randomized controlled trial, Obstet Gynecol 101:539, 2003.

72. **Grady WR, Klepinger DH, Billy JOG, Tanfer K,** Condom characteristics: the perceptions and preferences of men in the United States, Fam Plann Perspect 25:67, 1993.

73. **Trussell J, Warner DL, Hatcher RA,** Condom slippage and breakage rates, Fam Plann Perspect 24:20, 1992.

74. **Sparrow MJ, Lavill K,** Breakage and slippage of condoms in family planning clients, Contraception 50:117, 1994.

75. **Rosenberg MJ, Waugh MS,** Latex condom breakage and slippage in a controlled clinical trial, Contraception 56:17, 1997.

76. **Population Information Program,** Population Reports, Condoms, now more than ever, The Johns Hopkins University, Baltimore, Maryland, Report No. H-81, 1990.

77. **Walsh TL, Frezieres RG, Peacock K, Nelson AL, Clark VA, Bernstein L, Wraxall BGD,** Use of prostate-specific antigen (PSA) to measure semen exposure resulting from male condom failures: implications for contraceptive efficacy and the prevention of sexually transmitted disease, Contraception 67:139, 2003.

78. **Platt R, Rice PA, McCormack WM,** Risk of acquiring gonorrhea and prevalence of abnormal adnexal findings among women recently exposed to gonorrhea, JAMA 250:3205, 1983.

79. **Hooper RR, Reynolds GM, Jones OG, Zaidi A, Wiesner RJ, Latimer KP, Lester A, Campbell AF, Harrison WO, Karney WW, Holmes KK,** Cohort study of venereal disease. I. The risk of gonorrhea transmission from infected women to men, Am J Epidemiol 108:136, 1978.

80. **Anderson RM, Medley GF,** Epidemiology of HIV infection and AIDS: incubation and infectious periods, survival and vertical transmissions, AIDS 2(Suppl 1):557, 1988.

81. **Cameron DW, Simonsen JN, D'Costa LJ, Ronald AR, Maitha GM, Gakinya MN, Cheang M, et al,** Female to male transmission of human immunodeficiency virus type 1: risk factors for seroconverison in men, Lancet ii:403, 1989.

82. **Soper DE, Brockwell NJ, Dalton JP,** Evaluation of the effects of a female condom on the female lower genital tract, Contraception 44:21, 1991.

83. **Drew WL, Blair M, Miner RC, Conant M,** Evaluation of the virus permeability of a new condom for women, Sex Transm Dis 17:110, 1990.

84. **Beksinska M, Rees HV, Dickson-Tetteh KE, Mqoqi N, Kleinschmidt I, McIntyre JA,** Structural integrity of the female condom after multiple uses, washing, drying, and re-lubrication, Contraception 63:33, 2001.

85. **Bounds W, Guillebaud J, Newman GB,** Female condom (Femidom). A clinical study of its use-effectiveness and patient acceptability, Br J Fam Plann 18:36, 1992.

86. **Trussell J, Sturgen K, Strickler J, Dominik R,** Comparative contraceptive efficacy of the female condom and other barrier methods, Fam Plann Perspect 26:66, 1994.

87. **Farr G, Gabelnick H, Sturgen K, Dorflinger L,** Contraceptive efficacy and acceptability of the female condom, Am J Public Health 84:1960, 1994.

88. **Trussell J,** Contraceptive efficacy of the Reality® female condom, Contraception 58:147, 1998.

9

Periodic
Abstinence

Periodic abstinence as a method of contraception (also called natural
family planning) is keyed to the observation of naturally occurring
signs and symptoms of the fertile phase of the menstrual cycle. This
method must take into account the viability of sperm in the female reproductive tract (2–7 days) and the lifespan of the ovum (1–3 days). The
variability in the timing of ovulation is the reason why the period of abstinence must be relatively lengthy unless barrier methods are used during the
fertile days.

The period of maximal fertility begins 5 days before the day of ovulation
and ends on the day of ovulation.[1,2] The probability of conception plum-
mets the day after ovulation; however, conception occasionally occurs
more than 6 days before ovulation or immediately following ovulation.[3]
The likelihood of pregnancy steadily increases during this period of
fertility and is highest the day of ovulation and the preceding 2 days.[1,3,4]
Ovulation occurs at the following median times (note the relatively wide
ranges):[5]

- 16 hours after the LH peak (range 8–40 hours).
- 24 hours after the estradiol peak (range 17–32 hours).
- 8 hours after the rise in progesterone (range 12.5 hours before
  to 16 hours after).

Implantation occurs from 6–12 days after ovulation.[6] In the great majority
of instances, hormonal evidence of implantation can be detected 8–10
days after ovulation. The chance of early miscarriage increases when
implantation occurs later than day 10 after ovulation.

293

Approximately 2.3% of reproductive age contracepting women in the United States utilized some method of fertility timing in 1995.[7] This represented a dramatic decline since the 1960s.[8] Worldwide, it is estimated that 2.6% of reproductive age couples (27 million couples) use a method of periodic abstinence, with a high prevalence that reaches over 25% in parts of South America.[9, 10] Adherence to this method requires commitment from both partners; it is a way of life. Unsuccessful use can be predicted in couples who are unable to part with sexual spontaneity, women with irregular menses, disorganized people who cannot keep good records, and women with chronic problems of vaginitis or cervicitis. The advantage of periodic abstinence as a method of contraception is the availability of this method regardless of economic status or the accessibility of other methods. Users of this method also avoid religious proscription and the need to use "unnatural" substances.

Methods

There are several specific methods, and most teachers of periodic abstinence advocate the incorporation of features from more than one method.[11] Printed forms facilitate the careful record-keeping required to accurately estimate the fertile days each month. The sophistication of these methods was made possible by the tremendous increase in the scientific knowledge of the events in the human menstrual cycle. The time of ovulation (the fertile period) was identified in the 1930s, but it wasn't until the 1960s with the advent of the radioimmunoassay, that relatively precise timing of the various events became possible.

The Rhythm or Calendar Method

This method of periodic abstinence is based on the assumption that menstrual cycles are relatively constant, and therefore, the fertile period of the subsequent month could be predicted by the timing of the past cycle.

The general rule is to record the length of 6 cycles, then estimate the beginning of the fertile period by subtracting 18 days from the length of the shortest cycle and to estimate the end of the fertile period by subtracting 11 days from the length of the longest cycle. Thus a woman with cycles varying from 26–32 days practices periodic abstinence from the 8th day until the 21st day, a formidable requirement of 14 days of abstinence per cycle. Indeed, because of the normal variation in menstrual cycles, the average couple would practice periodic abstinence 16 days each month.

This method is useful only for women who have relatively regular and consistant menstrual cycles. This method has a pregnancy rate of about 40 per 100 woman-years, and, therefore, it is not advocated without combining it with other techniques. However, the utilization of programmed electronic devices to record temperatures, keep track of cycles, and provide a signal to the patient during the fertile period can reduce pregnancy rates to 5–10 per 100 woman-years.[12, 13]

The Cervical Mucus Method

The effectiveness of periodic abstinence has been improved by the development of methods that allow decisions to be made within each cycle. The cervical mucus method is also called the ovulation method, the Billings method, the Creighton Model Fertility Care System, or the TwoDay method.[14–16] This method requires sensing or observing the cervical mucus changes over time.[17] A woman successfully practicing this method must become aware of the estrogen-induced changes in cervical mucus that occur at midcycle: an increase in the amount of clear, thin, stringy mucus. Practitioners of this method describe these changes as wet, sticky (but slippery), and moist. The day of ovulation corresponds closely to the day of peak mucus.[18] This method requires the maintenance of a daily record, at least in the beginning.

The rules for intercourse are as follows:

1. Not on consecutive days during the postmenstrual preovulatory period so that seminal fluid does not obscure observation of cervical mucus changes, although assessment in the evening after intercourse that morning or the previous night should be reliable.
2. Abstinence when the mucus becomes sticky and moist.
3. Intercourse is permitted beginning on the 4th day after the last day of sticky, wet mucus. Most women (95%) have 4–12 days of observable secretions; thus the method requires a lengthy period of abstinence for many women.[19]

The Symptothermal Method

This method utilizes at least two indicators to identify the fertile period, usually combining the cervical mucus method with the basal body temperature (BBT). The BBT is recorded with any thermometer before getting out of bed. Prior to ovulation the temperature is usually below the normal body temperature. It rises about 0.2–0.4° C or 0.4–0.8° F in response to the increasing levels of progesterone after ovulation. The BBT method is so variable that, if practiced alone, it requires abstinence until the night of the 3rd day of a shift in temperature.

Combining the BBT with the mucus method, abstinence begins when the mucus becomes sticky and moist. Intercourse resumes the night of either the 3rd day of a temperature shift or the 4th day after the last day of sticky, wet mucus, whichever is later. Although this method is more complicated, the efficacy is slightly better, approaching only 2 failures per 100 woman-years when practiced by experienced couples who follow all the rules.[20] The performance of this method was superior in a comparison of the symptothermal method with various hormone-monitoring devices.[21]

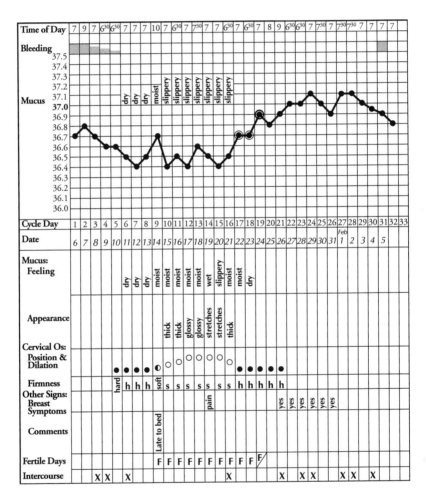

Individual women can be taught to incorporate other signals into their periodic abstinence method. For many women these additional signs and symptoms can add accuracy. These signals include mittleschmerz, breast tenderness, and changes in cervical position and texture.

Hormone Monitoring

Urinary concentrations of estrone-glucuronide and luteinizing hormone (LH) can be measured with disposable test sticks and a hand-held monitor. The Persona Monitor (Unipath and Inverness Medical Innovations, Waltham, Massachusets) indicates fertile days (the first rise in estrone-glucuronide) by displaying a red light after the insertion of the test stick, and the light changes to green at the end of the fertile period (4 days after the rise in LH). With a 6-day fertile period, this method was 94% effective (a 6% pregnancy rate over 1 year), although a criticism of this study concluded that the pregnancy rate is higher.[22, 23] In an Italian evaluation of several methods (salivary ferning, basal body temperature, salivary glucuronidase, and urinary LH), self-measurement of urinary LH levels was the best method to accurately minimize the number of days of abstinence.[24] The Clearplan Easy Fertility Monitor (Unipath Diagnostics Co., Princeton, New Jersey) is an electronic device that measures urinary LH and metabolites of estrogen.[25] It is marketed as an aid to achieve pregnancy, not as a method of family planning, and it should be emphasized that it underestimates the window of fertility; the device would have to be used in conjunction with one of the other measures of the fertile period.

The Standard Days Method

The Standard Days Method was developed by the Institute for Reproductive Health of Georgetown University in Washington, DC.[26] This method simply incorporates the avoidance of unprotected intercourse on days 8 through 19 of each menstrual cycle. CycleBeads, also developed by the Institute for Reproductive Health of Georgetown University, are a string of color-coded beads used with the Standard Days method to monitor cycle days and lengths. Users of this method are advised that efficacy is reduced even if only one menstrual cycle is out of the 26–32-day range, and to abandon the method if two cycles are out of the range.[26]

Resources

It is too much to expect the average clinician to provide the necessary instruction and support for these methods. Referral to a trained instructor is both appropriate and recommended. The local affiliate of the Planned Parenthood Federation of America can direct a clinician to a community program.

Most teachers of this method utilize detailed charts for recording changes and signals. The following resources can be contacted for advice, charts, and teaching plans:

The Couple to Couple League Foundation
http://www.ccli.org/

The National Fertility Awareness and Natural Family Planning Service for the United Kingdom
http://www.fertilityuk.org/
(charts available for download, including charts for Microsoft Excel)

The Natural Family Site, BYG Publishing Inc.
http://www.bygpub.com/natural/

Efficacy

The World Health Organization (WHO) completed a remarkable clinical trial of the periodic abstinence method of contraception in 725 couples in 5 countries: New Zealand, India, Ireland, the Phillipines, and El Salvador.[20, 27-30] The objectives were to determine whether the method could be taught to women of widely different educational and socioeconomical status and to document the effectiveness. Of the subjects, (97%) learned the method well.

The WHO defined failures with periodic abstinence as follows:

- Method-related (pregnancies that occur despite correct application of the rules).
- Inadequate teaching.
- Inaccurate application of instructions.
- Conscious departure from the rules.
- Uncertain.

Among those who learned the method, the pregnancy rate was 22.5 per 100 woman-years; however, almost all failures could be attributed to a conscious departure from the rules. Abstinence was necessary for about 17 days in each cycle.

Using the WHO data and a strict application of the definitions for method and use failure, method failure during the first year was associated with only a 3.1% pregnancy rate, but imperfect use with a 86.4% rate.[30] **Thus, if used perfectly, the method is very effective, but all methods of periodic abstinence are extremely unforgiving of imperfect use.** For this reason, the lowest achievable failure rate is considerably lower than the typical rate.

The probability of pregnancy is greatest when any of the following 3 rules are broken:[31]

- No intercourse during mucus days.
- No intercourse within 3 days after peak fecundity.
- No intercourse during times of stress.

Analysis of the periodic abstinence experience provides these conclusions:[31]

1. Periodic abstinence is associated with good efficacy when used correctly and consistently, but the method is very unforgiving of imperfect use.
2. There is an increased risk of pregnancy during periods of stress.
3. Couples with a poor attitude towards the rules are more likely to take risks.
4. Those couples who get away with taking risks are more likely to take risks again.

A multicenter trial in the 1970s of the cervical mucus method in the United States documented over a 2-year period of time a method failure rate of 1.2 pregnancies per 100 woman-years and a user failure rate of 19.3 pregnancies per 100 woman-years.[32] In the 1990s, the pregnancy rates of dedicated programs reported throughout the world have ranged from 2 to 20 pregnancies per 100 woman-years.[33, 34]

The cervical mucus method has been compared to the symptothermal method.[35, 36] Again, most pregnancies came from conscious departure from the rules. The two methods were comparable, with pregnancy rates of 20–24%. Better rates have been reported with newer methods that emphsize patient teaching and provide techniques to assess and record the window of fertility. Correct use of the TwoDay method yielded a pregnancy rate of 3.5% in 1 year, with a typicial use rate of 13.7%.[37] The Standard Days Method, used by women with regular 26- to 32-day cycles, produced a perfect use pregnancy rate of 4.75% and a typical use rate of 12% in 1 year.[38]

Prolonged sexual abstinence can be avoided by incorporating a barrier method during the fertile period into the overall program. Indeed, this is a relatively common practice, and it produces greater efficacy.[41]

Couples who do practice periodic abstinence successfully report no significant increase in marital-domestic friction, and some argue that the cooperation and communication required for the use of this method improve a relationship.

Failure Rates During the First Year of Use, United States[37-40]

Method	Percent of Women with Pregnancy Lowest Expected	Typical
Periodic abstinence		20.5
Calendar	9.0	
Ovulation method	3.0	
Symptothermal	2.0	
Postovulation	1.0	
Standard Days	4.8	
TwoDay	3.5	

Concerns

A lingering concern is that because of periodic abstinence, inadvertent fertilization could occur with aged gametes. Is pregnancy from aged gametes more likely to result in birth defects, spontaneous miscarriages, and chromosomal abnormalities?

No differences have been noted in the frequency of monosomic or trisomic abnormalities in relation to the timing of conception; however, conceptions with postovulatory aged ova appear to be at increased risk of polyploidy.[42] Furthermore, there is evidence, although not conclusive, to suggest that aged gametes have an increased risk of spontaneous miscarriages, as well as chromosomal defects.[43] In one cohort of women, an effect of aging sperm or oocytes on the risk of spontaneous miscarriage was present only in women who had a history of recurrent pregnancy losses.[44] In what is regarded as a well-designed, case-control study, increased relative risks for cleft lip and palate and congenital hydrocele were associated with periodic abstinence.[45] However, because of small numbers and the very difficult problem of recall bias, it is uncertain if this observation was real or due to chance.

It is worth emphasizing that the large, well-controlled WHO prospective trial observed no increase in congenital malformations, stillbirths, or spontaneous miscarriages.[29] A specific assessment of Down syndrome could not find an increase in the offspring of natural family planning users.[46] An analysis of pregnancy outcomes in 5 worldwide natural family planning centers could not detect an increased risk of spontaneous miscarriage, low birthweight, preterm birth, or other complications of pregnancy.[47, 48]

Evidence supports the idea that the further away from the time of highest fertility fertilization occurs, the more likely a male child conceived.[49] If this is true, the effect is not great, a ratio of approximately 58 males to 42 females. The WHO prospective clinical trial and another large multicenter, prospective study failed to detect any difference in the normal male to female ratio.[29, 50] Others have also reported that the day of conception does not influence the sex ratio.[1]

Conclusion

In our view, periodic abstinence is best suited for married couples who are united in their motivation to practice this method. Use of periodic abstinence is possible during lactation, but scrupulous attention is required to detect impending ovulation. With typical practice of the method, the pregnancy rate is about the same as with diaphragm and spermicides.

The problem of a long period of abstinence can be overcome by using a barrier method and/or spermicides during the fertile period. This combination is associated with an efficacy rate that is surpassed only by oral contraception, the IUD, and the long-acting methods.[51]

References

1. **Wilcox AJ, Weinberg CR, Baird DD,** Timing of sexual intercourse in relation to ovulation. Effects on the probability of conception, survival of the pregnancy, and sex of the baby, New Engl J Med 333:1517, 1995.

2. **Dunson DB, Baird DD, Wilcox AJ, Weinberg CR,** Day-specific probabilities of clinical pregnancy based on two studies with imperfect measures of ovulation, Hum Reprod 14:1835, 1999.

3. **Simpson JL, Gray RH, Queenan JT, Mena P, Perez A, Kambic RT, Paredo F, Barbato M, Spieler J,** Timing of intercourse, Hum Reprod 10:2176, 1995.

4. **Stanford JB, Smith KR, Dunson DB,** Vulvar mucus observations and the probability of pregnancy, Obstet Gynecol 101:1285, 2003.

5. **WHO,** Temporal relationships between ovulation and defined changes in the concentration of plasma estradiol-17beta, luteinizing hormone, follicle-stimulating hormone and progesterone. I. Probit analysis, Am J Obstet Gynecol 138:383, 1980.

6. **Wilcox AJ, Baird DD, Weinberg CR,** Time of implantation of the conceptus and loss of pregnancy, New Engl J Med 340:1796, 1999.

7. **Piccinino LJ, Mosher WD,** Trends in contraceptive use in the United States: 1982–1995, Fam Plann Perspect 30:4, 1998.

8. **Forrest JD, Fordyce RR,** U.S. women's contraceptive attitudes and practice: How have they changed in the 1980s? Fam Plann Persp 20:112, 1988.

9. **United Nations,** World Contraceptive Use 2001, United Nations Department of Social and Economic Affairs, New York, 2001.

10. **Che Y, Cleland JG, Ali MM,** Periodic abstinence in developing countries: an assessment of failure rates and consequences, Contraception 69:15, 2004.

11. **Labbok MH, Queenan JT,** The use of periodic abstinence for family planning, Clin Obstet Gynecol 32:387, 1989.

12. **Drouin J, Guilbert EE, Désaulniers G,** Contraceptive application of the Bioself fertility indicator, Contraception 50:229, 1994.

13. **Freundl G, Frank-Herrmann P, Godehardt E, Klemm R, Bachhofer M,** Retrospective clinical trial of contraceptive effectiveness of the electronic fertility indicator Ladycomp/Babycomp, Adv Contracept 14:97, 1998.

14. **Billings EL, Billings JJ, Catarinich M,** Atlas of the Ovulation Method, 2nd Edition, Advocate Press, Melbourne, 1974.

15. **Hilgers TW, Stanford JB,** Creighton-Model NaProEducation Technology for avoiding pregnancy, J Reprod Med 43:495, 1998.

16. **Jennings V, Sinai I,** Further analysis of the theoretical effectiveness of the TwoDay method of family planning, Contraception 64:149, 2001.

17. **Dunson DB, Sinai I, Colombo B,** The relationship between cervical secretions and the daily probabilities of pregnancy: effectiveness of the TwoDay Algorithm, Hum Reprod 16:2278, 2001.

18. **Fehring RJ,** Accuracy of the peak day of cervical mucus as a biological marker of fertility, Contraception 66:231, 2002.

19. **Sinai I, Jennings V, Arévalo M,** The TwoDay algorithm: a new algorithm to identify the fertile time of the menstrual cycle, Contraception 60:65, 1999.

20. **WHO,** A prospective multicenter trial of the ovulation method of natural family planning. I. The teaching phase, Fertil Steril 36:152, 1981.

21. **Freundl G, Godehardt E, Kern PA, Frank-Herrmann P, Koubenec HJ, Gnoth C,** Estimated maximum failure rates of cycle monitors using daily conception probabilities in the menstrual cycle, Hum Reprod 18:2628, 2003.

22. **Bonnar J, Flynn A, Freundl G, Kirkman R, Royston R, Snowden R,** Personal hormone monitoring for contraception, Br J Fam Plann 24:128, 1999.

23. **Trussell J,** Contraceptive efficacy of the personal hormone monitoring system Persona, Br J Fam Plann 25:178, 1999.

24. **Guida M, Tommaselli GA, Palomba S, Pellicano M, Moccia G, Di Carlo C, Nappi C,** Efficacy of methods for determing ovulation in a natural family planning program, Fertil Steril 72:900, 1999.

25. **Fehring RJ, Raviele K, Schneider M,** A comparison of the fertile phase as determined by the Clearplan Easy Fertility Monitor and self-assessment of cervical mucus, Contraception 69:9, 2004.

26. **Sinai I, Jennings V, Arévalo M,** The importance of screening and monitoring: the Standard Days Method and cycle regularity, Contraception 69:201, 2004.

27. **WHO,** A prospective multicenter trial of the ovulation method of natural family planning. II. The effectiveness phase, Fertil Steril 36:591, 1981.

28. **WHO,** A prospective multicenter trial of the ovulation method of natural family planning. III. Characteristics of the menstrual cycle and of the fertile phase, Fertil Steril 40:773, 1983.

29. **WHO,** A prospective multicenter trial of the ovulation method of natural family planning. IV. The outcome of pregnancy, Fertil Steril 41:593, 1984.

30. **WHO,** A prospective multicenter trial of the ovulation method of natural family planning. V. Psychosexual aspects, Fertil Steril 47:765, 1987.

31. **Trussell J, Grummer-Strawn L,** Contraceptive failure of the ovulation method of periodic abstinence, Fam Plann Perspect 22:65, 1990.

32. **Klaus H, Goebel JM, Muraski B, Egizio MT, Wetzel D, Taylor RS, Fagan MU, Ek K, Hobday K,** Use-effectiveness and client satisfaction in six centers teaching the Billings ovulation method, Contraception 19:613, 1979.

33. **Ryder B, Campbell H,** Natural family planning in the 1990s, Lancet 346:233, 1995.

34. **Howard MP, Stanford JB,** Pregnancy probabilities during use of the Creighton Model Fertility Care System, Arch Fam Med 8:391, 1999.

35. **Medina JE, Cifuentes A, Abernathy JR, Speiler SM, Wade ME,** Comparative evaluation of two methods of natural family planning in Columbia, Am J Obstet Gynecol 138:1142, 1980.

36. **Wade ME, McCarthy P, Braunstein GD, Abernathy JR, Suchindram CM, Harris GS, Danzer HC, Vricchio WA,** A randomized prospective study of the use-effectiveness of two methods of natural family planning, Am J Obstet Gynecol 141:368, 1981.

37. **Arévalo M, Jennings V, Nikula M, Sinai I,** Efficacy of the new TwoDay method of family planning, Fertil Steril 82:885, 2004.

38. **Arévalo M, Jennings V, Sinai I,** Efficacy of a new method of family planning: the Standard Days Method, Contraception 65:333, 2002.

39. **Trussell J, Vaughan B,** Contraceptive failure, method-related discontinuation and resumption of use: results from the 1995 National Survey of Family Growth, Fam Plann Perspect 31:64, 1999.

40. **Fu H, Darroch JE, Haas T, Ranjit N,** Contraceptive failure rates: new estimates from the 1995 National Survey of Family Growth, Fam Plann Perspect 31:58, 1999.

41. **Gnoth C, Frank-Hermann P, Freundl G, Kunert J, Godehart E,** Sexual behaviour of natural family planning users in Germany and its changes over time, Adv Contracept 11:173, 1995.

42. **Boue J, Boue A, Lazar P,** Retrospective and prospective epidemiological studies of 1500 karyotyped spontaneous human abortions, Teratology 12:11, 1975.

43. **Gray RH, Kambic RT,** Epidemiological studies of natural family planning, Hum Reprod 3:693, 1988.

44. **Gray RH, Simpson JL, Kambic RT, Queenan JT, Mena P, Perez A, Barbato M,** Timing of conception and the risk of spontaneous abortion among pregnancies occurring during the use of natural family planning, Am J Obstet Gynecol 172:1567, 1995.

45. **Bracken MB, Vita K,** Frequency of non-hormonal contraception around conception and association with congenital malformations in offspring, Am J Epidemiol 117:281, 1983.

46. **Castilla EE, Simpson JL, Queenan JT,** Down syndrome is not increased in offspring of natural family planning users (case control analysis), Am J Med Genet 59:525, 1995.

47. **Bitto A, Gray RH, Simpson JL, Queenan JT, Kambic RT, Perez A, Mena P, Barbato M, Li C, Jennings V,** Adverse outcomes of planned and unplanned pregnancies among users of natural family planning: a prospective study, Am J Public Health 87:338, 1997.

48. **Mena P, Bitto A, Barbato M, Perez A, Gray RH, Simpson JL, Queenan JT, Kambic RT, Pardo F, Stevenson W, Tagliabue G, Jennings V, Li C,** Pregnancy complications in natural family planning users, Adv Contracept 13:229, 1997.

49. **Kambic R, Gray RH, Simpson JL,** Outcome of pregnancy in users of natural family planning, Int J Gynecol Obstet (Suppl) 1:99, 1989.

50. **Gray RH, Simpson JL, Bitto AC, Queenan JT, Li C, Kambic RT, Perez A, Mena P, Barbato M, Stevenson W, Jennings V,** Sex ratio associated with timing of insemination and length of the follicular phase in planned and unplanned pregnancies during use of natural family planning, Hum Reprod 13:1397, 1998.

51. **Rogow D, Rintoul EJ, Greenwood S,** A year's experience with a fertility awareness program: a report, Adv Plann Parenthood 15:27, 1980.

303

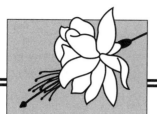

10

The Postpartum Period, Breastfeeding and Contraception

Breastfeeding protects infants against infection, offers an inexpensive supply of nutrition, contributes to maternal-infant bonding, and provides contraception. The relationship between lactation and fertility is an important public health issue. A birth interval of two or more years improves infant survival and reduces maternal morbidity.[1] In developing countries, breastfeeding provides protection from pregnancy and is important for achieving the two-year birth interval that advances good maternal and infant health.

Giving up breastfeeding was a misguided notion of civilized times. Urbanization, education, and modernization all contributed to a decline in breastfeeding, which, fortunately, has been somewhat reversed. Even in ancient Greek and Roman societies, breastfeeding was disdained by the elite. The tradition of wet nursing (the practice of breastfeeding by someone other than the mother) was popular from the days of the ancient Greeks to the time of medieval Europe.[2] A further decline in breastfeeding came with the introduction of bottle feeding.

The domestication of cattle dates back thousands of years, but the use of animal milk for infant feeding is recent. In the United States, modification of cow's milk for infant feeding was not established until 1900. In the early 1900s, milk banks were popular, using freezing techniques to keep the milk sterile. But it wasn't until the 1930s that the preparation of infant "formulas" moved from the home kitchen to commercial production and promotion. Breast milk substitutes were initially developed to meet specific needs (allergies and intolerance with cow's milk), but eventually came to be viewed as a means to free women from the responsibility of breastfeeding.

A decline in breastfeeding began in the 1930s (in 1922, about 90% of infants were still being breastfed at 1 year of age). By the 1950s, the prevalence of breastfeeding on discharge from the hospital fell to 30%, and the downward trend reached its nadir (22%) in 1972.[3] This trend was followed in Europe a decade or two later.

A higher mortality rate in artifically fed infants was observed in the 1900s. By the 1940s, the mortality difference between early and late weaned infants was recognized to be due to conditions of hygiene and general care. In the developed parts of the world, where infants receive good health supervision, the mortality difference is no longer a significant problem. However, in the developing world, excess mortality due to early weaning continues to be high.

The revival of breastfeeding can be attributed to the growth of knowledge regarding the health of infants.[4] The following reasons emerged as motivations to encourage breastfeeding:

1. Breastfeeding has a child-spacing effect, which is very important in the developing world as a means of limiting family size and providing good nutrition for infants.
2. Human milk prevents infections in infants, both by the transmission of immunoglobulins and by modifying the bacterial flora of the infant's gastrointestinal tract. However, avoidance of breastfeeding by HIV-infected women is strongly recommended.[5]
3. Breastfeeding enhances the bonding process between mother and child.
4. Breastfeeding provides some protection for the mother against breast cancer and protects against ovarian cancer.

Breastfeeding is a personal choice, but one influenced by custom and social and economic circumstances. Beginning in the 1960s, breastfeeding became more popular in the United States, Sweden, Canada, and the United Kingdom[3, 6] Even in the developing world there was evidence of increased breastfeeding. In general, the knowledge that breastfeeding is superior was spreading. But this upward trend in the United States peaked in 1982 (at 61% for initiation and 40% for 3 or more months).[3]

Unfortunately, and somewhat perplexing (does it represent more women in the workforce?), is the fact that during the 1980s, there was a steady decline in breastfeeding, reaching 52% for initiation by 1989.[3] By age 6 months, only 19.6% of infants were still breastfeeding. The average duration remains short, usually under 6 months, and most often only 2–3 months. This still provides a significant benefit for the infant, but as we shall see, it is not so good from a contraceptive point of view. Since 1990, breastfeeding has increased slightly, but the rates are still lower than the early 1980s peak (59.4% initiation in 1995 vs 61% in 1982).[4, 7]

Breast Physiology

The basic component of the breast lobule is the hollow alveolus or milk gland lined by a single layer of milk-secreting epithelial cells, derived from an ingrowth of epidermis into the underlying mesenchyme at 10–12 weeks of gestation. Each alveolus is encased in a crisscrossing mantle of contractile myoepithelial strands. Also surrounding the milk gland is a rich capillary network. The lumen of the alveolus connects to a collecting intralobular duct by means of a thin nonmuscular duct. Contractile muscle cells line the intralobular ducts that eventually reach the exterior via 15–20 collecting ducts in a radial arrangement, corresponding to the 15–20 distinct mammary lobules in the breast, each of which contains many alveoli.

Growth of this milk-producing system is dependent on numerous hormonal factors that occur in two sequences, first at puberty and then in pregnancy. Although there is considerable overlapping of hormonal influences, the differences in quantities of the stimuli in each circumstance and the availability of entirely unique inciting factors (human placental lactogen and prolactin) during pregnancy permit this chronologic distinction.

The major influence on breast growth at puberty is estrogen. In most girls, the first response to the increasing levels of estrogen is an increase in size and pigmentation of the areola and the formation of a mass of breast tissue just underneath the areola. Breast tissue binds estrogen in a manner similar to the uterus and vagina. The human breast expresses both estrogen receptors, ER-α and ER-β.[8] The development of estrogen receptors in the breast does not occur in the absence of prolactin. The primary effect of estrogen in subprimate mammals is to stimulate growth of the ductal portion of the gland system. Progesterone in these animals influences growth of the alveolar components of the lobule.[9] However, neither hormone alone, or in combination, is capable of yielding optimal breast growth and development. Full differentiation of the gland requires insulin, cortisol, thyroxine, prolactin, and growth hormone.[10] Of course, the ubiquitous growth factors are also involved, but the molecular mechanisms remain to be determined. Nevertheless, experimental evidence in mice indicates that progesterone is the key hormone required for mammary growth and differentiation; estrogen is necessary because the synthesis of progesterone receptors requires the critical presence of estrogen.[9]

307

Changes occur routinely in response to the estrogen-progesterone sequence of a normal menstrual cycle. Maximal size of the breast occurs late in the luteal phase. Fluid secretion, mitotic activity, and DNA production of nonglandular tissue and glandular epithelium peak during the luteal phase.[11–13] This accounts for cystic and tender premenstrual changes. During the normal menstrual cycle, estrogen receptors in mammary gland epithelium decrease in number during the luteal phase, whereas progesterone receptors remain at a high level throughout the cycle.[14] Studies using tissue from reduction mammoplasties or from breast tissue near a benign or malignant lesion have demonstrated a peak in mitotic activity during the luteal phase.[12, 15, 16] Using fine-needle biopsy tissue, an immunocytochemical marker of proliferation was higher in the luteal phase than in the proliferative phase.[14] And in this study there was a direct correlation with serum progesterone levels. However, important studies indicate that with increasing duration of exposure, progesterone imposes a limitation on breast cell proliferation.[17–19] Therefore, breast and endometrium epithelial cells may be more similar than initially proposed.

Final differentiation of the alveolar epithelial cell into a mature milk cell is accomplished by the gestational increase in estrogen and progesterone, combined with the presence of prolactin, but only after prior exposure to cortisol and insulin. The complete reaction depends on the availability of minimal quantities of thyroid hormone. Thus, the endocrinologically intact individual in whom estrogen, progesterone, thyroxine, cortisol, insulin, prolactin, and growth hormone are available can have appropriate breast growth and function. During the first trimester of pregnancy, growth and proliferation are maximal, changing to differentiation and secretory activity as pregnancy progresses.

Breast tissue changes with aging. During teenage years the breasts are dense and predominantly glandular. As the years go by, the breasts contain progressively more fat, but after menopause, this process accelerates so that soon into the postmenopausal years, the breast glandular tissue is mostly replaced by fat.

Lactation

During pregnancy, prolactin levels rise from the normal level of 10–25 ng/mL to high concentrations, beginning about 8 weeks and reaching a peak of 200–400 ng/mL at term.[20, 21] The increase in prolactin parallels the increase in estrogen beginning at 7–8 weeks' gestation, and the mechanism for increasing prolactin secretion is believed to be estrogen suppression of the hypothalamic prolactin-inhibiting factor, dopamine, and direct stimulation of prolactin gene transcription in the pituitary.[22, 23] There is marked variability in maternal prolactin levels in pregnancy, with pulsatile secretion and a diurnal variation similar to that found in nonpregnant subjects. The peak level occurs 4–5 hours after the onset of sleep.[24]

Made by the placenta and actively secreted into the maternal circulation from the sixth week of pregnancy, human placental lactogen (hPL) rises progressively, reaching a level of approximately 6,000 ng/mL at term. Human placental lactogen, though displaying less activity than prolactin, is produced in such large amounts that it may exert a lactogenic effect.

Although prolactin stimulates significant breast growth and is available for lactation, only colostrum (composed of desquamated epithelial cells and transudate) is produced during gestation. Full lactation is inhibited by progesterone, which interferes with prolactin action at the alveolar cell prolactin receptor level. Both estrogen and progesterone are necessary for the expression of the lactogenic receptor, but progesterone antagonizes the positive action of prolactin on its own receptor while progesterone and pharmacologic amounts of androgens reduce prolactin binding.[25–27] In the mouse, inhibition of milk protein production is due to progesterone suppression of prolactin receptor expression.[28] The effective use of high doses of estrogen to suppress postpartum lactation indicates that pharmacologic amounts of estrogen also block prolactin action.

The principal hormone involved in milk biosynthesis is prolactin. Without prolactin, synthesis of the primary protein, casein, does not occur, and true milk secretion is impossible. The hormonal trigger for initiation of milk production within the alveolar cell and its secretion into the lumen of the gland is the rapid disappearance of estrogen and progesterone from the circulation after delivery. The clearance of prolactin is much slower, requiring 7 days to reach nonpregnant levels in a nonbreastfeeding woman. These discordant hormonal events result in removal of the estrogen and progesterone inhibition of prolactin action on the breast. Breast engorgement and milk secretion begin 3–4 days postpartum when steroids have been sufficiently cleared. Maintenance of steroidal inhibition or rapid reduction of prolactin secretion (with a dopamine agonist) are effective in preventing postpartum milk synthesis and secretion. Augmentation of prolactin (by thyrotropin-releasing hormone [TRH] or sulpiride, a dopamine receptor blocker) results in increased milk yield.

In the first postpartum week, prolactin levels in breastfeeding women decline approximately 50% (to about 100 ng/mL). Suckling elicits increases in prolactin, which are important in initiating milk production. Until 2–3 months postpartum, basal levels are approximately 40–50 ng/mL, and there are large (about 10–20-fold) increases after suckling. Throughout breastfeeding, baseline prolactin levels remain elevated, and suckling produces a 2-fold increase that is essential for continuing milk production.[29, 30] The pattern or values of prolactin levels do not predict the postpartum duration of amenorrhea or infertility.[31]

Maintenance of milk production at high levels is dependent on the joint action of both anterior and posterior pituitary factors. By mechanisms to be described shortly, suckling causes the release of both prolactin and oxytocin as well as thyroid-stimulating hormone (TSH).[32, 33] Prolactin sustains the secretion of casein, fatty acids, lactose, and the volume of secretion, while oxytocin contracts myoepithelial cells and empties the alveolar lumen, thus enhancing further milk secretion and alveolar refilling. The increase in TSH with suckling suggests that thyrotropin-releasing hormone (TRH) may play a role in the prolactin response to suckling. The optimal quantity and quality of milk are dependent upon the availability of thyroid, insulin and the insulin-like growth factors, cortisol, and the dietary intake of nutrients and fluids.

Secretion of calcium into the milk of lactating women approximately doubles the daily loss of calcium.[34] In women who breastfeed for 6 months or more, this is accompanied by significant bone loss even in the presence of a high calcium intake.[35] However, bone density rapidly returns to base line levels in the 6 months after weaning.[36, 37] The bone loss is due to increased bone resorption, probably secondary to the relatively low estrogen levels associated with lactation. It is possible that recovery is impaired in women with inadequate calcium intake; total calcium intake during lactation should be at least 1,500 mg per day. Nevertheless, calcium supplementation has no effect on the calcium content of breast milk or on bone loss in lactating women who have normal diets.[38] Furthermore, studies indicate that any loss of calcium and bone associated with lactation is rapidly restored, and, therefore, there is no impact on the risk of post menopausal osteoporosis.[39–42]

Antibodies are present in breast milk and contribute to the health of an infant. Human milk prevents infections in infants both by transmission of immunoglobulins and by modifying the bacterial flora of the infant's gastrointestinal tract. Viruses are transmitted in breast milk, and although the actual risks are unknown, women infected with cytomegalovirus, hepatitis B, or human immunodeficiency virus are advised not to breastfeed. Vitamin A, vitamin B12, and folic acid are significantly reduced in the breast milk of women with poor dietary intake. As a general rule approximately 1% of any drug ingested by the mother appears in breast milk. In a study of Pima Indians, exclusive breastfeeding for at least 2 months was associated with a lower rate of adult-onset noninsulin-dependent diabetes mellitus, partly because overfeeding and excess weight gain are more common with bottlefeeding.[43]

Frequent emptying of the lumen is important for maintaining an adequate level of secretion. Indeed, after the fourth postpartum month, suckling appears to be the only stimulant required; however, environmental and emotional states also are important for continued alveolar activity. Vigorous aerobic exercise does not affect the volume or composition of breast milk, and, therefore, infant weight gain is normal.[44]

The ejection of milk from the breast does not occur as the result of a mechanically induced negative pressure produced by suckling. Tactile sensors concentrated in the areola activate, via thoracic sensory nerve roots 4, 5, and 6, an afferent sensory neural arc that stimulates the paraventricular and supraoptic nuclei of the hypothalamus to synthesize and transport oxytocin to the posterior pituitary. The efferent arc (oxytocin) is blood borne to the breast alveolus-ductal systems to contract myoepithelial cells and empty the alveolar lumen. Milk contained in major ductal repositories is ejected from openings in the nipple. This rapid release of milk is called "let-down." This important role for oxytocin is evident in knockout mice lacking oxytocin who undergo normal parturition but fail to nurse their offspring.[45]

In many instances, the activation of oxytocin release leading to let-down does not require initiation by tactile stimuli. The central nervous system can be conditioned to respond to the presence of the infant, or to the sound of the infant's cry, by inducing activation of the efferent arc. These messages are the result of many stimulating and inhibiting neurotransmitters. Suckling, therefore, acts to refill the breast by activating both portions of the pituitary (anterior and posterior) causing the breast to produce new milk and to eject milk. The release of oxytocin is also important for uterine contractions that contribute to involution of the uterus.

The oxytocin effect is a release phenomenon acting on secreted and stored milk. Prolactin must be available in sufficient quantities for continued secretory replacement of ejected milk. This requires the transient increase in prolactin associated with suckling. The amount of milk produced correlates with the amount removed by suckling. The breast can store milk for a maximum of 48 hours before production diminishes.

Cessation of Lactation

Lactation can be terminated by discontinuing suckling. The primary effect of this cessation is loss of milk let-down via the neural evocation of oxytocin. With passage of a few days, the swollen alveoli depress milk formation probably via a local pressure effect (although milk itself may contain inhibitory factors). With resorption of fluid and solute, the swollen engorged breast diminishes in size in a few days. In addition to the loss of milk let-down the absence of suckling reactivates dopamine (prolactin-inhibiting factor, PIF) production so that there is less prolactin stimulation of milk secretion.

Contraceptive Effect of Lactation

In primitive human societies, the duration of the birth interval has been very important for the survival of the young. Throughout human history, no preliterate society has achieved a fertility rate at the maximal level possible. The hunter-gatherer, nomadic !Kung women had a high suckling frequency and gave birth about every 4 years.[46] Lactational amenorrhea, lasting up to 2 years, has been nature's most effective form of contraception.[47] Indeed, lactation is the mechanism that maintains a reasonable interval between pregnancies in all nonseasonally breeding animals. In Africa and Asia, breastfeeding reduces the fertility rate by an average of about 30%.[1] Birth intervals of less than 2 years are associated with a greater incidence of low birth weight, preterm birth, and neonatal death for the new infant and malnutrition, infection, and increased second year mortality for the previous child.[48]

The contraceptive effectiveness of lactation, i.e., the length of the interval between births, depends on the level of nutrition of the mother (if low, the longer the contraceptive interval; however, well-nourished and undernourished women resume ovulating at the same time postpartum[49]), the intensity of suckling, and the extent to which supplemental food is added to the infant diet. If suckling intensity and/or frequency is diminished, contraceptive effect is reduced. Only amenorrheic women who exclusively breastfeed (full breastfeeding) at regular intervals, including nighttime, during the first 6 months have the contraceptive protection equivalent to that provided by oral contraception (98% efficacy); with menstruation or after 6 months, the chance of ovulation increases.[50, 51] With full or nearly full breastfeeding, approximately 70% of women remain amenorrheic through 6 months and only 37% through 1 year; nevertheless, with exclusive breastfeeding, the contraceptive efficacy at 1 year is high at 92%.[51] Fully breastfeeding women commonly have some vaginal bleeding or spotting in the first 8 postpartum weeks, but this bleeding is not due to ovulation.[52]

Mechanism of Action

Earlier experimental evidence suggested that the ovaries might be refractory to gonadotropin stimulation during lactation, and, in addition, the anterior pituitary might be less responsive to gonadotropine-releasing hormone (GnRH) stimulation. Other studies, done later in the course of lactation, indicated, however, that the ovaries as well as the pituitary were responsive to adequate tropic hormone stimulation.[53] These observations suggest that high concentrations of prolactin can work at both central and ovarian sites to produce lactational amenorrhea and anovulation. Prolactin appears to affect granulosa cell function in vitro by inhibiting the synthesis of progesterone. It also may change the testosterone:dihydrotestosterone ratio, thereby reducing aromatizable substrate and increasing local antiestrogen concentrations. Nevertheless, a direct effect of prolactin on ovarian follicular development does not appear to be a major factor. The central action predominates.

Elevated levels of prolactin inhibit the pulsatile secretion of GnRH.[54, 55] Prolactin excess has short loop positive feedback effects on dopamine. Increased dopamine reduces GnRH by suppressing arcuate nucleus function, perhaps in a mechanism mediated by endogenous opioid activity.[56, 57] However, blockade of dopamine receptors with a dopamine antagonist or the administration of an opioid antagonist in breastfeeding women does not always affect gonadotropin secretion.[58] The exact mechanism for the suppression of GnRH secretion remains to be unraveled. The principle of GnRH suppression by prolactin is reinforced by the demonstration that treatment of amenorrheic, lactating women with pulsatile GnRH fully restores pituitary secretion and normal ovarian cyclic activity.[59]

At weaning, as prolactin concentrations fall to normal, gonadotropin concentrations increase, and estradiol secretion rises. This prompt resumption of ovarian function is also indicated by the occurrence of ovulation within 14–30 days of weaning.

Prolactin concentrations are increased in response to the repeated suckling stimulus of breastfeeding. Given sufficient intensity and frequency, prolactin levels remain elevated. Under these conditions, follicle-stimulating hormone (FSH) concentrations are in the normal range (having risen from extremely low concentrations at delivery to follicular range in the 3 weeks postpartum) and luteinizing hormone (LH) values are in the low normal range. Despite the presence of gonadotropins, the ovary during lactational hyperprolactinemia does not display follicular development and does not secrete estrogen. Therefore, vaginal dryness and dyspareunia are commonly reported by breastfeeding women. The use of vaginal estrogen preparations is discouraged because absorption of the estrogen can lead to inhibition of milk production. Vaginal lubricants should be used until ovarian function and estrogen production return.

Postpartum Resumption of Ovulation

The resumption of ovulation in the postpartum period has been well studied in recent times.

Nonbreastfeeding Women

In nonbreastfeeding women, gonadotropin levels remain low during the early puerperium and return to normal concentrations during the 3rd to 5th week when prolactin levels have returned to baseline. In an assessment of this important physiologic event (in terms of the need for contraception), the mean delay before first ovulation was found to be approximately 45 days, while no woman ovulated before 25 days after delivery.[50, 60] Of the 22 women, 11 ovulated before the 6th postpartum week, underscoring the need to move the traditional postpartum medical visit to the 3rd week after delivery. In addition, two-thirds of the women ovulated before their first menses. The suppression of prolactin secretion with a dopamine agonist (e.g., bromocriptine), not surprisingly, is associated with the return of gonadotropin secretion in the 2nd postpartum week, and an earlier return to ovulation and menses.[61] In women who receive dopamine agonist treatment at or immediately after delivery, contraception is required a week earlier, in the 2nd week postpartum.[62]

Breastfeeding Women

In Scotland, no ovulation could be detected in women during exclusive breastfeeding.[63] However, in Chile, 14% of women ovulated during full breastfeeding, although full nursing provided effective contraception up to 3 months postpartum.[64, 65] It has been argued that the threshold for suppression of ovulation is at least 5 feedings for a total of at least 65 minutes per day suckling duration.[66] However in the studies from Chile, the frequency of nursing was the same in breastfeeders who ovulated and those who did not.

In Mexico, a study of 29 breastfeeding mothers and 10 nonbreastfeeders observed that in the absence of bleeding and supplementary feedings, 100% of the breastfeeders remained anovulatory for 3 months postpartum, and 96% up to 6 months.[67] The median time from delivery to first ovulation was 259 days for breastfeeders compared to 119 days for nonbreastfeeders. However, by the third postpartum month, 18% of the breastfeeders had ovulated.

In a well-nourished population in Australia, less than 20% of breastfeeding women ovulated by the 6th postpartum month, and less than 25% menstruated.[68] Neither time of first supplement nor the amount of supplement predicted the return of ovulation or menstruation. In other words, even in women giving their infants supplemental feedings, there is effective inhibition of ovulation during the first 6 months of breastfeeding.

Risk of Pregnancy

Over the years, Roger Short, more than anyone, has increased our appreciation for the importance of breastfeeding. He has documented from Australia that among women who have unprotected intercourse during lactation amenorrhea and use contraception when menses resume, 1.7%

become pregnant in the first 6 months of breastfeeding, 7% after 12 months, and 13% after 24 months.[69]

In a study of 422 middle-class women in Santiago, Chile, there was only one pregnancy (in month 6) when lactational amenorrhea was consciously relied upon for contraception.[70] This was equal to a cumulative 6-month life-table pregnancy rate of 0.45%. However, this accomplishment required an extensive program of education and support. In this study, 9% of exclusively breastfeeding women had resumption of menses by the end of 3 months and 19% by the end of 6 months. This increased suppression of fertility undoubtedly reflected the intensity of the breastfeeding program and the motivation of the participants.

In Chile, the probability of pregnancy in breastfeeding women has been measured as follows:[71]

Amenorrheic women:	**0.9% at 6 months;**
	17% at 12 months.
Menstruating women:	**36% at 6 months;**
	55% at 12 months.

In Pakistan, women who deliberately chose lactational amenorrhea as a method of contraception experienced a pregnancy rate of only 1.1% at 12 months if they remained amenorrheic.[72] It is apparent that while lactation provides a contraceptive effect, it is variable and not reliable for every woman, especially in view of the variablity in intensity of breastfeeding and the use of supplemental feeding.

An international group of researchers in the area of lactational infertility reached the following consensus in 1989, called the Bellagio Consensus (after the site of the conference at Bellagio, Italy):[73]

"The maximum birth spacing effect of breastfeeding is achieved when a mother 'fully' or nearly fully breastfeeds and remains amenorrheic. When these two conditions are fulfilled, breastfeeding provides more than 98% protection from pregnancy in the first six months."

Full breastfeeding means that the infant's total suckling stimulus is directed to the mother. There is no diminution of suckling by supplementation or the use of a pacifier. The Bellagio degree of protection in the first 6 months of full or nearly full breastfeeding has been demonstrated in clinical studies.[51, 74]

The World Health Organization (WHO) conducted a large prospective study examining the relationship between infant feeding and amenorrhea, as well as the rate of pregnancy during lactational amenorrhea.[75-78] Women who were still breastfeeding and remained amenorrheic had pregnancy rates of 0.8% at 6 months and 4.4% at 12 months, again confirming the Bellagio Consensus.

The duration of postpartum lochia is variable and can make it difficult to detect the onset of menstrual bleeding. In the WHO study, postpartum lochia was present from a minimum of 2 days to a maximum of 90 days, with an average duration of 27 days.[78] Most women with lactational amenorrhea do not experience true menstrual bleeding before postpartum day 56 (8 weeks). Breastfeeding frequency has no effect on the duration of postpartum lochia.

Only amenorrheic women who exclusively breastfeed at regular intervals, including nighttime, during the first 6 months have the contraceptive protection equivalent to that provided by oral contraception; with menstruation or after 6 months, the risk of ovulation increases.[50, 51, 79] Supplemental feeding increases the risk of ovulation (and pregnancy) even in amenorrheic women.[71] Total protection against pregnancy is achieved by the exclusively breastfeeding woman for a duration of only 10 weeks.[52]

Postpartum Choice of Contraception

When to Start

Additional contraception is necessary during lactation for most women. That is not to say that full breastfeeding shouldn't be encouraged and that the protection obtained in the first 6 months of breastfeeding shouldn't be emphasized. But after 3 months, the first ovulation can precede the first menstrual bleed. Half of women studied who are not fully breastfeeding ovulate before the 6th week, the time of the traditional postpartum visit; a visit during the 3rd postpartum week is strongly recommended for contraceptive counseling.

The Rule of 3's.

In the presence of FULL breastfeeding, a contraceptive method should be used beginning in the *3rd postpartum month*.

With PARTIAL breastfeeding or NO breastfeeding, a contraceptive method should begin during the *3rd postpartum week*.

After the termination of a pregnancy of less than 12 weeks, oral contraception can be started immediately. After a pregnancy of 12 or more weeks, the 3rd postpartum week rule should be followed if the pregnancy is term or near term. The latter delay has been based on a theoretical concern over an increased risk of thrombosis early in the postpartum period. This is probably no longer an issue with low-dose oral contraception. *We believe that oral contraception can be initiated immediately after a second trimester abortion or premature delivery.*

The Postpartum Visit

Contraception is usually on the mind of both patient and clinician at the first postpartum visit. A recent pregnancy and a new infant provide strong motivation to consider contraception. Traditionally, the first medical visit after delivery has been scheduled at 6 weeks, a time when good involution of the uterus and healing have occurred. Unfortunately in nonbreastfeeding women, ovulation can occur during the 4th postpartum week. We urge clinicians and patients to start a new tradition: schedule the first postpartum visit during the **3rd week after delivery**. Even breastfeeding women should be evaluated at this time, to consider whether breastfeeding is full and exclusive, or whether an additional contraceptive method is necessary.

Oral Contraception

Oral contraception even in low-dose formulations has been demonstrated to diminish the quantity and quality of lactation in postpartum women. Although there has been concern regarding the potential hazard of transfer of contraceptive steroids to the infant (a significant amount of the progestational component is secreted into breast milk),[80, 81] no adverse effects have thus far been identified. Because iron is an important factor in the bacteriostatic activity of breast milk, it is good to know that iron and copper concentrations in breast milk are not affected by the use of oral contraceptives.[82]

Women who use oral contraception have a lower incidence of breastfeeding after the 6th postpartum month, regardless of whether oral contraception is started at the 1st, 2nd, or 3rd postpartum month.[83–85] In adequately nourished women, no impairment of infant growth and development can be detected; presumably compensation is achieved either through supplementary feedings or increased suckling.[86–88] In an 8-year follow-up study of children breastfed by mothers using oral contraceptives, no effect could be detected on diseases, intelligence, or psychological behavior.[89] This study also found that mothers on birth control pills lactated a significantly shorter period of time than controls, a mean of 3.7 months vs 4.6 months in controls.

317

Because of the concerns regarding the impact of oral contraceptives on breastfeeding, a useful alternative is to combine the contraceptive effect of lactation with the progestin-only minipill (see Chapter 3); there is no evidence for any adverse effect on breastfeeding as measured by milk volume and infant growth and development.[86–88]

In contrast to the combined oral contraceptive, the progestin-only mini pill even provides a modest boost to milk production, and women using the minipill breastfeed longer and add supplementary feeding at a later time.[86, 90, 91] The combination of lactation and the progestin-only minipill is associated with near total contraceptive efficacy. In addition, the minipill can protect against the bone loss associated with lactation, a potential advantage in undernourished women.[92] In breastfeeding, overweight, Latina women with prior gestational diabetes, the progestin-only minipill was associated with a 3-fold increased risk of noninsulin dependent diabetes mellitus.[93] It is not known whether this might be a risk in all women who have experienced gestational diabetes; a prudent course would be to advise other methods for this special group of women.

Because of the slight positive impact on lactation, the minipill can be started immediately after delivery. A study investigating the impact of early initiation found no adverse effects on breastfeeding.[94]

In breastfeeding patients who insist on standard low-dose combined oral contraception, the full breastfeeder should begin during the 3rd postpartum month; all others during the 3rd postpartum week. Starting oral contraception during the 3rd postpartum week safely avoids the hypercoaguable state immediately after delivery. ***These considerations and recommendations also apply to the vaginal and transdermal methods of estrogen-progestin contraception.***

Depot-Medroxyprogesterone Acetate

Depot-medroxyprogesterone acetate does not affect breastfeeding or infant growth.[95, 96] Medroxyprogsterone acetate is transferred into the infant circulation; however, no adverse effects have been reported. A large WHO study failed to find any effects on infant growth or development with any progestin-only contraceptive method, including depot-medroxyprogesterone acetate.[87, 88] This is an excellent choice for postpartum contraception. Although studies have not been reported with use within 30 days after delivery, there are no effects associated with this method that require caution. Depot-medroxyprogesterone acetate can be administered immediately postpartum and certainly should be utilized no later than the 3rd postpartum week. Because the oral progestin-only minipill increased the risk of diabetes mellitus in breastfeeding, overweight Latino women with prior gestational diabetes,[93] depot-medroxyprogesterone acetate should be used with caution in all women with previous gestational diabetes.

Contraceptive Implants

Studies in Egypt indicate that when Norplant is inserted at least 30–42 days postpartum, the only difference in lactation or infant growth and development comparing Norplant users and controls is that infant weight gain in the first few months with exclusively breastfeeding Norplant users

Discontinuation of Breastfeeding Due to No Milk Secretion [97]

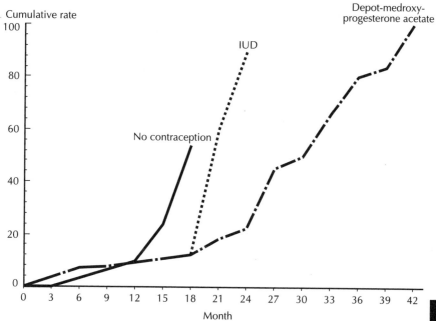

is slightly less.[98, 99] In Indonesian women whose infants were followed for 6 months after their mothers received Norplant 4–6 weeks postpartum, there was no adverse effect on infant growth.[100] A study of 100 Chilean women who received Norplant from 52–58 days postpartum was associated, as in Egypt, with a slightly lower infant weight gain in the first 4–6 months of breastfeeding, but after 6 months, weights were similar comparing Norplant users to controls.[101] However, in a subsequent study in Chile, Norplant had no effect on breastfeeding performance or infant growth.[96]

These findings with Norplant can be compared to those from studies of the effects of progestin-only minipills on lactation because the serum concentrations of levonorgestrel are comparable in the two methods. As noted above, women using levonorgestrel-only minipills have a better breastfeeding experience, beginning supplementary feeding about 1 month later and one-third are as likely to discontinue breastfeeding compared with women using nonhormonal contraceptives.[89, 90] We believe the experience with Implanon will be similar to that of Norplant.

The transfer of progestin from the mother's circulation to her milk and thence to the infant's blood has been studied with 3 delivery systems for levonorgestrel (minipill, implant, and intrauterine contraception).[80, 81] Transfer from maternal serum to breast milk was highest for the levonorgestrel intrauterine device (IUD) (12%) and lower for Norplant and the oral minipill, 7% and 8%, respectively. Transfer from breast milk to the infants' sera averaged 75% for the levonorgestrel IUD, 75% for Norplant, and only 32% for the Minipill.[80] These infant sera concentrations are about 25% of those reported for levonorgestrel-containing combination oral contraceptives.[81] This transfer is relatively low, and no adverse effects have been reported.

As noted above, the oral progestin-only minipill increased the risk of noninsulin-dependent diabetes mellitus in breastfeeding, overweight Latino women with prior gestational diabetes.[93] For this reason, all progestin-only methods, including implants, should be used with caution in women with previous gestational diabetes.

No studies have been reported examining the effects of implant administered prior to 30 days after delivery, and, therefore, the package advisory insert cautions against immediate postpartum use. In some situations, however, the delivery may provide the only opportunity to receive implant contraception. Since another pregnancy within a year of delivery poses a far greater health hazard to both mother and infant, in our view such caution is not warranted. If the new mother does not have access to implant contraception 30 days after delivery, we believe it is appropriate to provide it immediately postpartum.

Periodic Abstinence

Women skilled in the cervical mucus method can detect evidence of fertile type mucus prior to the first menses in the postpartum period. However, there are many false-postive and false-negative interpretations.[102] This method cannot be used with a great deal of confidence until regular menses are resumed.

Barrier Methods

Barrier methods, of course, have no impact on breastfeeding, and they are an excellent choice for motivated couples. Lubricated condoms are especially helpful for the vaginal dryness experienced by some breastfeeding women. Spermicides and foam products can also help with the dryness and dyspareunia. It is difficult to fit a diaphragm or cervical cap before healing and involution are complete (about 6 weeks), and it is not advisable to use a sponge, cap, or diaphragm while still bleeding. Therefore spermicides, foam, and condoms should be used in the immediate postpartum period, and use of the sponge, cap, or diaphragm can be started about the 6th postpartum week.

The Postpartum IUD

Expulsion rates were higher when the older, large plastic IUDs were inserted sooner than 8 weeks postpartum; however, studies indicate that the copper IUDs can be inserted between 4 and 8 weeks postpartum without an increase in pregnancy rates, expulsion, uterine perforation, or removals for bleeding and/or pain.[103, 104] Insertion can even occur immediately after a vaginal delivery; it is not associated with an increased risk of infection, uterine perforation, postpartum bleeding, or uterine subinvolution.[105] This is not recommended if intrauterine infection is present, and a slightly higher expulsion rate is to be expected compared to insertion 4–8 weeks postpartum. The IUD should be inserted within 15 minutes after delivery of the placenta. Administration of oxytocin or uterine massage ensures a well-contracted uterus. The angle between the cervix and the corpus is quickly reestablished after delivery. This angle should be straightened by traction with a sponge forceps (not a toothed tenaculum) placed on the anterior cervical lip. The IUD, held in a second sponge forceps, is advanced into the uterine cavity until it touches the fundus. This can be felt by abdominal palpation. The IUD is released and the strings are cut flush with the external os. The strings can be shortened as required at the postpartum visit. Expulsion usually occurs in the first 3 months and is less common with cooper devices and the frameless FlexiGard than with the Lippes Loop. The IUD can also be inserted at cesarean section; the expulsion rate is slightly lower than that with insertion immediately after vaginal delivery.[106]

Device	Expulsion Rate After Immediate Postpartum Insertion[107–110]
Lippes Loop	22.6 %
TCu-380A	9.8
TCu-220C	9.0
Nova T	6.2
FlexiGard	3.1

Insertion of an IUD in breastfeeding women is relatively easier and is associated with a lower removal rate for bleeding or pain.[105] An early suggestion that uterine perforation is more common in lactating women has not been substantiated.[105, 111]

An IUD can be inserted immediately after a first trimester abortion; but, after a second trimester abortion, one should wait until uterine involution occurs.[112, 113]

References

1. **Thapa S, Short RV, Potts M,** Breastfeeding, birthspacing and their effects on child survival, Nature 335:679, 1988.

2. **Davidson WD, Durham NC,** A brief history of infant feeding, J Pediatrics 43:74, 1953.

3. **National Academy of Sciences,** Nutrition During Lactation, Academy Press, Washington, DC, 1991.

4. **American Academy of Pediatrics,** Breastfeeding and the use of human milk, Pediatrics 100:1035, 1997.

5. **Read JS, American Academy of Pediatrics Committee on Pediatric AIDS,** Human milk, breastfeeding, and transmission of human immunodeficiency virus type 1 in the United States, Pediatrics 112:1196, 2003.

6. **Ryan AS, Pratt WF, Wysong JL, Lewandowski G, McNally JW, Krieger FW,** A comparison of breast-feeding data from the National Surveys of Family Growth and the Ross Laboratories Mothers Surveys, Am J Public Health 81:1049, 1991.

7. **Ryan AS,** The resurgence of breastfeeding in the United States, Pediatrics 99:E12, 1997.

8. **Enmark E, Pelto-Huikko M, Grandien K, Lagercrantz S, Lagercrantz J, Fried G, Nordenskjöld M, Gustafsson J-Å,** Human estrogen receptor β-gene structure, chromosomal localization, and expression pattern, J Clin Endocrinol Metab 82:4258, 1997.

9. **Shyamala G,** Roles of estrogen and progesterone in normal mammary gland development. Insights from progesterone receptor null mutant mice and in situ localization of receptor, Trends Endocrinol Metab 8:34, 1997.

10. **Klineberg DL, Niemann W, Flamm E, Cooper P, Babitsky G,** Primate mammary development, J Clin Invest 75:1943, 1985.

11. **Ferguson DP, Anderson TJ,** Morphological evaluation of cell turnover in relation to menstrual cycle in the "resting" human breast, Br J Cancer 44:177, 1988.

12. **Longacre TA, Bartow SA,** A correlative morphologic study of human breast and endometrium in the menstrual cycle, Am J Surg Path 10:382, 1986.

13. **Going JJ, Anderson TJ, Battersby S, MacIntyre CC,** Proliferative and secretory activity in human breast during natural and artificial menstrual cycles, Am J Path 130:193, 1988.

14. **Söderqvist G, Isaksson E, von Schoultz B, Carlström K, Tani E, Skoog L,** Proliferation of breast epithelial cells in healthy women during the menstrual cycle, Am J Obstet Gynecol 176:123, 1997.

15. **Potten CS, Watson RJ, Williams GT, Tickle S, Roberts SA, Harris M, Howell A,** The effect of age and menstrual cycle upon proliferative activity of the normal human breast, Br J Cancer 58:163, 1988.

16. **Vogel PM, Georgiade NG, Fetter BF, Vogel FS, McCarty KS,** The correlation of histologic changes in the human breast with the menstrual cycle, Am J Pathol 104:23, 1981.

17. **Chang K-J, Lee TTY, Linarez-Cruz G, Fournier S, de Ligniéres B,** Influences of percutaneous administration of estradiol and progesterone on human breast epithelial cell cycle in vivo, Fertil Steril 63:785, 1995.

18. **Laidlaw IJ, Clarke RB, Howell A, Owen AW, Potten CS, Anderson E,** The proliferation of normal human breast tissue implanted into athymic nude mice is stimulated by estrogen but not progesterone, Endocrinology 136:164, 1996.

19. **Foidart J-M, Colin C, Denoo X, Desreux J, Béliard A, Fournier S, de Ligniéres B,** Estradiol and progesterone regulate the proliferation of human breast epithelial cells, Fertil Steril 69:963, 1998.

20. **Tyson JE, Hwang P, Guyda H, Friesen HG,** Studies of prolactin secretion in human pregnancy, Am J Obstet Gynecol 113:14, 1972.

21. **Kletzky OA, Marrs RP, Howard WF, McCormick W, Mishell Jr DR,** Prolactin synthesis and release during pregnancy and puerperium, Am J Obstet Gynecol 136:545, 1980.

22. **Tyson JE, Friesen HG,** Factors influencing the secretion of human prolactin and growth hormone in menstrual and gestational women, Am J Obstet Gynecol 116:377, 1973.

23. **Barberia JM, Abu-Fadil S, Kletzky OA, Nakamura RM, Mishell Jr DR,** Serum prolactin patterns in early human gestation, Am J Obstet Gynecol 121:1107, 1975.

24. **Ehara Y, Siler TM, Yen SSC,** Effects of large doses of estrogen on prolactin and growth hormone release, Am J Obstet Gynecol 125:455, 1976.

25. **Murphy LJ, Murphy LC, Stead B, Sutherland RL, Lazarus L,** Modulation of lactogenic receptors by progestins in cultured human breast cancer cells, J Clin Endocrinol Metab 62:280, 1986.

26. **Simon WE, Pahnke VG, Holzel F,** In vitro modulation of prolactin binding to human mammary carcinoma cells by steroid hormones and prolactin, J Clin Endocrinol Metab 60:1243, 1985.

27. **Kelly PA, Kjiane J, Postel-Vinay M-C, Edery M,** The prolactin/growth hormone receptor family, Endocr Rev 12:235, 1991.

28. **Haslam SZ, Shyamala G,** Progesterone receptors in normal mammary gland: receptor modulations in relation to differentiation, J Cell Biol 86:730, 1980.

29. **Battin DA, Marrs RP, Fleiss PM, Mishell Jr DR,** Effect of suckling on serum prolactin, luteinizing hormone, follicle-stimulating hormone, and estradiol during prolonged lactation, Obstet Gynecol 65:785, 1985.

30. **Stern JM, Konner M, Herman TN, Reichlin S,** Nursing behaviour, prolactin, and postpartum amenorrhoea during prolonged lactation in American and !Kung mothers, Clin Endocrinol 25:247, 1986.

31. **Tay CCK, Glasier AF, McNeilly AS,** Twenty-four hour patterns of prolactin secretion during lactation and the relationship to suckling and the resumption of fertility in breast-feeding women, Hum Reprod 11:950, 1996.

32. **Dawood MY, Khan-Dawood FS, Wahl RS, Fuchs F,** Oxytocin release and plasma anterior pituitary and gonadal hormones in women during lactation, J Clin Endocrinol Metab 52:678, 1981.

33. **McNeilly AS, Robinson KA, Houston MJ, Howe PW,** Release of oxytocin and prolactin in response to suckling, Br Med J 286:257, 1983.

34. **Kumar R, Cohen WR, Epstein FH,** Vitamin D and calcium hormones in pregnancy, New Engl J Med 302:1143, 1980.

35. **Sowers M, Corton G, Shapiro B, Jannausch ML, Crutchfield M, Smith ML, Randolph JF, Hollis B,** Changes in bone density with lactation, JAMA 269:3130, 1993.

36. **Kalkwarf HJ, Specker BL,** Bone mineral loss during lactation and recovery after weaning, Obstet Gynecol 86:26, 1995.

37. **Kovacs CS,** Calcium and bone metabolism in pregnancy and lactation, J Clin Endocrinol Metab 86:2344, 2001.

38. **Kalkwarf HJ, Specker BL, Bianchi DC, Ranz J, Ho M,** The effect of calcium supplementation on bone density during lactation and after weaning, New Engl J Med 337:523, 1997.

39. **Laskey MA, Prentice A, Hanratty LA, Jarjou LM, Dibba B, Beavan SR, Cole TJ,** Bone changes after 3 mo of lactation: influence of calcium intake, breast-milk output, and vitamin D-receptor genotype, Am J Clin Nutr 67:685, 1998.

40. **Ritchie LD, Fung EB, Halloran BP, Turnlund JR, Van Loan MD, Cann CE, King JC,** A longitudinal study of calcium homeostasis during human pregnancy and lactation and after resumption of menses, Am J Clin Nutr 67:693, 1998.

41. **Polatti F, Capuzzo E, Viazzo F, Colleoni R, Klersy C,** Bone mineral changes during and after lactation, Obstet Gynecol 94:52, 1999.

42. **Kojima N, Douchi T, Kosha S, Nagata Y,** Cross-sectional study of the effects of parturition and lactation on bone mineral density later in life, Maturitas 41:203, 2002.

43. **Pettitt DJ, Forman MR, Hanson RL, Knowler WC, Bennett PH,** Breastfeeding and incidence of non-insulin-dependent diabetes mellitus in Pima Indians, Lancet 350:166, 1997.

44. **Dewey KG, Lovelady CA, Nommsen-Rivers LA, McCrory MA, Lönnerdal B,** A randomized study of the effects of aerobic exercise by lactating women on breast-milk volume and composition, New Engl J Med 330:449, 1994.

45. **Nishimori K, Young LJ, Guo Q, Wang Z, Insel TR, Matzuk MM,** Oxytocin is required for nursing but is not essential for parturition or reproductive behavior, Proc Natl Acad Sci USA 93:11699, 1996.

46. **Kolata G,** !Kung hunter-gatherers: feminism, diet and birth control, Science 185:932, 1974.

47. **Short RV,** Lactation — The central control of reproduction, Ciba Found Sympos 45:73, 1976.

48. **Miller JE,** Birth intervals and perinatal health: an investigation of three hypotheses, Fam Plann Perspect 23:62, 1991.

49. **Wasalathanthri S, Tennekoon KH,** Lactational amenorrhea/anovulation and some of their determinants: a comparison of well-nourished and undernourished women, Fertil Steril 76:317, 2001.

50. **Campbell OM, Gray RH,** Characteristics and determinants of postpartum ovarian function in women in the United States, Am J Obstet Gynecol 169:55, 1993.

51. **Labbok MH, Hight-Laukaran V, Peterson AE, Fletcher V, von Hertzen H, Van Look PFA,** Multicenter study of the lactational amenorrhea method (LAM): I. Efficacy, duration, and implications for clinical application, Contraception 55:327, 1997.

52. **Visness CM, Kennedy KI, Gross BA, Parenteau-Carreau S, Flynn AM, Brown JB,** Fertility of fully breast-feeding women in the early postpartum period, Obstet Gynecol 89:164, 1997.

53. **Tyson JE, Carter JN, Andreassen B, Huth J, Smith B,** Nursing mediated prolactin and luteinizing hormone secretion during puerperal lactation, Fertil Steril 30:154, 1978.

54. **Sauder SE, Frager M, Case GD, Kelch RP, Marshall JC,** Abnormal patterns of pulsatile luteinizing hormone secretion in women with hyperprolactinemia and amenorrhea: responses to bromocriptine, J Clin Endocrinol Metab 59:941, 1984.

55. **Tay CCK, Glasier A, McNeilly AS,** Twenty-four hour secretory profiles of gonadotropins and prolactin in breastfeeding women, Hum Reprod 7:951, 1992.

56. **Ishizuka B, Quigley ME, Yen SSC,** Postpartum hypogonadotrophinism: evidence for increased opioid inhibition, Clin Endocrinol 20:573, 1984.

57. **Petraglia F, De Leo V, Nappi C, Facchinetti F, Montemagno U, Brambilla F, Genazzani AR,** Differences in the opioid control of luteinizing hormone secretion between pathological and iatrogenic hyperprolactinemic states, J Clin Endocrinol Metab 64:508, 1987.

58. **Tay CCK, Glasier AF, McNeilly AS,** Effect of antagonists of dopamine and opiates on the basal and GnRH-induced secretion of luteinizing hormone, follicle stimulating hormone and prolactin during lactational amenorrhea in breastfeeding women, Hum Reprod 8:532, 1993.

59. **Zinaman MJ, Cartledge T, Tomai T, Tippett P, Merriam GR,** Pulsatile GnRH stimulates normal cyclic ovarian function in amenorrheic lactating postpartum women, J Clin Endocrinol Metab 80:2088, 1995.

60. **Gray RH, Campbell OM, Zacur HA, Labbok MH, MacRae SL,** Postpartum return of ovarian activity in nonbreastfeeding women monitored by urinary assays, J Clin Endocrinol Metab 64:645, 1987.

61. **Kremer JAM, Thomas CMG, Rolland R, van der Heijden PF, Thomas CM, Lancranjan I,** Return of gonadotropic function in postpartum women during bromocriptine treatment, Fertil Steril 51:622, 1989.

62. **Haartsen JE, Heineman MJ, Elings M, Evers JLH, Lancranjan I,** Resumption of pituitary and ovarian activity post-partum: endocrine and ultrasonic observations in bromocriptine-treated women, Hum Reprod 7:746, 1992.

63. **Howie PW, McNeilly AS, Houston MJ, Cook A, Boyle H,** Effect of supplementary food on suckling patterns and ovarian activity during lactation, Br Med J 283:757, 1981.

64. **Perez A, Vela P, Masnick GS, Potter RG,** First ovulation after childbirth: the effect of breastfeeding, Am J Obstet Gynecol 114:1041, 1972.

65. **Diaz S, Peralta O, Juez G, Salvatierra AM, Casado ME, Duran E, Croxatto HB,** Fertility regulation in nursing women. I. The probablity of conception in full nursing women living in an urban setting, J Biosoc Sci 14:329, 1982.

66. **McNeilly AS, Glasier A, Howie PW,** Endocrine control of lactational infertility, In: Dobbing J, ed. Maternal Nutrition and Lactational Infertility, Nevey/Raven Press, New York, 1985, pp 177.

67. **Rivera R, Kennedy KI, Ortiz E, Barrera M, Bhiwandiwala PP,** Breast-feeding and the return to ovulation in Durango, Mexico, Fertil Steril 49:780, 1988.

68. **Lewis PR, Brown JB, Renfree MB, Short RV,** The resumption of ovulation and menstruation in a well-nourished population of women breastfeeding for an extended period of time, Fertil Steril 55:529, 1991.

69. **Short RV, Lewis PR, Renfree MB, Shaw G,** Contraceptive effects of extended lactational amenorrhoea: beyond the Bellagio Consensus, Lancet 337:715, 1991.

70. **Pérez A, Labbok MH, Queenan JT,** Clinical study of the lactational amenorrhoea method for family planning, Lancet 339:968, 1992.

71. **Diaz S, Aravena R, Cardenas H, Casado ME, Miranda P, Schiappacasse V, Croxatto HB,** Contraceptive efficacy of lactational amenorrhea in urban Chilean women, Contraception 43:335, 1991.

72. **Kazi A, Kennedy KI, Visness CM, Khan T,** Effectiveness of the lactational amenorrhea method in Pakistan, Fertil Steril 64:717, 1995.

73. **Kennedy KI, Rivera R, McNeilly AS,** Consensus statement on the use of breastfeeding as a family planning method, Bellagio, Italy, Contraception 39:477, 1989.

74. **Ramos R, Kennedy KI, Visness CM,** Effectiveness of lactational amenorrhoea in preventing pregnancy in Manila, The Phillipines, Br Med J 313:909, 1996.

75. **World Health Organization Task Force on Methods for the Natural Regulation of Fertility,** The World Health Organization multinational study of breast-feeding and lactational amenorrhea. I. Description of infant feeding patterns and the return of menses, Fertil Steril 70:448, 1998.

76. **World Health Organization Task Force on Methods for the Natural Regulation of Fertility,** The World Health Organization multinational study of breast-feeding and lactational amenorrhea. II. Factors associated with the length of amenorrhea, Fertil Steril 70:461, 1998.

77. **World Health Organization Task Force on Methods for the Natural Regulation of Fertility,** The World Health Organization multinational study of breast-feeding and lactational amenorrhea. III. Pregnancy during breast-feeding, Fertil Steril 72:431, 1999.

78. **World Health Organization Task Force on Methods for the Natural Regulation of Fertility,** The World Health Organization multinational study of breast-feeding and lactational amenorrhea. IV. Postpartum bleeding and lochia in breast-feeding women, Fertil Steril 72:441, 1999.

79. **Gray RH, Campbell OM, Apelo R, Eslami SS, Zacur H, Ramos RM, Gehret JC, Labbok MH,** Risk of ovulation during lactation, Lancet 335:25, 1990.

80. **Shikary ZK, Bertrabet S, Patel ZM, Paytel S, Joshi JV, Toddywala VA, Toddywala SP, Patel DM, Jhaveri K, Saxena BN,** ICMR task force study on hormonal contraception. Transfer of levonorgestrel administered through different drug delivery systems from the maternal circulation into the newborn's circulation via breast milk, Contraception 35:477, 1987.

81. **Betrabet SS, Shikary ZK, Toddywalla VS, Toddywalla SP, Patel D, Saxena BN,** Transfer of norethisterone (NET) and levonorgestrel (LNG) from a single tablet into the infant's circulation through the mother's milk, Contraception 35:517, 1987.

82. **Dorea JG, Miazaki ES,** The effects of oral contraceptiveuse on iron and copper concentrations in breast milk, Fertil Steril 72:297, 1999.

83. **Diaz S, Peralta O, Juez G, Herreros C, Casado ME, Salvatierra AM, Miranda P, Durn E, Croxatto HB,** Fertility regulation in nursing women: III. Short-term influence of a low-dose combined oral contraceptive upon lactation and infant growth, Contraception 27:1, 1982.

84. **Croxatto HB, Diaz S, Peralta O, Juez G, Herreros C, Casado ME, Salvatierra AM, Miranda P, Durn E,** Fertility regulation in nursing women: IV. Long-term influence of a low-dose combined oral contraceptive initiated at day 30 postpartum upon lactation and child growth, Contraception 27:13, 1983.

85. **Peralta O, Diaz S, Juez G, Herreros C, Casado ME, Salvatierra AM, Miranda P, Durn E, Croxatto HB,** Fertility regulation in nursing women: V. Long-term influence of a low-dose combined oral contraceptive initiated at day 90 postpartum upon lactation and infant growth, Contraception 27:27, 1983.

86. **WHO, Special Programme of Research, Development, and Research Training in Human Reproduction, Task Force on Oral Contraceptives,** Effects of hormonal contraceptives on milk volume and infant growth, Contraception 30:505, 1984.

87. **WHO Task Force for Epidemiological Research on Reproductive Health, Special Programme of Research, Development and Research Training in Human Reproduction,** Progestogen-only contraceptives during lactation. I. Infant growth, Contraception 50:35, 1994.

88. **WHO Task Force for Epidemiological Research on Reproductive Health, Special Programme of Research, Development and Research Training in Human Reproduction,** Progestogen-only contraceptives during lactation. II. Infant development, Contraception 50:55, 1994.

89. **Nilsson S, Melbin T, Hofvander Y, Sundelin C, Valentin J, Nygren KG,** Long-term follow-up of children breast-fed by mothers using oral contraceptives, Contraception 34:443, 1986.

90. **McCann MF, Moggia AV, Hibbins JE, Potts M, Becker C,** The effects of a progestin-only oral contraceptive (levonorgestrel 0.03 mg) on breast-feeding, Contraception 40:635, 1989.

91. **Moggia AV, Harris GS, Dunson TR, Diaz R, Moggia MS, Ferrer MA, McMullen SL,** A comparative study of a progestin-only oral contraceptive versus non-hormonal methods in lactating women in Buenos Aires, Argentina, Contraception 44:31, 1991.

92. **Caird LE, Reid-Thomas V, Hannan WJ, Gow S, Glasier AF,** Oral progestogen-only contraception may protect against loss of bone mass in breast-feeding women, Clin Endocrinol 41:739, 1994.

93. **Kjos SL, Peters RK, Xiang A, Thomas D, Schaefer U, Buchanan TA,** Contraception and the risk of type 2 diabetes in Latino women with prior gestational diabetes, JAMA 280:533, 1998.

94. **Halderman LD, Nelson AL,** Impact of early postpartum administration of progestin-only hormonal contraceptives compared with nonhormonal contraceptives on short-term breast-feeding patterns, Am J Obstet Gynecol 186:1250, 2002.

95. **Jimenez J, Ochoa M, Soler MP, Portales P,** Long-term follow-up of children breast-fed by mothers receiving depot-medroxyprogesterone acetate, Contraception 30:523, 1984.

96. **Díaz S, Zepeda A, Maturana X, Reyes MV, Miranda P, Casado ME, Peralta O, Croxatto HB,** Fertility regulation in nursing women. IX. Contraceptive performance, duration of lactation, infant growth, and bleeding patterns during use of progesterone vaginal rings, progestin-only pills, Norplant® implants, and copper T 380-A intrauterine devices, Contraception 56:223, 1997.

97. **Zacharias S, Aguilena J, Assanzo JR, Zanatu J,** Effects of hormonal and non-hormonal contracepters on lactation and incidence of pregnancy, Contraception 33:203, 1986.

98. **Shaaban MM, Salem HT, Abdullah KA,** Influence of levonorgestrel contraceptive implants, Norplant, initiated early postpartum, upon lactation and infant growth, Contraception 32:623, 1985.

99. **Shaaban MM,** Contraception with progestogens and progesterone during lactation, J Steroid Biochem Mol Biol 40:705, 1991.

100. **Affandi B, Karmadibrata S, Prihartono J, Lubis F, Samil RS,** Effect of Norplant on mother and infants in the postpartum period, Adv Contracept 2:371, 1986.

101. **Diaz S, Herreros C, Juez G, Casado ME, Salvatierra AM, Miranda P, Peralta O, Croxatto HB,** Fertility regulation in nursing women: influence of Norplant levonorgestrel implants upon lactation and infant growth, Contraception 32:53, 1985.

102. **Gross BA,** Natural family planning indicators of ovulation, Clin Reprod Fertil 5:91, 1987.

103. **Mishell Jr DR, Roy S,** Copper intrauterine contraceptive device event rates following insertion 4 to 8 weeks post partum, Am J Obstet Gynecol 143:29, 1982.

104. **Zhuang L, Wang H, Yang P,** Observations of the clinical efficacies and side effects of six different timings of IUD insertions, Clin J Obstet Gynecol 22:350, 1987.

105. **Chi I-c, Farr G,** Postpartum IUD contraception—A review of an international experience, Adv Contracept 5:127, 1989.

106. **Zhou S, Chi I-c,** Immediate postpartum IUD insertions in a Chinese hospital—A two-year follow-up, Int J Gynaecol Obstet 35:157, 1991.

107. **Thiery M, Laufe L, Parewijck W, van der Pas H, van Kets H, Derom R, Defoort P,** Immediate postplacental IUD insertion: a randomized trial of sutured (Lippes Loop and TCu220c) and non-sutured (TCu220c) models, Contraception 28:299, 1983.

108. **Van Kets M, Kleinhout J, Osler M, Parewijck W, Zighelboim I, Tatum JH,** Clinical experience with the Gyne-T380 postpartum intrauterine device, Fertil Steril 55:1144, 1991.

109. **Chi I-c, Wilkens LR, Rogos S,** Expulsions in immediate postpartum insertion of Lippes Loop D and copper IUDs and their counterpart Delta devices — an epidemiologic analysis, Contraception 32:119, 1985.

110. **Van Kets H, Parewijck W, Van der Pas H, Batar I, Creatsas G, Koumantakis K, Thiery M,** Immediate postplacental insertion and fixation of the CuFix postpartum implant system, Contraception 48, 1993.

111. **Chi I-c, Potts M, Wilkens L, Champion C,** Performance of the TCu-380A device in breastfeeding and non-breastfeeding women, Contraception 39:603, 1989.

112. **Nielsen NC, Nygren K-G, Allonen H,** Three years of experience after post-abortal insertion of Nova-T and Copper-T-200, Acta Obstet Gynecol Scand 63:261, 1984.

113. **Querido L, Ketting E, Haspels AA,** IUD insertion following induced abortion, Contraception 31:603, 1985.

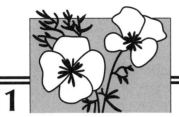

11

Clinical Guidelines for Contraception at Different Ages: Early and Late

Modern society is coping with two contraceptive problems, each at the opposite end of the reproductive lifespan. In the early years, we are struggling with the high rate of unwanted teenage pregnancies. In the later years, we face a growing demand for reversible contraception as the post–World War II baby boom generation ages. It is entirely appropriate, therefore, that we give special attention to these age groups: adolescence and the transition years (ages 35 to menopause).

Contraception for Adolescents

Providing contraception or information about contraception for young people under age 20 is an important obligation for clinicians. More young women (nearly 1 million teenagers per year) become pregnant in the United States than do their contemporaries in other developed parts of the world, and young American women have a higher induced abortion rate than young European women.[1] More than 50% of the 1.3 million induced abortions per year in the United States are obtained by women younger than age 25, about 33% in teenagers with the rate peaking at ages 18–19.[2-4] The differences among developed countries (and the unenviable highest teenage pregnancy rates in the United States) are not the consequence of differences in sexual activity but reflect effective sex education programs combined with easy access to contraception.

There was a marked increase in teenage sexual activity in the United States during the time period 1960–1990, and contrary to common opinion, much of that increase occurred among white and nonpoor adolescents.[5] Today, approximately 60% of young women and 70% of young men have had sexual intercourse by age 18.[1, 6] Within a relatively short period of time after becoming sexually active, 58% of adolescent females have had sex with 2 or more partners (and thus, increase their risk of sexually transmitted diseases). The good news is that the use of oral contraceptives and condoms increased in the 1990s; however, at least half of sexually active teenagers do not use condoms, placing them at increased risk for sexually transmitted infections (STIs). In 1995, only 49% of female and 61% of male high school students reported using a condom with their last coital experience.[7] Furthermore, teenagers are nearly twice as likely to experience contraceptive failure than women age 30 years or older.

The number of adolescent pregnancies in the United States has declined steadily for more than a decade since peak levels were reached in 1990.[1, 4, 9] The teenage pregnancy rate has reached the lowest rate since estimates began in 1976, a 21% decline from 1990 to 1997 for teenagers 15–17 years and a 13% decline for older teenagers.[10] Overall, there has been a 17% decline in teenage birth rates and a 12.8% decline in teenage induced abortions from 1990 through 1999. Nevertheless, approximately 78% of teenage pregnancies are unintended.[1, 11] Adolescents who have a much older partner (about 7% of women younger than age 18 have a partner 6 or more years older) represent a very high risk group, with a low rate of contraceptive use and high rates of pregnancy.[12] Unfortunately, adolescent mothers have a high rate of repeat pregnancy and are more likely to use ineffective methods and to use effective methods inconsistently.

Characteristics of Teen Pregnancy in the United States[4, 13–17]

1. 4,500 teen pregnancies occur every day.
2. One of every 10 teens aged 15–19 get pregnant.
3. Half of teen pregnancies occur in the first 6 months after first intercourse.
4. 20% of teen pregnancies occur in the first month after first intercourse.
5. Half who give birth do not graduate from high school.
6. Teen pregnancies are associated with increased risks of obstetrical and neonatal complications and mortality.
7. The children of teen mothers are more likely to have behavioral and social problems when they are adolescents.

Adolescence is a time for "trying your wings," a time for experimenting and testing. Most of the 25 million teenagers in the United States achieve good health, but unfortunately for some, the consequences of this time of trying things are lasting problems for health and life. Unwanted pregnancy (premature parenthood) and the STIs are the risks of sexual experimentation. Teenage girls carry the burdens of unprotected sexual activity:

unwanted pregnancy, undetected STIs, and pelvic inflammatory disease. Their male partners, who are often not teenagers themselves, must be made aware of these consequences through public education that reaches all young people, not just those in school, and through social programs that promote male responsibility for child support and disease prevention.

Teenagers are noted for their sense of invincibility and their risk-taking behavior, both of which denote the inability of immature people to connect present action with future consequences. It is not surprising that adolescents often have sex and do not use contraception. Contraception takes planning and premeditation about having sex, but television and movies present teenagers with unrealistic examples of romantic liaisons that disconnect sex from pregnancy, STIs, and contraception. More than half of female teenagers have risked pregnancy, infertility, and AIDS by having unprotected intercourse at least once. The onset of fertility following menarche cannot be predicted for individuals; any sexually active teenager is at risk for pregnancy and STIs. Approximately 48% of the new STI cases in the United States occur in the 15–24 age group, a group that accounts for only 25% of the sexually active population.[18] It is worth emphasizing that there is no evidence that provision of contraception leads to adolescents having sex earlier or more frequently. Studies have repeatedly documented a consistent finding: most adolescents seeking contraception usually do so many months to a year or more after initiating sexual activity.[1] Nevertheless, once teenagers begin using contraception, many are consistent users; more than two-thirds of U.S. young women, aged 15–19, report long-term uninterrupted contraceptive use.[19]

Among the obstacles to earlier use of contraception are exaggerated perceptions about the risks of contraceptive methods, as well as a deep dread of the misunderstood "pelvic exam."[20] We clinicians can do much to remove these obstacles by talking with teenagers and adjusting our practices to suit their special needs.

Our objective is to get adolescents to assess realistically their sexual futures, not just to let sex "happen." The fact that European adolescents use contraception at a rate higher than in the United States argues that we can do better. Unfortunately, secrecy usually surrounds a young person's decision to use contraception. Adolescent involvement in sex often occurs without an opportunity for discussion with family, other adults, peers, or even the partner. Access to contraception (physical and psychological) and motivation to use it are the keys to success in achieving our goals. Good communication with adolescents requires specific approaches and skills. Greater openness about sexual discussion in the family, church, or school can all lead to a better consideration of the health and social risks of early sexual activity by a teenager. Contraceptive education must be combined with an emphasis on overall life issues and interventions, including the decision to become sexually active; no single message or approach, by itself, is broadly effective for all adolescents.

School-Based Programs. Many school-based (or school-linked) educational programs and clinics have been developed to prevent adolescent pregnancies. These vary in focus and content, including abstinence and contraception. Unfortunately, the overall impact of these programs is questionable. Reviews of school-based programs have concluded that a focus on abstinence is ineffective.[21-23] Thirty-five percent of all school districts in the United States allow only the teaching of abstinence, and 51% teach abstinence as the preferred method of contraception (these percentages are higher than those of the past decade).[1] Although most school districts provide some contraceptive education (a development of the 1990s), approximately 33% of public school districts do not have a policy to teach sex education.[1] Current information on state policies is available at www.guttmacher.org/pubs/spib_SSEP.pdf.

Fortunately 86% of U.S. students live in districts that have a sex education policy, and even in those districts without a policy, individual schools and teachers can provide sex education. An emphasis on education is very important because although school clinics by themselves do not lower pregnancy rates, an associated community educational effort is effective.[21, 24, 25] A comprehensive community-wide program that includes school interventions, public education, and emphasis of both abstinence and contraception results in a reduction of the teenage pregnancy rate.[26-28] To again counter a common criticism, school-based programs and clinics do not affect the initiation or frequency of sexual activity.[1, 21, 25, 29]

Communication with Adolescents

Teenagers want to talk about STIs and contraception, but clinicians usually don't bring these subjects up for discussion.[30] Clinicians can be sure that by age 15 most adolescents are interested in discussing STIs and contraception. No matter what brings an adolescent into the office, contraception and continuation (compliance) are issues that should be addressed. Unfortunately, the younger a teenager is the more likely it is that she believes an unwanted pregnancy or STI cannot happen to her.[31]

Our goals are to promote abstinence among teenagers who are not yet ready to cope with sex and its consequences and to promote behavior that prevents pregnancy and STIs in sexually active adolescents. Building trust is a requirement for a successful interaction between clinician and adolescent. A teenager must be assured that a discussion about sexuality and contraception is strictly confidential. This must be stated in plain words. One reason European countries are able to provide better contraceptive services to adolescents is the guarantee by law of complete confidentiality (other reasons are dissemination of information via public media and distribution of contraceptives through free or low-cost services).[32] Research confirms that requiring parental notification or consent deters young people from using contraception and protecting themselves from STIs.[33] That is not to say that secrecy is encouraged; rather, communication with parents should be promoted because it yields better use of contraception. However, the clinician must receive permission from the adolescent for parental involvement.

Successful use of contraception (continuation) requires teenager involvement, not just passive listening. The clinician should frequently interrupt talking by asking questions and seeking opinions. Don't wait until the physical examination to initiate conversation. It is a good practice to see all patients first in an office setting prior to examination, and this is especially true with adolescents. Give some thought to body language and position. It is helpful to sit next to a patient; avoid the formality (and obstacle) of a desk between clinician and patient. A teenager should be asked about success in school, family life, and behaviors indicative of risk taking.

Don't miss the chance to point out the wisdom of abstinence to a young person who is not yet sexually active, but leave the door open for protection against pregnancy and STIs. Be careful to be nonjudgmental. Sometimes it is hard to keep disapproval over a teenager's activity from showing. A teenager who senses disapproval won't listen to instructions or advice.

A good way to introduce the subject of contraception is to ask an adolescent when he or she would like to have children. Then follow with: what plans do you have to avoid getting pregnant until then? Elicit objections, concerns, fears, and address each of them. The clinician must anticipate those concerns and fears that lead to poor continuation. They must be identified and addressed in advance.

Contraceptive use is a private matter, and therefore, instruction comes from the clinician, not from peers. Be very concrete; demonstrate the use of pill packages, the skin patch, the vaginal ring, foam aerosols, and condom application. This seems like oversimplification, but clinicians working with adolescents have found that this approach is both necessary and appreciated by their young patients. If possible, family involvement that results in improved emotional support of a teenager is worthwhile because it is associated with better contraceptive behavior.[34]

Adolescents must be convinced that having sex means you are at risk of becoming pregnant. Adolescents are immersed in conflicting messages about sexuality in our society. A clinician may be the only resource for

333

information and guidance, but clinicians must give the right signals to adolescents and must initiate communication. No matter what the chief complaint, any interaction with an adolescent is an opportunity to discuss sexuality and contraception.

Useful Web Sites for Adolescents and Clinicians

Center for Young Women's Health, Children's Hospital, Boston: http://youngwomenshealth.org

Planned Parenthood: http://Teenwire.com/index.asp

Columbia University Health Education Program: http://goaskalice.columbia.edu/

Princeton University Emergency Contraception Site: http://ec.princeton.edu

Choice of Method

Oral, Vaginal, and Transdermal Estrogen-Progestin Contraception

The combined oral contraceptive is the most popular and most requested method of contraception by teenagers.[35] This is appropriate because oral contraceptives are almost never medically contraindicated in healthy adolescents. The risk of death from oral contraceptive use by adolescents is virtually nil. This is a good match; adolescents are at highest risk for unwanted pregnancies and are at lowest risk for complications. Thus, the high efficacy of combined oral contraception is an excellent choice for teenagers.

Adolescents certainly don't know the history of oral contraception. It is important to point out the change in dosage and the new safety. But teenagers do have concerns regarding oral contraception, citing most often a fear of cancer, concern with impact on future fertility, and problems with weight gain and acne.[36]

The cancer issue is a difficult one to discuss with teenagers. We believe it is appropriate to state that there is no definitive evidence demonstrating a link between breast cancer and oral contraception.[37] Cervical cancer, especially adenocarcinoma, continues to be a concern (Chapter 2), although confounding factors have been difficult to control. Teens must be made aware that Pap smear surveillance detects premalignant conditions.

By the time of menarche, growth and reproductive development are essentially complete. There is no evidence that early use of oral contraception has any inhibiting impact on growth or any adverse effects on the reproductive tract. With great confidence, a clinician can tell adolescents that there is no impact on future fertility with the use of oral contraception.[38] Indeed, one can emphasize that oral contraception preserves future fertility by its protection against PID and ectopic pregnancies. Whereas oral contraception protects against PID, it does not protect against contracting STIs, hence the recommendation to combine oral contraception use with barrier methods. *Because younger women change partners more frequently than older women, a dual approach is recommended, combining the contraceptive efficacy offered by oral contraceptives with the use of a barrier method, especially for teenagers, so that they can prevent PID and viral STIs, including HIV.*

It is worth emphasizing repeatedly to adolescents that studies with low-dose oral contraception,[39–46] even studies in adolescents,[39] do not indicate a problem of weight gain and that acne is usually improved. Weight gain as it is perceived by the teenager deserves attention at every visit.[47] In placebo-controlled randomized trials of low-dose oral contraceptives and acne, the incidence of weight gain was identical in both the treated and the placebo groups.[44, 46] The beneficial impact of oral contraceptives on acne can be especially motivating for adolescents.

Adolescents are very receptive to hearing about the beneficial impact of oral contraception on menstrual problems: cramps, bleeding, and iron-deficiency anemia. Relief of dysmenorrhea in teenagers has been documented to be associated with better and more consistent use of oral contraceptives.[48] Although irregular bleeding on oral contraceptives can distress teenagers, it does not by itself cause improper use if teenagers are well prepared and instructed.

Oral Contraceptive Benefits to Emphasize with Teenagers

> **Safety with low dosage.**
> **Lack of weight gain.**
> **Acne improvement and prevention.**
> **Reduction in menstrual flow and dysmenorrhea.**
> **Preservation of fertility.**
> **Reduced risk of pelvic inflammatory disease.**

Although decreasing in prevalence, teenage smoking continues to be a big problem. In the year 2003, approximately 22% of people in the United States who had not obtained a high school diploma were smokers, but only 11% of those with higher education were smokers. Currently, approximately 25% of men and 21% of women are smokers.[49] Smoking initiation has decreased markedly in men but unfortunately has changed less in women. In addition, female smokers begin smoking at a younger age. Smoking appears to have a greater adverse effect on women compared to men.[50, 51] Women who smoke only 1 to 4 cigarettes per day have a 2.5-fold increased risk of fatal coronary heart disease.[52]

The relative risk of cardiovascular events is increased for women of all ages who smoke and use oral contraceptives. However, because the actual incidence of cardiovascular events is so low at a young age, the real risk is very, very low for young women. Smoking produces a shift to hypercoagulability.[53] A 20-μg estrogen formulation has been reported to have no effect on clotting parameters, even in smokers.[53, 54] One study comparing a 20-μg product with a 30-μg product found similar mild pro-coagulant and fibrinolytic activity, although there was a trend toward increased fibrinolytic activity with the lower dose.[55] It is worth considering a 20-μg formulation for all smoking women, regardless of age. This recommendation also applies to all women using nicotine-containing products as an aid to stop smoking. Exsmokers (for at least 1 year) should be regarded as nonsmokers. However, keep in mind that the theoretical greater safety of 20-μg estrogen has not been confirmed by epidemiologic data.

Adolescents with diabetes mellitus uncomplicated with vascular changes can use oral contraception. Other conditions with which oral contraception is acceptable include cystic fibrosis and sickle cell disease but not systemic lupus erythematosus.

Unfortunately, the failure rate of oral contraceptives among adolescents is higher compared with all typical users.[8] This is the reason that adolescents require special attention at every opportunity. Education and support are necessary to maximize efficacy and continuation. Serial monogamy is usual among younger women, and this often is associated with episodic use of contraception. With oral contraception, it is helpful to instruct the adolescent that the minor side effects diminish in frequency with use, and, therefore, there is an advantage to staying on the oral contraceptive. It is also good advice to tell teenagers to continue taking oral contraceptives for at least 2 months after "breaking up" with a boyfriend, because by then a new relationship is likely to have begun.

One reason the average teenager waits months to a year after initiating sexual activity before seeking contraception is fear about the pelvic exam. Furthermore, anxiety over the pelvic exam is a barrier to comprehending contraceptive instructions. Thus, letting teenagers know that the pelvic exam can be delayed until the 3rd or 6th month or even later encourages them to seek contraceptive advice. This approach requires a completely normal history (an absence of risk factors for STIs) and a limited prescription. We advocate the elimination of the pelvic examination as a requirement for teenagers to obtain contraceptives. Demonstration projects have indicated that this approach is safe and effective.[56, 57]

We believe that the risks, benefits, and considerations associated with oral contraception are similar for the vaginal and transdermal estrogen-progestin contraceptive methods. However, the contraceptive patch (Ortho-Evra) and the vaginal ring (NuvaRing) have an important advantage. Avoiding the necessity of daily pill-taking yields better compliance rates (Chapter 4).[58–61] Adolescents have used the transdermal contraceptive patch with good compliance, but difficulties with patch detachments underscore the need for good instruction (see Chapter 4).[62]

Barrier Methods

Teenagers have the highest rates of hospitalization for PID. Because of the following statistics cited about adolescent women, sexually active young women should be examined every 6 months, with Pap smear and STI screening:[63–65]

1. 5–25% of sexually active adolescent females are infected with *Chlamydia trachomatis*.
2. 0.4–12% are infected with *Neisseria gonorrhoeae*.
3. 15–38% have human papillomavirus infection.
4. 16% of adolescents have abnormal Pap smears.

For these reasons, combined with the AIDS scare, there has been an increase in the use of condoms among adolescents. After steroid contraception, in our view, the condom is the next best choice for adolescents. And this obviously is the only choice for male adolescents. *Indeed, we strongly advocate combining condoms with oral contraception to provide maximum protection against pregnancy and STIs.* Approximately 20% of American adolescent women do combine condom use with another method.[66]

The advantage of condoms is that neither a prescription nor a consultation with a clinician is required. The problem, then, is achieving sufficient education and motivation without the intervention of clinicians. We believe this is a social problem, not a medical problem, and we are strongly supportive of public education efforts in schools and the media to accomplish this important public and individual health objective.

Many teenagers rely only on condoms (a close second in use to oral contraceptives), and of course their contribution to preventing STIs is important.[67] Indeed, among the youngest teenagers, condoms are the most commonly used method of contraception.[67] Condom failures, unfortunately, are about 10 times as high among teenagers as among older, married couples. Don't assume that teenagers know how to use a condom;

use a model and demonstrate. Furthermore, young women need to know that they are in charge; they can insist on condom use.

The female condom provides a young woman with a female-controlled method, but its expense and complexity are obstacles for teenagers. Its use by teenagers has not been studied, and its effects on STIs are not documented.

Diaphragms or cervical caps are not good choices for adolescents. Adolescents are not comfortable with body interventions, and the insertion before coitus is too willful an act for most teens. Furthermore, these methods require privacy for insertion. Adolescents are discouraged by complicated methods. The diaphragm and cervical cap should be reserved for very motivated and mature young people.

Intrauterine Contraception

Traditionally, IUDs have not been recommended for nulligravid women and those who have a high risk of STIs. This eliminates it from consideration for most teenagers. However, we wish to emphasize that age and parity are not the critical factors; the risk for STIs is the most important consideration. The IUD can and should be considered for the older teenager who is in a stable monogamous relationship and has had a child, and even in the appropriate nulligravid young woman, although increased menstrual pain and bleeding can be a problem. It is also a good choice in a patient with a chronic illness, such as diabetes mellitus or systemic lupus erythematosus, or in mentally retarded individuals. The levonorgestrel-releasing IUD (Mirena) performs as well as oral contraceptives when used by young nulliparous women.[68]

Vaginal Nonsteroid Contraceptives

The creams, foams, suppositories, and jellies are not ideal for adolescents. They require proper timing before coitus, careful placement, and consistent use to achieve good efficacy, approaching that of hormonal methods or condoms. Their effects on STIs, including HIV, are not certain.

Long-Acting Methods for Adolescents

Although long-acting methods are an excellent answer for continuation problems, the many minor side effects present difficult problems for teenagers. Acne, weight change, and irregular bleeding are more common among implant and injectable users compared with oral contraception (however, the differences are not great). In addition the cost and the surgical procedure with implants are major difficulties for adolescents.[69] Nevertheless, both implants and injectables have proved to be relatively popular and successful with teenagers, especially among those who have experienced previous pregnancies or have used oral contraception in the past.[70–72] The long-acting feature and the ease of continuation are attractive to teenagers.[73] Effective counseling and education are critical for the successful use of these long-acting methods. The problems experienced with contraceptive implants are identical in adolescent and adult women.[74] In properly prepared adolescent mothers, the use of Norplant has been reported to have a higher continuation rate and a lower failure rate compared with oral contraceptives, and the rate of condom use continued unchanged (in other words, condom use for protection against STIs was not diminished in Norplant users).[75, 76] However, in a group of urban adolescents, followed for 2 years, Norplant users were less likely to use condoms compared with those who used oral contraceptives or condoms alone, but this was partly because teenagers in this cohort who chose Norplant were in longer relationships and less exposed to STIs.[77] Continuation and repeat pregnancy rates are similar comparing oral contraceptive and depot-medroxyprogesterone acetate use by postpartum adolescents.[78]

There are special candidates to consider for long-acting contraception: teens who have failed oral contraception and teens who are mentally retarded or who have chronic illnesses.

The contraceptive use of depot-medroxyprogesterone acetate is associated with the loss of bone. (This issue is discussed fully in Chapter 6.) Bone density increases rapidly and significantly during adolescence. Almost all of the bone mass in the hip and the vertebral bodies is accumulated in young women by age 18, and the years immediately following menarche are especially important.[79, 80] For this reason any drug that prevents this increase in bone density may increase the risk of osteoporosis later in life. Studies in adolescents have documented bone loss compared to normal controls and young women using oral contraceptives.[81, 82] Do adolescents who use depot-medroxyprogesterone acetate regain bone density after discontinuing this method of contraception, or are adolescents at greater risk for osteoporosis compared with women who use depot-medroxyprogesterone acetate later in life?

The degree of bone loss is not as severe as that observed in the early postmenopausal years. Furthermore, this amount of bone loss is not so great that it cannot be regained. Bone density measurements in women who stopped using depot-medroxyprogesterone acetate indicated that the loss was regained in the lumbar spine but not in the femoral neck within 2 years even after long-term use, but in another cohort of past users, both spinal density and hip density were restored 30 months after discontinuation. [83, 84] Most importantly, cross-sectional studies of postmenopausal women in New Zealand and a large multicenter, worldwide population could not detect a difference in bone density comparing former users of depot-medroxyprogesterone acetate to never users, indicating that any loss of bone during use is regained.[85, 86]

A definitive response to this clinical concern is not possible because not all studies are in agreement. Indeed, there are an equal number of studies finding no bone loss with the use of depot-medroxyprogesterone acetate (see Chapter 6). Furthermore, the degree of bone loss is similar to that associated with lactation, also secondary to relatively low estrogen levels. This bone loss rapidly turns to baseline levels in the 6 months after weaning.[87]

The mixed results, the degree of bone loss, some evidence that the bone loss is regained, and the similarity to the benign bone loss associated with lactation all argue that the use of depot-medroxyprogesterone acetate should not be limited by this concern and that supplemental estrogen treatment is not indicated (and would influence and complicate compliance). This concern requires ongoing surveillance of past users. However, at the present time, in our view, this should not be a reason to avoid this method of contraception. *It is unlikely that bone loss occurs sufficiently to raise the risk of osteoporosis later in life.*

Emergency Postcoital Contraception

Because adolescents often have unplanned sexual intercourse, access to emergency postcoital contraception is important. The failure rate is approximately 2% using oral contraceptives and 1% with levonorgestrel. Treatment should be initiated as soon after exposure as possible, but no later than 72 hours as indicated in Chapter 3. The following treatment regimens have been documented (Chapter 3) to be effective:

Ovral: 2 tablets followed by 2 tablets 12 hours later.

Alesse: 5 tablets followed by 5 tablets 12 hours later.

Lo Ovral, Nordette, Levlen, Triphasil, Tri-Levlen: 4 tablets followed by 4 tablets 12 hours later.

Levonorgestrel in a dose of 0.75 mg given twice, 12 hours apart, is more successful and better tolerated than the combination oral contraceptive method.[88, 89] In many countries, special packages of 0.75 mg levonorgestrel (Plan B, Norlevo, Vikela) are available for emergency contraception. Greater efficacy and fewer side effects make low-dose levonorgestrel the treatment of choice.

In the United States, a kit (Preven) is available containing 4 tablets, each containing 50 μg ethinyl estradiol and 0.250 mg levonorgestrel, to be used in the usual fashion, 2 tablets followed by 2 tablets 12 hours later. A package (Plan B) containing only levonorgestrel (two 0.75 mg tablets) is also available, one tablet taken within 72 hours of intercourse and the second 12 hours later. *The two tablets can be combined into a single, one-time dose of 1.5 mg levonorgestrel with no loss of efficacy or increase in side effects.*[90, 91] *This is the strongly recommended choice for drug and schedule of treatment.*

Clinicians should consider providing emergency contraceptive kits to adolescents (a kit can be a simple envelope containing instructions and the appropriate number of oral contraceptives or preferably levonorgestrel tablets) to be taken when needed. Experience with the use of emergency contraception by adolescents indicates that teenagers can use the medication correctly with a side effect profile similar to that in older women, and they have a favorable attitude toward its use.[92] It would be a major contribution to our efforts to avoid unwanted teenage pregnancies to have emergency contraception available for use when needed. A controlled trial among young women in San Francisco documented that those who received emergency contraception in advance were 3 times as likely to use it compared with those who received only counseling about its use.[93] In studies of self-administration, adult women in Scotland and younger women in San Francisco, Pittsburgh, and Mexico increased the use of emergency contraception without adverse effects such as increasing unprotected sex.[93-97]

It has been argued that the use of emergency contraception would reduce the rates of induced abortions; indeed, in the United States, it is estimated that emergency contraception could annually prevent 1.7 million unintended pregnancies and the number of induced abortions would decrease by about 40%.[98] However, studies do not agree. In two studies at abortion units, it was concluded that 50–60% of the patients would have been suitable for emergency contraception and would have used it if readily available.[99, 100] On the other hand, the advance provision of emergency contraception had no effect on the abortion rates in a community in Scotland.[101]

Adolescent Contraceptive Continuation

Knowing that contraception is available is not enough to prevent adolescent pregnancy. Adolescents have higher failure rates with all methods. Adolescent continuation with oral contraception has been particularly well-studied.[36, 102] Factors associated with good continuation include: older age, suburban residence, health care in a private practice, good payment ability, prior use of contraception, mother's unawareness of teen's oral contraception use, married parents, older boyfriend, and satisfaction with pill use. Good continuation is also associated with educational goals and an absence of side effects. Inner city teens express more concern with side effects and safety, while suburban patients are more worried about weight gain and the effect of smoking. Surprisingly, in a study of 214 patients, only 11 reported reading the written instruction sheets that were provided.[102]

These studies indicate the importance of verbal instructions and the need to allow for questions. Long-term continuation is associated with an adolescent's career goals; it is worth bringing this up in conversation. Because adolescents tend to switch methods, all methods should be discussed with adolescents at each visit. Studies demonstrate that the extra time and effort required to meet the needs of adolescents result in improved contraceptive use and lower pregnancy rates.[47, 103]

1. Establish and maintain confidentiality.
2. Do not lecture; make the patient visit a conversation; build trust.
3. Identify and address fears and concerns in advance.
4. Emphasize benefits.
5. Emphasize that minor side effects with steroid contraception diminish with use.
6. Give instructions for managing side effects.
7. Demonstrate package and pill taking (use the 28-day package), condom application, skin patches, and the vaginal ring.
8. Incorporate pill-taking into patient's daily routine.
9. Don't let patients run out of contraceptives.
10. Consider the transdermal and vaginal methods of estrogen-progestin contraception to achieve better compliance.
11. Request that you be called before contraception is discontinued.
12. Identify and educate office personnel to interact with adolescents.
13. Frequent visits (every 3 months the first year), short waiting time, convenient hours.

Contraception for Older Women

Women of the post–World War II generation faced a unique evolutionary change. They were the first to be able to exercise control over their fertility, and then as they aged and deferred pregnancy, they had to deal with the problem of unintended infertility. After World War II, the U.S. total fertility rate reached a modern high of 3.7 births per woman. The last women born in this period will not reach their 45th birthday until around 2010. For approximately a 20-year period, therefore, there will be an unprecedented number of women in the later child-bearing years. The aging of the post–World War II population boom is resulting in a greater number of women who are delaying marriage and childbirth. This demographic change has 3 specific impacts on couples.

1. A need for effective contraception.
2. The problem of achieving pregnancy later in life.
3. The problem of being pregnant later in life.

This combination of increasing numbers, deferment of marriage, and postponement of pregnancy in marriage is responsible for the fact that we will be seeing many older women who will need reversible contraception. This is underscored by the fact that from ages 20–44, American women have the highest proportion of pregnancies aborted compared with women in other countries, indicating an unappreciated, but real, problem of unintended pregnancy existing beyond the teenage years, especially after age 35.[104] More than half of all pregnancies in the United States are estimated to be unplanned, and more than half of these are aborted.[11] The best way to minimize the number of induced abortions is effective contraception.

From 1970 to 1986, the number of births in women over 30 quadrupled; however, since 1990, the fertility rate among women over 30 has remained relatively stable. For those couples deferring pregnancy until later in life, the use of sterilization under age 35 declines, and the need for reversible contraception increases. Between 1988 and 1995, oral contraceptive use decreased in women younger than 25 and increased in women aged 30–44.[35]

Steroid Contraception for the Transition Years

The years from age 35 to menopause can be referred to as the transition years. Preventive health care for women is especially important during the transition years. The issues of preventive health care are familiar ones. They include contraception, cessation of smoking, prevention of heart disease and osteoporosis, maintenance of mental well-being (including sexuality), and cancer screening. Management of the transition years should be significantly oriented to preventive health care, and the use of low-dose oral contraception can now legitimately be viewed as a component of preventive health care. A discussion of the noncontraceptive health benefits of low-dose oral contraception is especially important with patients in their transition years. This group of women appreciates and understands decisions made with the risk:benefit ratio in mind.

During this period of time, there are several medical needs that must be addressed: the need for contraception, the management of persistent anovulation, and finally, menopausal and postmenopausal hormone therapy.

At approximately 40 years of age, the frequency of ovulation decreases. This initiates a period of waning ovarian function called the climacteric, which lasts several years, carrying a woman through decreased fertility and menopause to the postmenopausal years. Prior to menopause, the remaining follicles perform less well. As cycles become irregular, vaginal bleeding occurs at the end of an inadequate luteal phase or after a peak of estradiol without subsequent ovulation and corpus luteum formation. Eventually, many women live through a period of anovulation. Occasionally, corpus luteum formation and function occur, and therefore the older woman is not totally safe from the threat of an unplanned and unexpected pregnancy.

Fortunately, clinicians and patients have recognized that low-dose oral contraception is very safe for healthy, nonsmoking older women. Besides fulfilling a need for contraception, we believe that this population of women has many benefits to be derived from oral contraception that tilt the risk:benefit ratio to the positive side. The benefits of oral contraceptives reviewed in Chapter 2 are especially pertinent for older women. An approach that emphasizes these benefits encourages greater use of oral contraceptives by older women.

Steroid Contraceptive Benefits to Emphasize with Older Women

Less endometrial cancer.
Less ovarian cancer.
More regular menses.
Increase in bone density.
Probably less endometriosis.
Possibly fewer fibroids.
Possibly less benign breast disease.
Possibly less rheumatoid arthritis.
Possibly protection against atherosclerosis.
Possibly fewer ovarian cysts.

An Austrian study concluded that osteoporosis occurs later and is less frequent in women who have used long-term oral contraception,[105] and most studies indicate that prior use of oral contraception is associated with higher levels of bone density and that the degree of protection is related to duration of exposure.[106-112] However, other studies reflecting modern use of low-dose products indicate little impact of oral contraceptive use on bone.[113-115] These measurements of bone density are not as important as the clinical outcome: fractures. The available evidence fails to provide a clear-cut picture. Retrospective studies indicated a reduction in fractures in postmenopausal women who had previously used oral contraceptives.[116-119] In the Royal College of General Practitioners Study, the overall risk of fractures long-term in users of oral contraceptives was actually slightly increased.[120] Similar results have been observed in the Oxford Family Planning Association Study.[121] It is likely that the increased risk reflects lifestyle effects among oral contraceptive users, but there was no evidence of a protective effect against fractures. In contrast, a case-control study from Sweden found a reduction in the risk of postmenopausal hip fractures when oral contraceptives (mostly older high dose products) were used after age 40 by women who were not overweight, with an increasing benefit with increasing duration of use.[122] Previous oral contraceptive users are just now becoming elderly and reaching the age of greatest fracture prevalence. Future studies of postmenopausal women should eventually reveal the accurate relationship between oral contraceptive use and osteoporotic fractures.

Despite the widespread teaching and publicity that smoking is a contraindication to oral contraceptive use over the age of 35, more older women who use oral contraceptives smoke and smoke heavily, compared with young women.[123] This strongly implies that older smokers are less than honest with clinicians when requesting oral contraception. *A former smoker must have stopped smoking for at least 12 consecutive months to be regarded as a nonsmoker. Women who have nicotine in their bloodstream obtained from patches or gum should be regarded as smokers.* Smokers over age 35 should continue to be advised that combined oral contraceptives are not a good choice, regardless of the number of cigarettes smoked. In view of the unreported high rate of smoking in older women who use oral contraceptives, clinicians should consider using 20-μg estrogen products for women over age 35.

A product containing 20 μg ethinyl estradiol and 150 μg desogestrel has been demonstrated in multicenter studies of women over age 30 to have the same efficacy and side effects as pills containing 30 and 35 μg of estrogen.[124-126] In a randomized study of women over age 30, this formulation was associated with the virtual elimination of any effects on coagulation factors.[127] Indeed, formulations with 20 μg ethinyl estradiol have no significant impact on the measurements of clotting factors, even in smokers.[53, 54, 127, 128]

Although it is true that the implied safety of the lowest estrogen dose remains to be documented by epidemiologic studies, it seems clinically prudent to maximize the safety margin in this older age group of women. Although there may be some increase in breakthrough bleeding, we believe that older women who understand the increased safety implicit in the lowest estrogen dose are more willing to endure breakthrough bleeding and maintain continuation. With avoidance of risk factors and use of lowest dose pills, health risks are negligible for healthy nonsmoking women. For healthy nonsmoking women, no specific laboratory screening is necessary beyond that which is usually incorporated in a program of preventive health care.

We should also mention the progestin-only minipill. Because of reduced fecundity, the minipill achieves near total efficacy in women over age 40. Therefore, the progestin-only minipill is a good choice for older woman, and especially for those women in whom estrogen is contraindicated. Older women are more accepting of irregular menstrual bleeding when they understand its mechanism and, thus, are more accepting of the progestin-only minipill.

Anovulation and Bleeding. Throughout the transitional period of life there is a significant incidence of dysfunctional uterine bleeding due to anovulation. While the clinician is usually alerted to this problem because of irregular bleeding, clinician and patient often fail to diagnose anovulation when bleeding is not abnormal in schedule, flow, or duration. As a woman approaches menopause, a more aggressive attempt to document ovulation is warranted. A serum progesterone level measured approximately 1 week before menses is simple enough to obtain and worth the cost. The prompt diagnosis of anovulation (serum progesterone less than 3 ng/mL) leads to appropriate therapeutic management that has a significant impact on the risk of endometrial cancer.

In an anovulatory woman with proliferative or hyperplastic endometrium (unaccompanied by atypia), periodic oral progestin therapy is mandatory, such as 5–10 mg medroxyprogesterone acetate daily the first 2 weeks of each month. If hyperplasia is already present, follow-up aspiration office curettage after 3–4 months is required. The follow-up biopsy should be performed 1–2 months after the progestin treatment to allow any progestin-induced masking of atypia to recede. If progestin treatment is ineffective and histologic regression is not observed, more aggressive treatment is warranted. Monthly progestin treatment should be continued until withdrawal bleeding ceases or menopausal symptoms are experienced. These are reliable signs (in effect, a bioassay) indicating the onset of estrogen deprivation and the need for the addition of estrogen in a postmenopausal hormone program.

When monthly progestin therapy reverses hyperplastic changes (which it does in 95–98% of cases) and controls irregular bleeding, treatment should be continued until withdrawal bleeding ceases. This is a reliable sign (in effect, a bioassay) indicating the onset of estrogen deprivation and the need for the addition of estrogen. If vasomotor disturbances begin before the cessation of menstrual bleeding, the combined estrogen-progestin program can be initiated as needed to control the flushes.

Two case-control studies, one using data from the WHO Collaborative Study and one using the data from the U.K. general practice research database, assessed the risk of idiopathic venous thrombosis in users of progestins alone for therapeutic purposes and concluded that therapeutic progestins alone may be associated with an increased risk of venous thromboembolism.[129, 130] These epidemiologic conclusions were based on extremely small numbers and had very wide confidence intervals. Patients who receive progestin-only for therapeutic reasons are probably older and are more likely to have family histories of cardiovascular disease. In addition, a problem of preferential prescribing is probably present in that clinicians are more likely to promote the use of progestin-only for women they perceive to be at greater risk of venous thromboembolism. Thus, it is likely that the case groups represented a higher risk group than the control groups in these reports. For these reasons, we do not believe progestins are associated with an increased risk of venous thromboembolism.

If contraception is desired, the clinician and patient should seriously consider the use of steroid contraception given orally, transdermally, or vaginally. The anovulatory woman cannot be guaranteed that spontaneous ovulation and pregnancy will not occur. The use of steroid contraception at the same time provides contraception and prophylaxis against irregular, heavy anovulatory bleeding and the risk of endometrial hyperplasia and neoplasia. In some patients, oral contraceptive treatment achieves better regulation of menses than monthly progestin administration.

Clinicians often prescribe a traditional postmenopausal hormone regimen to treat a woman with the kind of irregular cycles usually experienced in the perimenopausal years or to treat vasomotor symptoms. This addition of exogenous estrogen without a contraceptive dose of progestin when a woman is not amenorrheic or experiencing menopausal symptoms is inappropriate and even risky (exposing the endometrium to excessively high levels of estrogen). ***And most importantly, a postmenopausal hormonal regimen does not inhibit ovulation and provide contraception.***[131] The appropriate response is to regulate anovulatory cycles with monthly progestational treatment along with an appropriate contraceptive method or to utilize low-dose oral contraception. The oral contraceptive that contains 20 μg estrogen provides effective contraception, improves menstrual cycle regularity, diminishes bleeding, and relieves menopausal symptoms.[132] We would expect similar salutary clinical effects with the vaginal ring and the transdermal patch methods.

Long-Acting Methods for Older Women

The long-acting methods of hormonal contraception deserve consideration in those situations where combination estrogen-progestin is unacceptable because of health problems (where estrogen is contraindicated) or where oral contraception has already proved to be unsuccessful. These methods are especially advantageous for smokers and for women with a history of thromboembolic disease. Progestin-only contraception is a good choice for women with hypertriglyceridemia, for diabetic women (even if they are older and smoke), and for women with severe migraine headaches or hypertension. Oral and injectable progestin-only methods of contraception are not associated with increased risks of stroke, myocardial infarction, or venous thromboembolism.[130, 133, 134]

Older women, as they approach the menopause, may be more comfortable with the irregular bleeding or amenorrhea associated with the implants, injections, or progestin-only pills. However, the irregular bleeding patterns can worry some women about possible pathology. A study of Implanon in older women yielded results comparable to those reported in younger women.[135]

When to Change from Steroid Contraception to Postmenopausal Hormone Therapy

A common clinical dilemma is when to change from steroid contraception to postmenopausal hormone therapy. It is important to change because even with the lowest estrogen dose oral contraceptive available, the estrogen dose is 4-fold greater than the standard postmenopausal dose, and with increasing age, the dose-related risks with estrogen become significant. One approach to establish the onset of the postmenopausal years is to measure the follicle-stimulating hormone (FSH) level, beginning at age 50, on an annual basis, being careful to obtain the blood sample on day 6 or 7 of the hormone-free week (when steroid levels have declined sufficiently to allow FSH to rise). Friday afternoon works well for patients who start new packages on Sunday. When FSH is greater than 20 IU/L, it is time to change to a postmenopausal hormone program. Because of the variability in FSH levels experienced by women around the menopause, this method is not always accurate.[136, 137] Indeed, in some women, FSH does not rise until 2 weeks after the last dose of hormones. This is not very practical and places the patient at risk for an unwanted pregnancy. The hormone-free week method is practical and works for most women. Postmenopausal hormone treatment can be initiated if menopausal symptoms develop or when annual measurement of the FSH level, beginning at age 50, indicates a rise above 20 IU/L. This approach can be also be used in users of progestin-only contraceptive methods because pharmacologic amounts of progestins do not restore FSH to premenopausal levels, although greater reliability is achieved with injectable methods if the blood sample is obtained at the time of the next injection.[138] Some clinicians are comfortable allowing patients to enter their mid-50s on low-dose steroid contraception and then empirically switching to a postmenopausal hormone regimen.

The IUD for Older Women

The growing need for reversible contraception in older women would also be served by increased utilization of the IUD. The copper and levonorgestrel IUDs are among the most effective contraceptives, better than some sterilization operations. The decline in IUD use in the United States is in direct contrast to the experience in the rest of the world, a complicated response to publicity and litigation. An increased risk of pelvic infection with contemporary IUDs in use is limited to the insertion procedure and the transportation of pathogens to the upper genital tract. This risk is effectively minimized by careful screening for STI risks and the use of good aseptic technique.

The IUD is a good reversible contraceptive choice for older women. An older woman is more likely to be mutually monogamous and less likely to develop PID, and for those women who have already had their children, concern with fertility and problems with cramping and bleeding are both lesser issues. If protection from STIs is not a concern, insertion of a copper IUD can provide very effective contraception until menopause without the need to do anything other than check the string occasionally. On the other hand, because alterations of bleeding patterns become more common in this age group, it may be necessary to remove an IUD to avoid misinterpreting bleeding that could be due to endometrial disease. Because older women are more likely to have diabetes mellitus, it is worth emphasizing that no increase in adverse events has been observed with copper IUD use in women with either insulin-dependent or noninsulin-dependent diabetes.[139, 140] The IUD is not a good choice when the uterine cavity is distorted by leiomyomas. There are epidemiologic data indicating that both the copper IUD and the inert IUD reduce the risks of endometrial cancer and invasive cervical cancer,[141–145] presumably because of the induced biochemical alterations that affect cellular responses.

The levonorgestrel-releasing IUD (Mirena) is especially worth considering for older women. The levonorgestrel IUD lasts up to 10 years and reduces menstrual blood loss and pelvic infection rates.[146–148] Indeed, the levonorgestrel IUD is about as effective as endometrial ablation for the treatment of menorrhagia.[149] The local progestin effect directed to the endometrium can be utilized in patients on tamoxifen,[150] patients with dysmenorrhea,[151] and in postmenopausal women receiving estrogen therapy.[152]

Barrier Methods for Older Couples

Some women use barrier methods throughout their reproductive years, but most change to easier, more effective methods as their sexual lives become more stable, their risk of STIs decreases accordingly, and they need contraception for avoiding rather than spacing pregnancies. Some women begin new relationships as they age and may require reminding about the risks of STIs and the need to use condoms with new partners whose sexual and drug use histories are unknown. Perimenopausal women whose earlier use of contraception was not directed at avoiding HIV infection may need to learn how and with whom to use condoms.

Preventive Health Care for Older Women

Preventive health care for women is especially important during the transition years. The issues of preventive health care are familiar ones. They include contraception, cessation of smoking, prevention of heart disease and osteoporosis, maintenance of mental well-being (including sexuality), and cancer screening. Management of the transition years should be significantly oriented to preventive health care, and the use of contraception can now legitimately be viewed as a constituent of preventive health care. A discussion of the noncontraceptive health benefits of low-dose steroid contraception is especially important with patients in their transition years. This group of women appreciates and understands decisions made with the risk:benefit ratio in mind. For example, a useful observation to bring to our patients' attention is the following: continuous use of oral contraception for 10 years by women with a positive family history for ovarian cancer can reduce the risk of epithelial ovarian cancer to a level equal to or less than that experienced by women with a negative family history.[153]

Contraceptive advice is a component of good preventive health care. The patient's informed choice is the key to good care in the transitional years. Patients deserve to know the facts and need help in dealing with the state of the art and the uncertainty expressed in the media's coverage of research findings. But there is no doubt that patients are influenced in their choice by their clinician's advice and attitude. While the role of a clinician is to provide the education necessary for the patient to make proper choices, one should not lose sight of the powerful influence exerted by the clinician in the choices ultimately made. An emphasis on safety and benefits can have a major impact on contraceptive decisions.

References

1. **The Alan Guttmacher Institute,** Facts in Brief: Sexuality Education, The Alan Guttmacher Institute, New York, 2002.

2. **Koonin L, Smith J, Ramick M,** Abortion surveillance—United States, 1993 and 1994, MMWR 46:23, 1997.

3. **Henshaw SK, Van Vort J,** Abortion services in the United States, 1991 and 1992, Fam Plann Perspect 26:100, 1994.

4. **The Alan Guttmacher Institute,** U.S. Teenage Pregnancy Statistics. Overall Trends, Trends by Race and Ethnicity and State-by-State Information, The Alan Guttmacher Institute, New York, 2004.

5. **Forrest JD, Singh S,** The sexual and reproductive behavior of American women, 1982–1988, Fam Plann Perspect 22:206, 1990.

6. **Grunbaum JA, Kann L, Kinchen S, Ross J, Hawkins J, Lowry R, Harris WA, McManus T, Chyen D, Collins J,** Youth risk behavior surveillance—United States, 2003, MMWR Surveil Summ 53:1, 2004.

7. **Centers for Disease Control and Prevention,** Youth risk behavior surveillance—United States, 1995, MMWR 45:1, 1996.

8. **Fu H, Darroch JE, Haas T, Ranjit N,** Contraceptive failure rates: new estimates from the 1995 National Survey of Family Growth, Fam Plann Perspect 31:58, 1999.

9. **The Alan Guttmacher Institute,** Facts in Brief: Teenagers' Sexual and Reproductive Health, The Alan Guttmacher Institute, New York, 2002.

10. **Ventura SJ, Mosher WD, Curtin SC, Abma JC, Henshaw S,** Trends in pregnancy rates for the United States, 1976–97: An update, Natl Vit Stat Rep 49:1, 2001.

11. **Henshaw SK,** Unintended pregnancy in the United States, Fam Plann Perspect 30:24, 1998.

12. **Darroch JE, Landry DJ, Oslak S,** Age differences between sexual partners in the United States, Fam Plann Perspect 31:160, 1999.

13. **Zabin LS, Kanatner JF, Zelnick M,** The risk of adolescent pregnancy in the first months of intercourse, Fam Plann Perspect 11:215, 1979.

14. **Trussell J,** Teenage pregnancy in the United States, Fam Plann Perspect 20:262, 1989.

15. **Ahn N,** Teenage childbearing and high school completion: accounting for individual heterogeneity, Fam Plann Perspect 26:17, 1994.

16. **McAnarney ER, Hendee WR,** Adolescent pregnancy and its consequences, JAMA 262:74, 1989.

17. **Furstenberg FF, Brooks-Gunn J, Morgan SP,** Adolescent mothers and their children in later life, Fam Plann Perspect 19:142, 1987.

18. **Weinstock H, Berman S, Cates W, Jr.,** Sexually transmitted diseases among American youth: incidence and prevalence estimates, 2000, Persp Sexual Reprod Health 36:6, 2004.

19. **Glei DA,** Measuring contraceptive use patterns among teenage and adult women, Fam Plann Perspect 31:73, 1999.

20. **Zabin LS, Stark HA, Emerson MR,** Reasons for delay in contraceptive clinic utilization, J Adolesc Health 12:225, 1991.

21. **Kirby D, Short L, Collins J, Rugg D, Kolbe L, Howard M, Miller B, Sonenstein F, Zabin LS,** School-based programs to reduce sexual risk behaviors: a review of effectiveness, Public Health Reports 109:339, 1994.

22. **Grunseit A, et al,** Sexuality education and young people's sexual behaviors: a review of studies, J Adolesc Res 12:421, 1997.

23. **DiCenso A, Guyatt G, Willan A, Griffith L,** Interventions to reduce unintended pregnancies among adolescents: systematic review of randomised controlled trials, Br Med J 324:1426, 2002.

24. **Kirby D, Waszak C, Ziegler J,** Six school-based clinics: their reproductive health services and impact on sexual behavior, Fam Plann Perspect 23:6, 1991.

25. **Kirby D, Resnick MD, Downes B, Kocher T, Gunderson P, Potthoff S, Zelterman D, Blum RW,** The effects of school-based health clinics in St. Paul on school wide birthrates, Fam Plann Perspect 25:12, 1993.

26. **Vincent ML, Clearie AF, Schluchter MD,** Reducing adolescent pregnancy through school and community-based education, JAMA 257:3382, 1987.

27. **Paine-Andrews A, Harris KJ, Fisher JL, Lewis RK, Williams EL, Fawcett SB, Vincent ML,** Effects of a replication of a multicomponent model for preventing adolescent pregnancy in three Kansas communities, Fam Plann Perspect 31:182, 1999.

28. **O'Donnell L, Stueve A, San Doval A, Duran R, Haber D, Atnafou R, Johnson N, Grant U, Murray H, Juhn G, Tang J, Piessens P,** The effectiveness of the Reach for Health Community Youth Service learning program in reducing early and unprotected sex among urban middle school students, Am J Public Health 89:176, 1999.

29. **Kirby D,** The impact of schools and school programs upon adolescent sexual behavior, J Sex Research 39:27, 2002.

30. **Burstein GR, Lowry R, Klein JD, Santelli JS,** Missed opportunities for sexually transmitted diseases, human immunodeficiency virus, and pregnancy prevention services during adolescent health supervision, Pediatrics 111:996, 2003.

31. **Davis AJ,** Adolescent contraception and the clinician: an emphasis on counseling and communication, Clin Obstet Gynecol 44:114, 2001.

32. **Jones EF, Forrest JD, Goldman N, Henshaw SK, Lincoln R, Rosoff J, Westoff CF, Wulf D,** Teenage pregnancy in developed countries: determinants and policy implications, Fam Plann Persect 17:53, 1985.

33. **Reddy DM, Fleming R, Swain C,** Effect of mandatory parental notification on adolescent girls' use of sexual health care services, JAMA 288:710, 2002.

34. **Hanson SL,** Involving families in programs for pregnant teens: consequences for teens and their families, J Appl Fam Child Stud 41:303, 1992.

35. **Piccinino LJ, Mosher WD,** Trends in contraceptive use in the United States: 1982–1995, Fam Plann Perspect 30:4, 1998.

36. **Jay MS, DuRant RH, Litt IF,** Female adolescents' compliance with contraceptive regimens, Ped Clinics N Am 36:731, 1989.

37. **Marchbanks PA, McDonald JA, Wilson HG, Folger SG, Mandel MG, Daling JR, Bernstein L, Malone KE, Ursin G, Strom BL, Norman SA, Wingo PA, Burkman RT, Berlin JA, Simon JS, Spirtas R, Weiss LK,** Oral contraceptives and the risk of breast cancer, New Engl J Med 346:2025, 2002.

38. **Bagwell MA, Coker AL, Thompson SJ, Baker ER, Addy CL,** Primary infertility and oral contraceptive steroid use, Fertil Steril 63:1161, 1995.

39. **Carpenter S, Neinstein LS,** Weight gain in adolescent and young adult oral contraceptive users, J Adolesc Health Care 7:342, 1986.

40. **Reubinoff BE, Wurtman J, Rojansky N, Adler D, Stein P, Schenker JG, Brzezinski A,** Effects of hormone replacement therapy on weight, body composition, fat distribution, and food intake in early postmenopausal women: a prospective study, Fertil Steril 64:963, 1995.

41. **Moore LL, Valuck R, McDougall C, Fink W,** A comparative study of one-year weight gain among users of medroxyprogesterone acetate, levonorgestrel implants, and oral contraceptives, Contraception 52:215, 1995.

42. **Rosenberg M,** Weight change with oral contraceptive use and during the menstrual cycle. Results of daily measurements, Contraception 58:345, 1998.

43. **Risser WL, Gefter L, Barratt MS, Risser JM,** Weight change in adolescents who used hormonal contraception, J Adolesc Health 24:433, 1999.

44. **Redmond G, Godwin AJ, Olson W, Lippman JS,** Use of placebo controls in an oral contraceptive trial: methodological issues and adverse event incidence, Contraception 60:81, 1999.

45. **Gupta S,** Weight gain on the combined pill—is it real? Hum Reprod Update 6:427, 2000.

46. **Thiboutot D, Archer DF, Lemay A, Washenik K, Roberts J, Harrison DD,** A randomized, controlled trial of a low-dose contraceptive containing 20 μg of ethinyl estradiol and 100 μg of levonorgestrel for acne treatment, Fertil Steril 76:461, 2001.

47. **Grace E, Emans SJ, Havens KK, Merola JL, Woods ER,** Contraceptive compliance with a triphasic and a monophasic norethindrone-containing oral contraceptive pill in a private adolescent practice, Adolesc Pediatr Gynecol 7:29, 1994.

48. **Robinson JC, Plichter S, Weisman CS, Nathanson CA, Ensminger M,** Dysmenorrhea and use of oral contraceptives in adolescent women attending a family planning clinic, Am J Obstet Gynecol 166:578, 1992.

49. **Centers for Disease Control,** Youth risk behavior surveillance—United States, 2003, MMWR 53:No. SS2, 2004.

50. **Risch HA, Howe GR, Jain M, Burch JD, Holowaty EJ, Miller AB,** Are female smokers at higher risk for lung cancer than male smokers? A case-control analysis by histologic type, Am J Epidemiol 138:281, 1993.

51. **Davis DL, Dinse GE, Hoel DG,** Decreasing cardiovascular disease and increasing cancer among whites in the United States from 1973 through 1987, JAMA 271:431, 1994.

52. **Willett WC, Green A, Stampfer MJ, Speizer FE, Colditz GA, Rosner B, Monson RR, Stason W, Hennekens CH,** Relative and absolute excess risks of coronary heart disease among women who smoke cigarettes, New Engl J Med 317:1303, 1987.

53. **Fruzzetti F, Ricci C, Fioretti P,** Haemostasis profile in smoking and nonsmoking women taking low-dose oral contraceptives, Contraception 49:579, 1994.

54. **Basdevant A, Conard J, Pelissier C, Guyene T-T, Lapousterle C, Mayer M, Guy-Grand B, Degrelle H,** Hemostatic and metabolic effects of lowering the ethinyl-estradiol dose from 30 mcg to 20 mcg in oral contraceptives containing desogestrel, Contraception 48:193, 1993.

55. **Winkler UH, Schindler AE, Endrikat J, Düsterberg B,** A comparative study of the effects of the hemostatic system of two monophasic gestodene oral contraceptives containing 20 μg and 30 μg ethinylestradiol, Contraception 53:75, 1996.

56. **Harper C, Balistreri E, Boggess J, Leon K, Darney P,** Provision of hormonal contraceptives without a mandatory pelivic examination: the first stop demonstration project, Fam Plann Perspect 33:13, 2001.

57. **Stewart FH, Harper CC, Ellertson CE, Grimes DA, Sawaya GF, Trussell J,** Clinical breast and pelvic examination requirements for hormonal contraception. Current practice vs evidence, JAMA 285:2231, 2001.

58. **Audet M-C, Moreau M, Koltun WD, Waldbaum AS, Shangold G, Fisher AC, Creasy GW, for the ORTHO EVRA/EVRA 004 Study Group,** Evaluation of contraceptive efficacy and cycle control of a transdermal contraceptive patch vs an oral contraceptive. A randomized controlled trial, JAMA 285:2347, 2001.

59. **Archer DF, Bigrigg A, Smallwood GH, Shangold GA, Creasy GW, Fisher AC,** Assessment of compliance with a weekly contraceptive patch (Ortho Evra™/Evra™) among North American women, Fertil Steril 77(Suppl 2):S27, 2002.

60. **Archer DF, Cullins V, Creasy GW, Fisher AC,** The impact of improved compliance with a weekly contraceptive transdermal system (Ortho Evra) on contraceptive efficacy, Contraception 69:189, 2004.

61. **Logsdon S, Richards J, Omar HA,** Long-term evaluation of the use of the transdermal contraceptive patch in adolescents, Scientific World Journal 4:512, 2004.

62. **Rubinstein ML, Halpern-Felsher BL, Irwin CE, Jr.,** An evaluation of the use of the transdermal contraceptive patch in adolescents, J Adolesc Health 34:395, 2004.

63. **Werner MJ, Biro FM,** Contraception and sexually transmitted diseases in adolescent females, Adolesc Pediatr Gynecol 3:127, 1990.

64. **Nsuami M, Cammarata CL, Brooks BN, Taylor SN, Martin DH,** Chlamydia and gonorrhea co-occurrence in a high school population, Sex Transm Dis 31:424, 2004.

65. **Nsuami M, Elie M, Brooks BN, Sanders LS, Nash TD, Makonnen F, Taylor SN, Cohen DA,** Screening for sexually transmitted diseases during preparticipation sports examination of high school adolescents, J Adolesc Health 32:336, 2003.

66. **Santelli JS, Warren CW, Lowry R, Sogolow E, Collins J, Kann L, Kaufmann RB, Celentano DD,** The use of condoms with other contraceptive methods among young men and women, Fam Plann Persp 29:261, 1997.

67. **Abma JC, Chandra A, Mosher WD, Peterson L, Piccinino L,** Fertility, family planning, and women's health: new data from the 1995 National Survey of Family Growth, Report No. 19, Series 23, Centers for Disease Control and Prevention, National Center For Heath Statistics, Washington, D.C., 1997.

68. **Suhonen S, Haukkamaa M, Jakobsson T, Rauramo I,** Clinical performance of a levonorgestrel-releasing intrauterine system and oral contraceptives in young nulliparous women: a comparative study, Contraception 69:407, 2004.

69. **Darney PD, Klaisle CM, Tanner S, Alvarado AM,** Sustained-release contraceptives, Curr Prob Obstet Gynecol Fertil 13:95, 1990.

70. **Smith RD, Cromer BA, Hayes JR, et al.,** Medroxyprogesterone acetate (Depo-Provera) use in adolescents: uterine bleeding and blood pressure patterns, patient satisfaction, and continuation rates, Adolesc Pediatr Gynecol 8:24, 1995.

71. **Berenson AB, Wiemann CM,** Use of levonorgestrel implants versus oral contraceptives in adolescence: a case-control study, Am J Obstet Gynecol 172:1128, 1995.

72. **Weisman CS, Plichta SB, Tirado DE, Dina KH,** Comprison of contraceptive implant adopters and pill users in a family planning clinic in Baltimore, Fam Plann Perspect 25:224, 1993.

73. **Cromer BA, Smith RD, Blair JM, Dwyer J, Brown RT,** A prospective study of adolescents who choose among levonorgestrel implant (Norplant), medroxyprogesterone acetate (Depo-Provera), or the combined oral contraceptive pill as contraception, Pediatrics 94:687, 1994.

74. **Cullins VE, Remsburg RE, Blumenthal PD, Huggins GR,** Comparison of adolescent and adult experience with Norplant levonorgestrel contraceptive implants, Obstet Gynecol 83:1026, 1994.

75. **Polaneczky M, Slap G, Forke C, Rappaport A, Sondheimer S,** The use of levonorgestrel implants (Norplant) for contraception in adolescent mothers, New Engl J Med 331:1201, 1994.

76. **Zibners A, Cromer BA, Hayes J,** Comparison of continuation rates for hormonal contraception among adolescents, J Pediatr Adolesc Gynecol 12:90, 1999.

77. **Darney PD, Callegari LS, Swift A, Atkinson ES, Robert AM,** Condom practices of urban teens using Norplant contraceptive implants, oral contraceptives, and condoms for contraception, Am J Obstet Gynecol 180:929, 1999.

78. **O'Dell CM, Forke CM, Polaneczky MM, Sondheimer SJ, Slap GB,** Depot-medroxyprogesterone acetate or oral contraception in postpartum adolescents, Obstet Gynecol 91:609, 1998.

79. **Theitz G, Buch B, Rizzoli R, Slosman D, Clavien H, Sizonko PC, Bonjour JPH,** Longitudinal monitoring of bone mass accumulation in healthy adolescents: evidence for a marked reduction after 16 years of age in the levels of lumbar spine and femoral neck in female subjects, J Clin Endocrinol Metab 75:1060, 1992.

80. **Matkovic V, Jelic T, Wardlaw GM, Ilich J, Goel PK, Wright JK, Andon MB, Smith KT, Heaney RP,** Timing of peak bone mass in caucasian females and its implication for the prevention of osteoporosis: inference from a cross-sectional model, J Clin Invest 93:799, 1994.

81. **Cromer BA, Blair JM, Mahan JD, Zibners L, Naumovski Z,** A prospective comparison of bone density in adolescent girls receiving depot-medroxyprogesterone acetate (Depo-Provera), levonorgestrel (Norplant), or oral contraceptives, J Pediatr 129:671, 1996.

82. **Lara-Torre E, Edwards CP, Perlaman S, Hertweck SP,** Bone mineral density in adolescent females using depot-medroxyprogesterone acetate, J Pediatr Adolesc Gynecol 17:17, 2004.

83. **Cundy T, Cornish J, Evans MC, Roberts H, Reid IR,** Recovery of bone density in women who stop using medroxyprogesterone acetate, Br Med J 308:247, 1994.

84. **Scholes D, LaCroix AZ, Ichikawa LE, Barlow WE, Ott SM,** Injectable hormone contraception and bone density: results from a prospective study, Epidemiology 13:581, 2002.

85. **Orr-Walker BJ, Evans MC, Ames RW, Clearwater JM, Cundy T, Reid IR,** The effect of past use of the injectable contraceptive depot-medroxyprogesterone acetate on bone mineral density in normal post-menopausal women, Clin Endocrinol 49:615, 1998.

86. **Petitti DB, Piaggio G, Mehta S, Cravioto MC, Meirik O, for the WHO Study of Hormonal Contraception and Bone Health,** Steroid hormone contraception and bone mineral density: a cross-sectional study in an international population, Obstet Gynecol 95:736, 2000.

87. **Kalkwarf HJ, Specker BL,** Bone mineral loss during lactation and recovery after weaning, Obstet Gynecol 86:26, 1995.

88. **Ho PC, Kwan MSW,** A prospective randomized comparison of levonorgestrel with the Yuzpe regimen in post-coital contraception, Hum Reprod 8:389, 1993.

89. **Task Force on Postovulatory Methods of Fertility Regulation,** Randomised controlled trial of levonorgestrel versus the Yuzpe regimen of combined oral contraceptives for emergency contraception, Lancet 352:428, 1998.

90. **von Hertzen H, Piaggio G, Ding J, Chen J, Song S, Bartfai G, Ng E, Gemzell-Danielsson K, Oyunbileg A, Wu S, Cheng W, Ludicke F, Pretnar-Darovec A, Kirkman R, Mittal S, Khomassuridze A, Apter D, Peregoudov A, WHO Research Group on Post-Ovulatory Methods of Fertility Regulation,** Low dose mifepristone and two regimens of levonorgestrel for emergency contraception: a WHO multicentre randomised trial, Lancet 360:1803, 2002.

91. **Arowojoulu AO, Okewole IA, Adekunie AO,** Comparative evaluation of the effectiveness and safety of two regimens of levonorgestrel for emergency contraception in Nigerians, Contraception 66:269, 2002.

92. **Harper CC, Rocca CH, Darney PD, von Hertzen H, Raine TR,** Tolerability of levonorgestrel emergency contraception in adolescents, Am J Obstet Gynecol 191:1158, 2004.

93. **Raine T, Harper C, Leon K, Darney P,** Emergency contraception: advance provision in a young, high-risk clinic population, Obstet Gynecol 96:1, 2000.

94. **Glasier A, Baird D,** The effects of self-administering emergency contraception, New Engl J Med 339:1, 1998.

95. **Jackson RD, Bimla Schwarz E, Freedman L, Darney P,** Advance supply of emergency contraception: effect on use and usual contraception—a randomized trial, Obstet Gynecol 102:8, 2003.

96. **Gold MA, Wolford JE, Smith KA, Parker AM,** The effects of advance provision of emergency contraception on adolescent women's sexual and contraceptive behaviors, J Pediatr Adolesc Gynecol 17:87, 2004.

97. **Walker DM, Torres P, Gtutierrez JP, Flemming K, Bertozzi SM,** Emergency contraception use is correlated with increased condom use among adolescents: results from Mexico, J Adolesc Health 35:329, 2004.

98. **Harper CC, Ellerton CE,** The emergency contraceptive pill: a survey of knowledge and attitudes among students at Princeton, Am J Obstet Gynecol 173:1438, 1995.

99. **Burton R, Savage W, Reader F,** The "morning after pill." Is this the wrong name for it? Br J Fam Plann 15:119, 1990.

100. **Young L, McCowan LM, Roberts HE, Farquhar CM,** Emergency contraception — why women don't use it, N Z Med J 108:145, 1995.

101. **Glasier A, Fairhurst K, Wyke S, Ziebland S, Seaman P, Walker J, Lakha F,** Advanced provision of emergency contraception does not reduce abortion rates, Contraception 69:361, 2004.

102. **Emans SJ, Grace E, Woods ER, Smith DE, Klein K, Merola J,** Adolescents' compliance with the use of oral contraceptives, JAMA 257:3377, 1987.

103. **Winter L, Breckenmaker LC,** Tailoring family planning services to the special needs of adolescents, Fam Plann Perspect 23:24, 1991.

104. **Centers for Disease Control and Prevention,** Abortion Surveillance—United States, 1999, MMWR 52:1, 2002.

105. **Enzelsberger H, Metka M, Heytmanek G, Schurz B, Kurz C, Kusztrich M,** Influence of oral contraceptive use on bone density in climacteric women, Maturitas 9:375, 1988.

106. **Lindsay R, Tohme J, Kanders B,** The effect of oral contraceptive use on vertebral bone mass in pre- and post-menopausal women, Contraception 34:333, 1986.

107. **Enzelberger H, Metka M, Heytmanek G, Schurz B, Kurz C, Kusztrich M,** Influence of oral contraceptive use on bone density in climacteric women, Maturitas 9:375, 1988.

108. **Kleerekoper M, Brienza RS, Schultz LR, Johnson CC,** Oral contraceptive use may protect against low bone mass, Arch Intern Med 151:1971, 1991.

109. **Kritz-Silverstein D, Barrett-Connor E,** Bone mineral density in postmenopausal women as determined by prior oral contraceptive use, Am J Public Health 83:100, 1993.

110. **Tuppurrainen M, Kröger H, Saarikoski S, Honkanen R, Alhava E,** The effect of previous oral contraceptive use on bone mineral density in perimenopausal women, Osteoporosis Int 4:93, 1994.

111. **Gambacciani M, Spinetti A, Taponeco F, Cappagli B, Piaggesi L, Fioretti P,** Longitudinal evaluation of perimenopausal vertebral bone loss: effects of a low-dose oral contraceptive preparation on bone mineral density and metabolism, Obstet Gynecol 83:392, 1994.

112. **Pasco JA, Kotowicz MA, Henry MJ, Panahi S, Seeman E, Nicholson GC,** Oral contraceptives and bone mineral density: a population-based study, Am J Obstet Gynecol 182:265, 2000.

113. **Mais V, Fruzzetti F, Aiossa S, Paoletti AM, Guerriero S, Melis GB,** Bone metabolism in young women taking a monophasic pill containing 20 μg ethinylestradiol, Contraception 48:445, 1993.

114. **Polatti F, Perotti F, Filippa N, Gallina D, Nappi RE,** Bone mass and long-term monophasic oral contraceptive treatment in young women, Contraception 51:221, 1995.

115. **Hartard M, Bottermann P, Bartenstein P, Jeschke D, Schwaiger M,** Effects on bone mineral density of low-dosed oral contraceptives compared to and combined with physical activity, Contraception 55:87, 1997.

116. **Mallmin H, Ljunghall S, Persson I, Bergstrom R,** Risk factors for fractures of the distal forearm: a population-based case-control study, Osteoporosis Int 4:97, 1994.

117. **Johansson C, Mellström D,** An earlier fracture as a risk factor for new fracture and its association with smoking and menopausal age in women, Maturitas 24:97, 1996.

118. O'Neill TW, Marsden D, Adams JE, Silman AJ, Risk factors, falls, and fracture of the distal forearm in Manchester, UK, J Epidemiol Community Health 50:288, 1996.

119. O'Neill TW, Silman AJ, Naves Diaz M, Cooper C, Kanis J, Felsenberg D, Influence of hormonal and reproductive factors on the risk of vertebral deformity in European women, Osteoporosis Int 7:72, 1997.

120. Cooper C, Hannaford P, Croft P, Kay CR, Oral contraceptive pill use and fractures in women: a prospective study, Bone 14:41, 1993.

121. Vessey M, Mant J, Painter R, Oral contraception and other factors in relation to hospital referral for fracture. Findings in a large cohort study, Contraception 57:231, 1998.

122. Michaëlsson K, Baron JA, Farahmand BY, Persson I, Ljunghall S, Oral contraceptive use and risk of hip fracture: a case-control study, Lancet 353:1481, 1999.

123. Barrett DH, Anda RF, Escobedo LG, Croft JB, Williamson DF, Marks JS, Trends in oral contraceptive use and cigarette smoking, Arch Fam Med 3:438, 1994.

124. Kirkman RJE, Pedersen JH, Fioretti P, Roberts HE, Clinical comparison of two low-dose oral contraceptives, Minulet and Mercilon, in women over 30 years of age, Contraception 49:33, 1994.

125. Fioretti P, Fruzzetti F, Navalesi R, Ricci C, Moccoli R, Cerri FM, Orlandi MC, Melis GB, Clinical and metabolic study of a new pill containing 20 mcg ethinylestradiol plus 0.150 mg desogestrel, Contraception 35:229, 1987.

126. Steffensen K, Evaluation of an oral contraceptive containing 0.150 mg desogestrel and 0.020 mg ethinylestradiol in women aged 30 years or older, Acta Obstet Gynecol Scand Suppl 144:23, 1987.

127. Melis GB, Fruzzetti F, Nicoletti I, Ricci C, Lammers P, Atsma WJ, Fioretti P, A comparative study on the effects of a monophasic pill containing desogestrel plus 20 μg ethinylestradiol, a triphasic combination containing levonorgestel and a monophasic combination containing gestodene on coagulatory factors, Contraception 43:23, 1991.

128. Gordon EM, Williams SR, Frenchek B, Mazur CH, Speroff L, Dose-dependent effects of postmenopausal estrogen/progestin on antithrombin III and factor XII, J Lab Clin Med 111:52, 1988.

129. Poulter NR, Chang CL, Farley TMM, Meirik O, Risk of cardiovascular diseases associated with oral progestagen preparations with therapeutic indications, Lancet 354:1610, 1999.

130. Vasilakis C, Jick H, del Mar Melero-Montes M, Risk of idiopathic venous thromboembolism in users of progestagens alone, Lancet 354:1610, 1999.

131. Gebbie AE, Glasier A, Sweeting V, Incidence of ovulation in perimenopausal women before and during hormone replacement therapy, Contraception 52:221, 1995.

132. Casper RF, Dodin S, Reid RL, and Study Investigators, The effect of 20 μg ethinyl estradiol/1 μg norethindrone acetate (MinnestrinÒ), a low-dose oral contraceptive, on vaginal bleeding patterns, hot flashes, and quality of life in symptomatic perimenopausal women, Menopause 4:139, 1997.

133. WHO, Multinational comparative clinical evaluation of two long-acting injectable contraceptive steroids: norethisterone enanthate and medroxyprogesterone acetate. Final report, Contraception 28:1, 1983.

134. World Health Organization Collaborative Study of Cardiovascular Disease and Steroid Hormone Contraception, Cardiovascular disease and use of oral and injectable progestogen-only contraceptives and combined injectable contraceptives. Results of an international, multicenter, case-control study, Contraception 57:315, 1998.

135. Booranabunyat S, Taneepanichskul S, Implanon use in Thai women above the age of 35 years, Contraception 69:489, 2004.

136. Castracane VD, Gimpel T, Goldzieher JW, When is it safe to switch from oral contraceptives to hormonal replacement therapy? Contraception 52:371, 1995.

137. Creinin MD, Laboratory criteria for menopause in women using oral contraceptives, Fertil Steril 66:101, 1996.

138. Beksinska ME, Smit JA, Kleinschmidt I, Rees H, Farley TMM, Guidozzi F, Detection of raised FSH levels among older women using depomedroxyprogesterone acetate and norethisterone enanthate, Contraception 68:339, 2003.

139. Kimmerle R, Weiss R, Bergert M, Kurz K, Effectiveness, safety, and acceptability of a copper intrauterine deivce (Cu Safe 300) in type I diabetic women, Diabetes Care 16:1227, 1993.

140. **Kjos SL, Ballagh SA, La Cour M, Xiang A, Mishell DR, Jr.,** The copper T380A intrauterine device in women with Type II diabetes mellitus, Obstet Gynecol 84:1006, 1994.

141. **Castellsague X, Thompson WD, Dubrow R,** Intra-uterine contraception and the risk of endometrial cancer, Int J Cancer 54:911, 1993.

142. **Lassise DL, Savitz DA, Hamman RF, Baron AE, Brinton LA, Levines RS,** Invasive cervical cancer and intrauterine device use, Int J Epidemiol 20:865, 1991.

143. **Parazzini F, La Vecchia C, Negri E,** Use of intrauterine device and risk of invasive cervical cancer, Int J Epidemiol 21:1030, 1992.

144. **Hill DA, Weiss NS, Voigt LF, Beresford SAA,** Endometrial cancer in relation to intrauterine device use, Int J Cancer 70:278, 1997.

145. **Sturgeon SR, Brinton LA, Berman ML, Mortel R, Twiggs LB, Barrett RJ, Wilbanks GD, Lurain JR,** Intrauterine device use and endometrial cancer risk, Int J Epidemiol 26:496, 1997.

146. **Sivin I, Stern J, Coutinho E, Mattos CER, El Mahgoub S, Diaz S, Pavéz M, Alvarez F, Brache V, Thevinin F, Diaz J, Faundes A, Diaz MM, McCarthy T, Mishell Jr DR, Shoupe D,** Prolonged intrauterine contraception: a seven-year randomized study of the levonorgestrel 20 mcg/day (LNg 20) and the copper T380 Ag IUDs, Contraception 44:473, 1991.

147. **Toivonen J, Luukkainen T, Alloven H,** Protective effect of intrauterine release of levonorgestrel on pelvic infection: three years' comparative experience of levonorgestrel and copper-releasing intrauterine devices, Obstet Gynecol 77:261, 1991.

148. **Bilian X, Liying Z, Xuling Z, Mengchun J, Luukkainen T, Allonen H,** Pharmacokinetic and pharmacodynamic studies of levonorgestrel-releasing intrauterine device, Contraception 41:353, 1990.

149. **Crosignani PG, Vercellini P, Mosconi P, Oldani S, Cortesi I, De Giorgi O,** Levonorgestrel-releasing intrauterine device versus hysteroscopic endometrial resection in the treatment of dysfunctional uterine bleeding, Obstet Gynecol 90:257, 1997.

150. **Gardner FJE, Konje JC, Abrams KR, Brown LJR, Khanna S, Al-Azzawi F, Bell SC, Taylor DJ,** Endometrial protection from tamoxifen-stimulated changes by a levonorgestrel-releasing intrauterine system: a randomised controlled trial, Lancet 356:1711, 2000.

151. **Vercellini P, Aimi G, Panazza S, De Giorgi O, Pesole A, Crosignani PG,** A levonorgestrel-releasing intrauterine system for the treatment of dysmenorrhea associated with endometriosis: a pilot study, Fertil Steril 72:505, 1999.

152. **Varila E, Wahlstrom T, Rauramo I,** A 5-year follow-up study on the use of a levonorgestrel intrauterine system in women receiving hormone replacement therapy, Fertil Steril 76:969, 2001.

153. **Gross TP, Schlesselman JJ,** The estimated effect of oral contraceptive use on the cumulative risk of epithelial ovarian cancer, Obstet Gynecol 83:419, 1994.

12

Sterilization

Contraceptive methods today are very safe and effective; however, we remain decades away from a perfect method of contraception for either women or men. Because reversible contraceptive methods are not perfect, more than one-third of American couples use sterilization instead, and sterilization is now the predominant method of contraception in the world.

Over the past 20 years, over 1 million Americans each year have undergone a sterilization operation, and recently, more women than men. Currently 36% of reproductive-aged American women rely on contraceptive sterilization: 27% undergo tubal occlusion (11 million women), and 9.2% depend on their partners' vasectomies (3.6 million men).[1] This same trend has occurred in Great Britain, where by age 40, more than 20% of men and women have had a sterilization procedure.[2] In Spain and Italy, sterilization rates are very low, but the use of oral contraceptives and the intrauterine device (IUD) is very high.[3]

Americans use sterilization for contraceptive purposes more than the people of most countries, in our view, partly because the IUD and oral contraception have a worse reputation here than in the rest of the world. Publicity about side effects and litigation have frightened prospective users, and it is little wonder that Americans turn to sterilization more often and at an earlier age and, we believe, before they really want to. A significant increase in both female and male sterilization occurred between 1973 and 1988, a period during which the use of IUDs declined, and the use of oral contraception decreased substantially, although since the late 1980s, oral contraception has regained some of its popularity (Chapter 1).

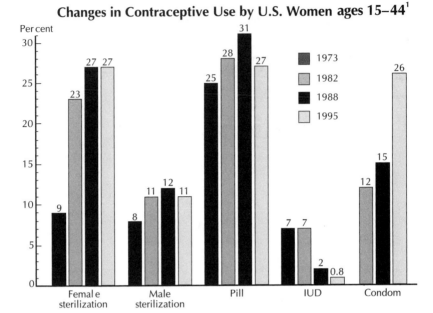

Changes in Contraceptive Use by U.S. Women ages 15–44[1]

History

James Blundell proposed in 1823, in lectures at Guy's Hospital in London, that tubectomy ought to be performed at cesarean section to avoid the need for repeat sections.[4] He also proposed a technique for sterilization, which he later described so precisely that he actually must have performed the operation, although he never wrote about it. The first report was published in 1881 by Samuel Lungren of Toledo, Ohio, who ligated the tubes at the time of cesarean section, as Blundell had suggested 58 years earlier.[5] The Madlener procedure was devised in Germany in 1910 and reported in 1919. Because of many failures, the Madlener technique was supplanted in the United States by the method of Ralph Pomeroy, a prominent physician in Brooklyn, New York. This method, still popular today, was not described to the medical profession by Pomeroy's associates until 1929, 4 years after Pomeroy's death. Frederick Irving of the Harvard Medical School described his technique in 1924, and the Uchida method was not reported until 1946.

Few sterilizations were performed until the 1930s when "family planning" was first suggested as an indication for surgical sterilization by Baird in Aberdeen. He required women to be older than 40 and to have had 8 or more children. Mathematical formulas of this kind persisted through the 1960s. In 1965, Sir Dugald Baird delivered a remarkable lecture, entitled "The Fifth Freedom," calling attention to the need to alleviate the fear of unwanted pregnancies and the important role of sterilization.[6] By the end of the 1960s, sterilization was a popular procedure.

The Pomeroy

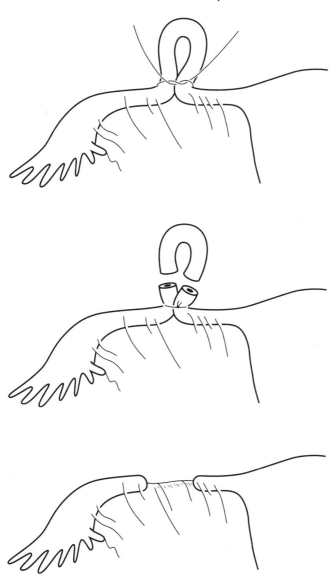

The Irving

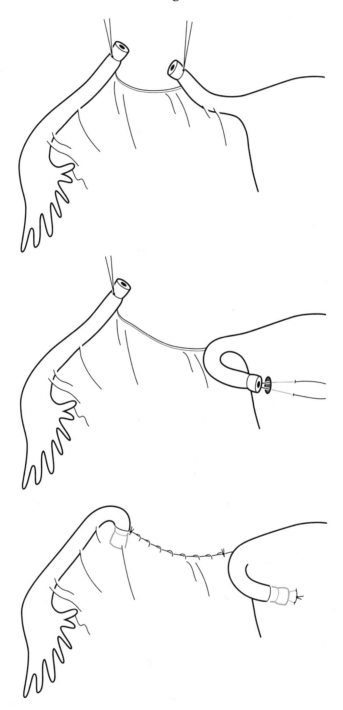

The Uchida

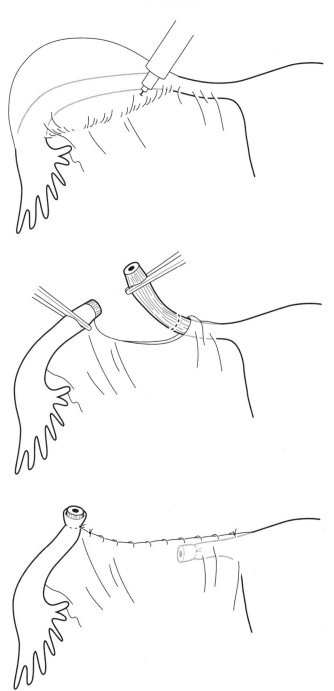

Laparoscopic methods were introduced in the early 1970s. The annual number of vasectomies began to decline, and the number of tubal occlusion operations increased rapidly. By 1973, more sterilization operations were performed for women than for men. This is accurately attributed to dramatic decreases in costs, hospital time, and pain because of the introduction of laparoscopy and minilaparotomy methods. The use of laparoscopy for tubal occlusion increased from only 0.6% of sterilizations in 1970 to more than 35% by 1975.[7] Since 1975, minilaparotomy, a technique popular in the less developed world, has been increasingly performed in the United States. These methods have allowed women to undergo sterilization operations at times other than immediately after childbirth or during major surgery.

Laparoscopy and minilaparotomy have led to a profound change in the convenience and cost of sterilization operations for women. In 1970, the average woman stayed in the hospital 6.5 days for a tubal sterilization. By 1975, this had declined to 3 days, and today, women rarely remain in the hospital overnight. The shorter length of stay achieved from 1970 to 1975 represented a savings of more than $200 million yearly in health care costs and a tremendous increase in convenience for women eager to return to work and their families.[8] Unlike some advances in technology, laparoscopy and minilaparotomy sterilization are technical innovations that have resulted in large savings in medical care costs.

The great majority of sterilization procedures are accomplished in hospitals by physicians in private practice, but a rapidly increasing proportion is performed outside of hospitals in ambulatory surgical settings, including physicians' offices. In either hospital or outpatient settings, female sterilization is a very safe operation. Deaths specifically attributed to sterilization now account for only 1.5 per 100,000 procedures, a mortality rate that is lower than that for childbearing (about 8 per 100,000 births in the United States).[9, 10] When the risk of pregnancy from contraceptive method failure is taken into account, sterilization is the safest of all contraceptive methods.

Vasectomy has long been more popular in the United States than anywhere else in the world, but why don't more men use it? One explanation is that women have chosen laparoscopic sterilization in increasing numbers. Another is that men have been frightened by reports, often from animal data, of associations with autoimmune diseases, atherosclerosis, and, most recently, prostatic cancer. Large epidemiologic studies have failed to confirm any definite adverse consequences.[11] When patients consider sterilization, we can assure them that vasectomy has not been demonstrated to have any harmful effects on men's health.[12] In addition, vasectomy is less expensive than tubal sterilization, morbidity is less, and mortality is essentially zero.

Efficacy of Sterilization

Laparoscopic and minilaparotomy sterilizations are not only convenient, they are almost as effective at preventing pregnancy as were the older, more complex operations. Vasectomy is also highly effective once the supply of remaining sperm in the vas deferens is exhausted. Approximately 50% of men reach azoospermia at 8 weeks and nearly 100% by 10 weeks.[13]

In addition to the specific operation used, the skill of the operator and characteristics of the patient make important contributions to the efficacy of female sterilization. Up to 50% of failures are due to technical errors. The methods using complicated equipment, such as spring-loaded clips and silastic rings, fail for technical reasons more commonly than do simpler procedures such as the Pomeroy tubal ligation.[15] Minilaparotomy failures, therefore, occur much less frequently from technical errors.

Failure Rates During the First Year, United States [14]

Method	Percent of Women with Pregnancy	
	Lowest Expected	Typical
Female sterilization	0.2	0.4
Male sterilization	0.1	0.15

It is hardly surprising that more complicated techniques of tubal occlusion have higher technical failure rates. What is surprising is the finding that characteristics of the patient influence the likelihood of failure even when technical problems are controlled for in analytical adjustments. In a careful study of this issue, two patient characteristics, age and lactation, demonstrated a significant impact.[16] Patients younger than 35 years were 1.7 times more likely to become pregnant, and women who were not breastfeeding following sterilization were 5 times more likely to become pregnant. These findings probably reflect the greater fecundity of younger women and the contraceptive contribution of lactation.

Significant numbers of pregnancies after tubal occlusion are present before the procedure. For this reason, some clinicians routinely perform a uterine evacuation or curettage prior to tubal occlusion. It seems more reasonable (and cost-effective) to exclude pregnancy by careful history-taking, physical examination, and an appropriate pregnancy test prior to the sterilization procedure.[17]

Because method, operator, and patient characteristics all influence sterilization failures, it is difficult to predict which individual will experience a pregnancy after undergoing a tubal occlusion. Therefore, during the course of counseling, all patients should be made aware of the possibility of failure as well as the intent to cause permanent, irreversible sterility. It is important to avoid giving patients the impression that the tubal occlusion procedure is foolproof or guaranteed. Individual clinicians must be cautious judging their own success in accomplishing sterilization because failure is infrequent and many patients who become pregnant after sterilization never reveal the failure to the original surgeon.

Ectopic pregnancies can occur following tubal occlusion, and the incidence is much higher with some types of tubal occlusion.[18–20] Bipolar tubal coagulation is more likely to result in ectopic pregnancy than is mechanical occlusion.[15, 21, 22] The probable explanation is that microscopic fistulae in the coagulated segment connected to the peritoneal cavity permit sperm to reach the ovum. Ectopic pregnancies following tubal ligation are more likely to occur 3 or more years after sterilization, rather than immediately after. The proportion of ectopic pregnancies is 3 times as high in the 4th through the 10th years after sterilization as in the first 3 years.[22] For laparoscopic methods, the cumulative rate of ectopic pregnancy continues to increase for at least 10 years after surgery, reaching 17 per 1,000 for bipolar coagulation.[22] Overall, however, the risk of an ectopic pregnancy in sterilized women is lower than if they had not been sterilized. Nevertheless, approximately one-third of the pregnancies that occur after tubal sterilization are ectopic.[22]

Vaginal procedures have higher failure rates than laparoscopy or minilaparotomy, but the principal disadvantage is a higher rate of infection. Intraperitoneal infection is a rare complication of minilaparotomy or laparoscopic techniques, but in vaginal procedures, abscess formation approaches 1%.[23] This risk can be reduced by the use of prophylactic antibiotics administered intraoperatively, but open laparoscopy is usually easier and safer than vaginal sterilization even in obese women.

Sterilization and Ovarian Cancer — A Benefit of Sterilization

Evidence from the Nurses' Health Study indicated that tubal sterilization was associated with a 67% reduced risk of ovarian cancer.[24] In the prospective mortality study, conducted by the American Cancer Society, women who had undergone tubal sterilization experienced about a 30% reduction in the risk of fatal ovarian cancer.[25] In addition, case-control data have consistently supported this finding.[26–28] The mechanism for such an effect is not clear, but this information is worth sharing with patients.

Female Sterilization Techniques

Because laparoscopy permits direct visualization and manipulation of the abdominal and pelvic organs with minimal abdominal disruption, it offers many advantages. Hospitalization is not required; most patients return home within a few hours, and the majority return to full activity within 24 hours. Discomfort is minimal, the incision scars are barely visible, and sexual activity need not be restricted. In addition, the surgeon has an opportunity to inspect the pelvic and abdominal organs for abnormalities. The disadvantages of laparoscopic sterilization include the cost; the expensive, fragile equipment; the special training required; and the risks of inadvertent bowel or vessel injury.

Laparoscopic sterilization can be achieved with any of these methods:

1. Occlusion and partial resection by unipolar electrosurgery.
2. Occlusion and transection by unipolar electrosurgery.
3. Occlusion by bipolar electrocoagulation.
4. Occlusion by mechanical means (clips or silastic rings).

All of these methods can use an operating laparoscope alone, the diagnostic laparoscope with operating instruments passed through a second trocar, or both the operating laparoscope and secondary puncture equipment. All can be used with the "open" laparoscopic technique in which the laparoscopic instrument is placed into the abdominal cavity under direct vision to avoid the risk of bowel or blood vessel puncture on blind entry. Patient acceptance and recovery are approximately the same with all methods.

It is now apparent that the long-term failure rates for all methods are higher than previous estimates; overall, 1.85% of sterilized American women experience a failure within 10 years.[29] As much as one-third of these failures are ectopic pregnancies.[22] The higher failure rates with silastic rings, clips, and bipolar coagulation reflect the greater degree of skill required for these methods. Because of the effect of declining fecundity with increasing age, younger sterilized women are more likely to have a failure, including ectopic pregnancy, compared with older women. For these reasons, younger women seeking sterilization should consider the use of the IUD or implants, reversible methods that offer very low failure rates.

Tubal Occlusion by Electrosurgical Methods

If electrons from an electrosurgical generator are concentrated in one location, heat within the tissue increases sharply and desiccates the tissue until resistance is so high that no more current can pass. Unipolar methods of sterilization create a dense area of current under the grasping forceps of the unipolar electrode. To complete the circuit, however, these electrons must

Female Tubal Sterilization Methods
Ten-Year Cumulative Failure Rates [29]

Unipolar coagulation	0.75%
Postpartum tubal excision	0.75%
Silastic (Falope or Yoon) ring	1.77%
Interval tubal excision	2.01%
Bipolar coagulation	2.48%
Hulka-Clemens clip	3.65%

Life Table Cumulative Probability of Pregnancy [29]

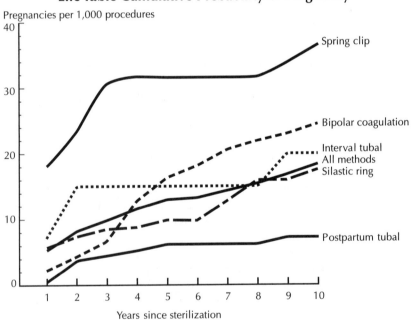

spread through the body and be returned to the generator via a return electrode (the ground plate) that has a broad surface to minimize the density of the current to avoid burns as the electrons leave the body. "Unipolar" refers to the method that requires the patient ground plate.

With the unipolar method, if tissue resistance is high and the electrical pressure (voltage) relatively low, current may cease to flow or may search out alternate pathways with lower resistance. When the voltage is increased, the electrons have more "push" to find another pathway; therefore, the surgeon must use the lowest possible voltage necessary to completely coagulate. The return electrode must be in good contact with the patient.

Unipolar electrosurgery can create a unique electrical "capacitance" problem. A capacitor is any device that can hold an electric charge and can exist wherever an insulated material separates two conductors that have different potentials. This property of capacitance explains some of the inadvertent bowel burns that have occurred with laparoscopic sterilization.[30] The operating laparoscope is a hollow metal tube surrounding an active electrode, the forceps used to grasp and coagulate the tubes. When current passes through the active electrode, the laparoscope itself becomes a capacitor. Up to 70% of the current passed through the active electrode can be induced into the laparoscope. If bowel or other structures touch a laparoscope, which is insulated from the abdominal incision (e.g., by a fiberglass cannula), the stored electrons are discharged at high density directly into the vital organ. This potential hazard is eliminated by using a metal trocar sleeve rather than a nonconductive sleeve such as fiberglass. Because there is little pressure behind the electrons from a low-voltage generator, not enough heat is generated to burn the skin as the capacitance current leaks out into the patient's body through the metal sleeve. Even if the active electrode comes in direct contact with the laparoscope, as when a two-incision technique is used, the current leaks harmlessly through the metal trocar sleeve. The risk of inadvertent coagulation of bowel or other organs cannot be completely eliminated because all body surfaces offer a path back to the ground plate.

The unipolar electrosurgical technique is straightforward. The isthmic portion of the fallopian tube is grasped and elevated away from the surrounding structures, and the electrical energy is applied until the tissue blanches, swells, and then collapses. The tube is then grasped, moving toward the uterus, recoagulated, and the steps repeated until 2–3 cm of tube have been coagulated. Some surgeons advise against cornual coagulation for fear it may increase the risk of ectopic pregnancy due to fistula formation.

The coagulation and transection technique is performed in a similar fashion with the same instruments. To transect the tube, however, an instrument designed to cut tissue must be used. The transection of tissue increases the risk of possible bleeding and does not, by itself, reduce the failure rate over coagulation alone. The specimens obtained by this method are usually coagulated beyond microscopic recognition and, therefore, do not provide pathologic evidence of successful sterilization.

The bipolar method of sterilization eliminates the ground plate required for unipolar electrosurgery and uses a specially designed forceps. One jaw of the forceps is the active electrode, and the other jaw is the ground electrode. Current density is great at the point of forceps contact with tissue, and the use of a low-voltage, high-frequency current prevents the spread of electrons. By eliminating the return electrode, the chance of an aberrant pathway through bowel or other structures is greatly reduced. There is, however, a disadvantage with this technique. Because electron spread is decreased, more applications of the grasping forceps are necessary to coagulate the same length of tube than with unipolar coagulation. As desiccation occurs at the point of high current density, tissue resistance increases, and the coagulated area eventually provides resistance to flow of the low-voltage current. Should the resistance increase beyond the voltage's capability to push electrons through the tissue, incomplete coagulation of the endosalpinx can result.[31] Bipolar coagulation is very effective only if 3 or more sites are coagulated on each tube.[32]

Bipolar cautery is safer than unipolar cautery with regard to burns of abdominal organs, but most studies indicate higher failure rates. Although the bipolar forceps do not burn tissues that are not actually grasped, care must be taken to avoid coagulating structures adherent to the tubes. For example, the ureter can be damaged when the tube is adherent to the pelvic side wall.

The bipolar method can be used with either a single-port operating laparoscope or with dual-port instruments. The forceps are, however, more delicate than unipolar equipment and must be kept meticulously clean. Damage to the instruments can alter the ability to coagulate, and inadequate or incomplete electrocoagulation is the main cause of failure. The bipolar forceps must be used with an amp meter so that accurate current flow can be confirmed.

Tubal Occlusion with Clips and Rings

Female sterilization by mechanical occlusion eliminates the safety concerns with electrosurgery. However, mechanical devices are subject to flaws in material, defects in manufacturing, and errors in design, all of which can alter efficacy. Three mechanical devices have been widely used and have low failure rates with long-term follow-up: the Hulka-Clemens (spring) clip, the Filshie Clip, and the silastic (Falope or Yoon) ring. Each of the three requires an understanding of its mechanical function, a working knowledge of the intricate applicator necessary to apply the device, meticulous attention to maintenance of the applicators, and skillful tubal placement. These devices are less effective when used immediately postpartum on dilated tubes.

Hulka-Clemens Spring Clip. The spring clip consists of two plastic jaws made of Lexan, hinged by a small metal pin 2 mm from one end. Each jaw has teeth on the opposed surface, and a stainless steel spring is pushed over the jaws to hold them closed over the tube. A special laparoscope for one-incision application is most commonly used, although the spring clip can also be used in a two-incision procedure. The spring clip is applied at a 90-degree angle to include some mesosalpinx at the proximal isthmus of a stretched fallopian tube. The spring clip destroys 3 mm of tube and has 1-year pregnancy rates of 2 per 1,000 women but the highest 10-year cumulative failure rate.[15, 29]

Complications unique to spring clip sterilization result from mechanical difficulties. If the clip is dislodged or dropped into the abdomen during the procedure, it should be retrieved. Usually, it can be removed laparoscopically, but sometimes laparotomy is necessary. Should incomplete occlusion or incorrect alignment of the clip occur, a second clip can be applied without hazard. This clip offers a good chance for reanastomosis, better than electrosurgical methods that destroy more tube.

The Hulka-Clemens Spring Clip

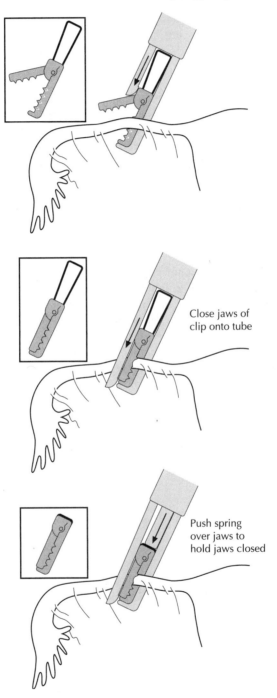

Close jaws of
clip onto tube

Push spring
over jaws to
hold jaws closed

The Filshie Clip

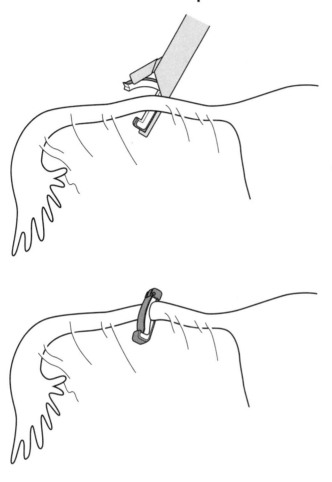

Filshie Clip. The Filshie clip is made of titanium lined with silicone rubber. The hinged clip is locked over the tube using a special applicator through a second incision or operating laparoscope. The rubber lining of the clip expands on compression to keep the tube blocked. Only 4 mm of the tube is destroyed. Failure rates 1 year after the procedure approximate 1 per 1,000 women.[20] Because the Filshie clip is longer, it is reported to occlude dilated tubes more readily than does the spring clip. Both the spring clip and the Filshie clip provide good chances for tubal reanastomosis.

The Silastic (Falope or Yoon) Ring

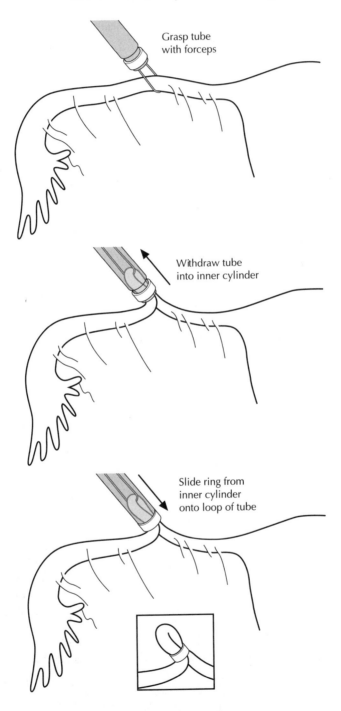

Grasp tube with forceps

Withdraw tube into inner cylinder

Slide ring from inner cylinder onto loop of tube

Silastic (Falope or Yoon) Ring. This nonreactive silastic rubber band has an elastic memory of 100% if stretched to no more than 6 mm for a brief time (a few minutes at most). A special applicator, 6 mm in diameter, can be placed through a second cannula or through a standard offset operating laparoscope. The applicator is designed to grasp a knuckle of tube and release the silastic band onto a 2.5 cm loop of tube. The avascular loop of tube can be resected with biopsy forceps to provide a pathology specimen, but this is rarely performed (it does not increase efficacy). Ten percent to 15% of patients experience severe postoperative pelvic cramping from the tight bands (which can be alleviated by the application of a local anesthetic to the tube before or after banding).

Mesosalpingeal bleeding is the most common complication of silastic ring application. It usually occurs when the forceps grab not only the tube but also a vascular fold of mesosalpinx. The mesosalpinx can also be torn on the edge of the stainless steel cylinder as the tube is drawn into the applicator. If bleeding is noted, application of the silastic band often controls it. If the placement of additional bands or electrocoagulation fails to stop bleeding, laparotomy may be required.

Silastic rings are occasionally placed on structures other than the tube. If this mistake is recognized, the band can usually be removed from the round ligament or mesosalpingeal folds by grasping the band with the tongs of the applicator and applying gradual, increasing traction. If a gentle attempt fails, removal is not necessary. If rings are inadvertently discharged into the peritoneal cavity, they can safely be left behind.

The ring applicator consists of two concentric cylinders. Within the inner cylinder is a forceps for grasping, elevating, and retracting a segment of the tube. The silastic ring is stretched around the exposed end of the inner cylinder by means of a special ring loader and ring guide. The outer cylinder moves the ring from the inner cylinder on to the tube, a loop of which is held within the inner cylinder by the forceps.

As with application of clips, the ring should be placed at the junction of the proximal and middle third of each fallopian tube. Once the tube is grasped, it is gently withdrawn into the inner cylinder by slowly squeezing the pistol-like handle of the applicator. A final strong pull is needed to slide the ring from the inner applicator cylinder onto the loop of tube. Necrosis occurs promptly and a 2–3 cm segment of the tube is destroyed. Failure rates are about 1% after 2 years, and the 10-year cumulative rate is only better with unipolar coagulation and postpartum tubal excision.[29]

Patients should be prepared for the use of electrosurgical instruments in case bands or clips cannot be applied (because of adhesions or bleeding). However, rings or clips are preferable to coagulation for sterilization under local anesthesia.[33]

Minilaparotomy

Tubal ligation, accomplished through a small suprapubic incision, minilaparotomy, is the most common method of interval female sterilization around the world. In the United States and most of the developed world, laparoscopy is more popular, but minilaparotomy is gaining in favor because of its safety, simplicity, and adaptability to ambulatory surgical settings (particularly when local anesthesia is used).[34, 35]

The fallopian tubes can be occluded through the minilaparotomy incision with bands or clips, but a simple Pomeroy tubal ligation is the method most commonly used. Patient characteristics, such as obesity, previous pelvic infection, or previous surgery, are the principal determinants of complications.[36]

Minilaparotomy is accomplished through an incision that usually measures 2–4 cm in length. Tubal ligation through a suprapubic incision can be accomplished for obese patients, but the incision necessarily exceeds the usual length. Forceful retraction increases the pain associated with the procedure and the time of recovery. For these reasons, we believe that minilaparotomy for ambulatory tubal occlusion should be limited to patients who are not obese (usually less than 150–160 pounds, 70 kg).

Tubal occlusion is difficult to accomplish through a minilaparotomy if the uterus is immobile. Laparoscopic tubal occlusion, on the other hand, does not require extreme uterine elevation or rotation and is a better choice for a patient with a uterus fixed in position.

Patients who are likely to have adhesions from previous surgery or pelvic infection probably have a shorter operating and recovery time (and less pain) with open laparoscopic tubal occlusion. In addition, the wide view provided by the laparoscope makes possible a precise description of the pelvic abnormalities that may be useful should the patient develop chronic pelvic pain or recurrent infection.

The Transcervical Approach

Essure is a coil device with polyester fibers, which when placed hysteroscopically within the proximal segments of the fallopian tubes, spanning the uterotubal junction, expands when released, anchoring itself in place. The device stimulates a tissue reaction, which is fibrotic and occlusive.

After backup contraception for 3 months, a hysterosalpingogram is performed to confirm occlusion. Short-term pregnancy rates (several years) have been comparable to other methods of sterilization.[37] Effective permanent sterilization is achieved in about 85–90% of women.[38] The procedure is quick, performed in the outpatient setting, often without analgesia.

The Vaginal Approach

Although vaginal techniques are still used for tubal sterilization, high rates of infection and occasional pelvic abscesses following these operations have caused most clinicians to abandon them.[23] An apparent advantage in obese patients is sometimes deceptive because omental fat can block access to the fallopian tubes. Open laparoscopy is usually easier and safer in obese women.

Counseling for Sterilization

All patients undergoing a surgical procedure for permanent contraception should be aware of the nature of the operation, its alternatives, efficacy, safety, and complications. The operation can be described using drawings or pelvic models, films, slides, or videotapes. The description of the operation should emphasize its similarities to and differences from laparoscopy and pelvic surgery, especially hysterectomy or ovariectomy that may be confused with simple tubal ligation. Women who undergo tubal sterilization by any method are 4–5-fold more likely to have a hysterectomy; no biologic explanation is apparent, and this may reflect patient attitudes toward surgical procedures.[39] Alternatives, including vasectomy, oral contraception, long-acting hormone methods, barrier methods, and IUDs, should be reviewed. It is important to emphasize to the patient that tubal ligation is not intended to be reversible, that it cannot be guaranteed to prevent intrauterine or ectopic pregnancy, and that failures can occur long after the sterilization procedure. Informed consent is best obtained at a time when a patient is not distracted or distraught; e.g., not immediately before or after an induced abortion.

Sexuality. There is no detrimental effect on sexuality specifically due to sterilization procedures.[40, 41] Indeed, sexual life is usually positively affected. Many couples are less inhibited and more spontaneous in lovemaking when they do not have to worry about an unwanted pregnancy.

Menstrual Function. The effects of tubal sterilization on menstrual function have been confusing and, therefore, difficult to explain. The first well-controlled studies of this issue demonstrated no change in menstrual patterns, volume, or pain.[42, 43] Subsequently these same authors reported an increase in dysmenorrhea and changes in menstrual bleeding.[44, 45] However, these authors failed to agree in their findings (a change found by one group

377

was not confirmed by the other). Adding to the confusion, the incidence of hysterectomy for bleeding disorders in women after tubal sterilization was reported to be increased by some,[46] but not by others.[47] In a large cohort of women in a group health plan, hospitalization for menstrual disorders was significantly increased; however, the authors believed this reflected bias by patient and physician preference for surgical treatment.[48] In the U.S. prospective long-term follow-up study of sterilization, the increased risk of hysterectomy after sterilization was concentrated in women who were treated for gynecologic disorders before tubal sterilization.[39] These discordant reports do not make patient counseling about the long-term effects of tubal sterilization an easy task.

It was initially speculated that extensive electrocoagulation of the fallopian tubes can cause ovarian tissue damage, changing ovarian steroid production. This was suggested as the reason why menstrual changes were detected with longer (4 years) follow-up, whereas no changes have been noted with the use of rings or clips.[48-50] However, attempts to relate post-sterilization menstrual changes with extent of tissue destruction fail to find a correlation, and an increase in hospitalization for menstrual disorders after unipolar cautery cannot be documented.[48, 50] A long-term follow-up study (3-4.5 years) failed to document any significant changes in menstrual cycles.[51] Another 5-year follow-up study of sterilization by bipolar coagulation could detect no changes in day 3 measures of ovarian reserve (gonadotropins, estradiol, and inhibin).[52]

The U.S. Collaborative Review of Sterilization, the largest and most comprehensive assessment of sterilization, could find no evidence that tubal sterilization is followed at 2 years and again at 5 years by a greater incidence of menstrual changes or abnormalities.[50, 53] *The best current information to provide patients is that the evidence indicates that tubal sterilization does not cause menstrual abnormalities.*

Reversibility. An important objective of counseling is to help couples make the right decision about an irreversible decision to become sterile. The active participation of both partners is a critical factor.[54] Not all couples are pleased following sterilization; in one series, 2% of U.S. women expressed regret 1 year later and 2.7% after 2 years.[55] At the 2-year mark, the main factors associated with regret were age under 30 and sterilization at the convenient time of a cesarean section. In a long-term follow-up study of U.S. women, women younger than the age of 30 at the time of sterilization were most likely to express regret, but no differences were observed comparing timing after cesarean delivery, vaginal delivery, or a year later.[56] In the 1995 National Survey of Family Growth, nearly 25% of U.S. women with a tubal ligation expressed a desire for reversal, by either one of the partners or both.[57] The U.S. Collaborative Review of

Sterilization reported that only 14.3% requested reversal information after 14 years of follow-up, but the percentage was nearly 4 times higher in women aged 18 to 24 at sterilization.[58] Overall, however, only 1.1% of women obtained reversal. In Canada, 1% of men and women obtained a reversal within 5 years after sterilization; in the United States reversal within 5 years was obtained by 0.2% of women and 0.4% of men, a difference that could reflect the lack of insurance coverage for this procedure in the United States.[59, 60]

In Europe where tubal sterilization is less common, the most important risk factor for regret was an unstable marriage.[61] A change in marital status is undoubtedly also an important reason for a desire to reverse sterilization.[62]

Young couples in unstable relationships need special attention in counseling. Furthermore, for many couples tubal occlusion at the time of cesarean section or immediately after a difficult labor and delivery is not the best time for the procedure. Sterilized women have not been observed to develop psychological problems at a greater than expected rate.[63, 64]

Microsurgery for tubal reanastomosis is associated with excellent results if only a small segment of the tube has been damaged. Pregnancy rates correlate with the length of remaining tube; a length of 4 cm or more is optimal. Thus, the pregnancy rates are lowest with electrocoagulation and reach 70–80% with clips, rings, and surgical methods such as the Pomeroy.[65, 66] About 2 per 1,000 sterilized women eventually undergo tubal reanastomosis.[62]

Male Sterilization: Vasectomy

Vasectomy is safer, easier, less expensive, and has a lower failure rate than female sterilization.[67] In the U.S. Collaborative Review of Sterilization, there were 6 pregnancies that occurred from 6 to 72 weeks after vasectomy.[68] This gave a failure rate equivalent to female sterilization, about 9 pregnancies per 1,000 procedures after 1 year, but half of the failures occurred within the first 3 months, a period when a backup method is strongly recommended. The absence of sperm should be documented (beginning 3 months after the procedure) before a couple can be reassured that reliable contraception is in place.

The operation is almost always performed under local anesthesia, usually by a urologist in a private office.[69] Surgeons who do more than 10 operations yearly have lower complication rates.[70]

379

Hematomas and infection occur rarely and are easily treated with heat, scrotal support, and antibiotics. Most men develop sperm antibodies following vasectomy, but no long-term sequelae have been observed, including no increased risk of cardiovascular disease.[12, 71, 72] Adverse psychological and sexual effects have not been reported. Because the other constituents of semen are made downstream from the testes, men do not notice a decreased volume or velocity of ejaculate.

Prostate cancer is the most frequent cancer among men, with a lifetime risk of 1 in 8 in the United States. An increased risk of prostate cancer after vasectomy has been reported in several cohort and case-control studies.[73-76] However, there is disagreement because other studies could not support an association between prostate or testicular cancer risk and vasectomy.[77-80] In a very large mixed racial/ethnic (black and white; Chinese-Americans and Japanese-Americans) case-control study of prostate cancer, no statistically significant increase in risk could be identified after vasectomy, including no effect of age at vasectomy or years since vasectomy.[81] Reviews of 6 cohort studies and 5 case-control studies concluded that there is no increased risk of cancer of the testis following vasectomy, and consideration of the studies examining the possible association between prostate cancer and vasectomy (6 cohort and 7 case-control studies), found the evidence to be equivocal and weak.[82, 83] A meta-analysis of the literature concluded that there is no increased risk of prostate cancer in men who have undergone vasectomy.[84] A case-control study from New Zealand found no increase in prostate cancer even after more than 25 years since the vasectomy.[85] Observational studies cannot totally avoid potential biases, and the disagreement regarding prostate cancer is consistent with either no effect or an effect too small to escape confounding biases. It is worth noting that the countries with the highest vasectomy rates (China and India) do not have the highest rates of prostate cancer. Screening for prostate cancer should be no different in men who have had a vasectomy.

Animal studies had indicated that vasectomy accelerates the process of atherosclerosis. In the U.S. Physicians' Heath Study (a large prospective cohort study), no increase in the risk of subsequent cardiovascular disease could be detected following vasectomy.[72] Indeed, vasectomy has not been demonstrated to have any adverse consequences or harmful effects on men's health.[11, 12]

Vasectomy does not change the secretion of human immunodeficiency virus (HIV) into semen, and vasectomy should not change the risk of HIV transmission.[86]

Vasectomy Methods

Providers of vasectomy worldwide have adopted the "no scalpel" technique perfected over the past 30 years by Li Shunqiang in Sichuan Province of China.[89] This approach is faster, less invasive, and requires only a few simple instruments.[90] In a 1-day comparison in Bangkok, 680 vasectomies were performed using the no scalpel method with 3 complications, and 523 vasectomies were performed with a standard technique with 16 complications.[91] The method is no easier to reverse than other vasectomies. A video tape and instruments for this method can be obtained from AVSC International, 440 Ninth Avenue, New York, NY 10001.

Reversibility

Vasectomy reversal is associated with pregnancy rates greater than 50%.[87, 88] The prospect for pregnancy diminishes with time elapsed from vasectomy, decreasing significantly to 30% after 10 years; the best results are achieved when reversal is performed within 3 years after vasectomy. In most cases, sperm can be collected at the time of the reversal procedure and frozen for future intracytoplasmic sperm injection in case of reversal failure.[92]

Medical Methods for the Male

A reversible method of contraception for men has been sought for years. Hormonal contraception for men is inherently a difficult physiologic problem because, unlike cyclic ovulation in women, spermatogenesis is continuous, dependent upon gonadotropins and high levels of intratesticular testosterone.[93] Investigational approaches to inhibit production of sperm include the administration of sex steroids, the use of gonadotropin-releasing hormone (GnRH) analogs, and the administration of gossypol, a derivative of cottonseed oil.[94, 95]

The sex steroids reduce testosterone synthesis, which leads to loss of libido and development of female secondary sexual characteristics. Furthermore, despite the use of large doses, sperm counts are not adequately reduced in all subjects. Levonorgestrel, cyproterone acetate, and medroxyprogesterone acetate all have been studied combined with testosterone, given intramuscularly to provide the desired systemic androgen effects. GnRH analogs also decrease the endogenous synthesis of testosterone, and supplemental testosterone must be provided. The overall metabolic and health consequences of these approaches have not been assessed, and frequent injections are required.

381

Gossypol effectively decreases sperm counts to contraceptive levels, apparently by incapacitating the sperm producing cells. Experience in China revealed that a substantial number of men remain sterile after exposure to gossypol, and animal studies in the United States indicated that gossypol, or contaminants of the preparation, were toxic; work on gossypol was discontinued.[96] Analogs of gossypol may offer potential but are years away from development.

Future Developments with Sterilization

Although current methods of sterilization are safe and effective, they require skillful surgeons and, in the case of laparoscopic operations, elaborate and expensive equipment. Simpler approaches could make sterilization available and acceptable to more people. Female transcervical methods have used electrocoagulation, cryosurgery, or laser to destroy the interstitial portion of the tube, to inject sclerosing agents or tissue adhesives through the tubal ostia, and to mechanically obstruct the tubal lumen. Most of these methods, and the formed-in-place silicone plugs applied either hysteroscopically or with the "Femcept" intrauterine device, are either too complicated or have high failure rates. The most practical approach is the application of sclerosing agents to the tubal openings using cannulae or an IUD. Transcervical insertion of quinicrine pellets during the proliferative phase of the menstrual cycle occludes the tubes and is the most promising of the "nonsurgical" approaches, but long-term safety and efficacy have not been assessed.[97]

Excellent Web Site for Sterilization (and Contraception)

AVSC International: http://www.avsc.org

References

1. **Mosher WD, Martinez GM, Chandra A, Abma JC, Willson SJ,** Use of contrception and use of family planning services in the United States: 1982–2002, Advance Data from Vital and Health Statistics, No. 350, December 10, 2004.

2. **Murphy M,** Sterilisation as a method of contraception: recent trends in Great Britain and their implications, J Biosoc Sci 27:31, 1995.

3. **Riphagen FE, Fortney JA, Koelb S,** Contraception in women over forty, J Biosoc Sci 20:127, 1988.

4. **Speert H,** Obstetric & Gynecologic Milestones Illustrated, The Parthenon Publishing Group, New York, 1996.

5. **Lungren SS,** A case of cesarean section twice successfully performed on the same patient, with remarks on the time, indications, and details of the operation, Am J Obstet 14:78, 1881.

6. **Baird D,** The Fifth Freedom, Br Med J i:234, 1966.

7. **Centers for Disease Control and Prevention,** Surgical sterilization surveillance: tubal sterilization 1976–1978, U.S. Department of Health and Human Services, Public Health Service, 1981.

8. **Layde PM, Ory HW, Peterson HB, Scally MJ, Greenspan JR, Smith JC, Fleming D,** The declining lengths of hospitalization for tubal sterilizations, JAMA 245:714, 1981.

9. **Escobedo LG, Peterson HB, Grubb GS, Franks AL,** Case fatality rates for tubal sterilization in U.S. hospitals, Am J Obstet Gynecol 160:147, 1989.

10. **U.S. National Center for Health Statistics,** Vital Statistics of the United States, www.cdc.gov/nchs/, 2003.

11. **Peterson HB, Huber DH, Belker AM,** Vasectomy: an appraisal for the obstetrician-gynecologist, Obstet Gynecol 76:568, 1990.

12. **Giovannucci E, Tosteson TD, Speizer FE, Vessey MP, Colditz GA,** A long-term study of mortality in men who have undergone vasectomy, New Engl J Med 326:1392, 1992.

13. **Cortes M, Flick A, Barone MA, Amatya R, Pollack AE, Otero-Flores J, Juarez C, McMullen S,** Results of a pilot study of the time to azoospermia after vasectomy in Mexico City, Contraception 56:215, 1997.

14. **Trussell J, Hatcher RA, Cates Jr W, Stewart FH, Kost K,** Contraceptive failure in the United States: an update, Stud Fam Plann 21:51, 1990.

15. **Chi I-c, Laufe L, Gardner SD, Tolbert M,** An epidemiologic study of risk factors associated with pregnancy following female sterilizations, Am J Obstet Gynecol 136:768, 1980.

16. **Cheng M, Wong YM, Rochat R, Ratnam SS,** Sterilization failures in Singapore: An examination of ligation techniques and failure rates, Stud Fam Plann 8:109, 1977.

17. **Lichterg E, Laff S, Friedman E,** Value of routine dilatation and curretage at the time of interval sterilization, Obstet Gynecol 67:763, 1986.

18. **WHO Special Programme of Research, Development and Research Training in Human Reproduction, Task Force on Intrauterine Devices for Fertility Regulation,** A multinational case-control study of ectopic pregnancy, Clin Reprod Fertil 3:131, 1985.

19. **Holt V, Chu J, Daling JR, Stergachis AS, Weiss NS,** Tubal sterilization and subsequent ectopic pregnancy, JAMA 266:242, 1991.

20. **Chick PH, Frances M, Paterson PJ,** A comprehensive review of female sterilisation tubal occlusion methods, Clin Reprod Fertil 3:81, 1985.

21. **McCausland A,** High rate of ectopic pregnancy following laparoscopic tubal coagulation failure, Am J Obstet Gynecol 136:977, 1980.

22. **Peterson HB, Xia Z, Hughes JM, Wilcox LS, Tylor LR, Trussell J, for the U.S. Collaborative Review of Sterilization Working Group,** The risk of ectopic pregnancy after tubal sterilization, New Engl J Med 336:762, 1997.

23. **Miesfeld R, Gaarontans R, Moyers T,** Vaginal tubal sterilization. Is infection a significant risk? Am J Obstet Gynecol 137:183, 1980.

24. **Hankinson SE, Hunter DJ, Colditz GA, Willett WC, Stampfer MJ, Rosner B, Hennekens CH, Speizer FE,** Tubal sterilization, hysterectomy, and risk of ovarian cancer. A prospective study, JAMA 270:2813, 1993.

25. **Miracle-McMahill HL, Calle EE, Kosinski AS, Rodriguez C, Wingo PA, Thun MJ, Heath CW, Jr.,** Tubal ligation and fatal ovarian cancer in a large prospective cohort study, Am J Epidemiol 145:349, 1997.

26. **Mori M, Harabuchi I, Miyake H, Casagrande JT, Henderson BE, Ross RK,** Reproductive, genetic, and dietary risk factors for ovarian cancer, Am J Epidemiol 128:771, 1988.

27. **Irwin KL, Weiss NS, Lee NC, Peterson HB,** Tubal sterilization, hysterectomy, and the subsequent occurrence of epithelial ovarian cancer, Am J Epidemiol 134:362, 1991.

28. **Whittemore AS, Harris R, Itnyre J, and the Collaborative Ovarian Cancer Group,** Characteristics relating to ovarian cancer risk: collaborative analysis of 12 US case-control studies. II: Invasive epithelial ovarian cancers in white women, Am J Epidemiol 136:1184, 1992.

29. **Peterson HB, Xia Z, Hughes JM, Wilcox LS, Tylor LR, Trussell J, for the U.S. Collaborative Review of Sterilization Working Group,** The risk of pregnancy after tubal sterilization: findings from the U.S. Collaborative Review of Sterilization, Am J Obstet Gynecol 174:1161, 1996.

30. **Centers for Disease Control and Prevention,** Deaths following female sterilization with unipolar electrocoagulating devices, MMWR 30:150, 1981.

31. **Soderstrom RM, Levy BS, Engel T,** Reducing bipolar sterilization failures, Obstet Gynecol 74:60, 1989.

32. **Peterson HB, Xia Z, Wilcox LS, Tylor LR, Trussell J, for the U.S. Collaborative Review of Sterilization Working Group,** Pregnancy after tubal sterilization with bipolar electrocoagulation, Obstet Gynecol 94:163, 1999.

33. **Lipscomb GH, Stovall TG, Ramanathan JA, Ling FW,** Comparison of silastic rings and electrocoagulation for laparoscopic tubal ligation under local anesthesia, Obstet Gynecol 80:645, 1992.

34. **McCann M, Cole L,** Laparoscopy and minilaparotomy: two major advances in female sterilization, Stud Fam Plann 11:119, 1980.

35. **Ruminjo JK, Lynam PF,** A fifteen-year review of female sterilization by minilaparotomy under local anesthesia in Kenya, Contraception 55:249, 1997.

36. **Layde PM, Peterson HB, Dicker RC, DeStefano F, Ruben GL, Ory HW,** Risk factors for complications of interval tubal sterilization by laparotomy, Obstet Gynecol 62:180, 1983.

37. **Kerin JF, Cooper JM, Price T, Herendael BJ, Cayuela-Font E, Cher D, Carignan CS,** Hysteroscopic sterilization using a micro-insert device: results of a multicentre Phase II study, Hum Reprod 18:1223, 2003.

38. **Cooper JM, Carignan CS, Cher D, Kerin JF, Group STOPI,** Microinsert nonincisional hysteroscopic sterilization, Obstet Gynecol 102:59, 2003.

39. **Hillis SD, Marchbanks PA, Tylor LR, Peterson HB, for the U.S. Collaborative Review of Sterilization Working Group,** Higher hysterectomy risk for sterilized than nonsterilized women: findings from the U.S. Collaborative Review of Sterilization, Obstet Gynecol 91:241, 1998.

40. **Kjer J,** Sexual adjustment to tubal sterilization, Eur J Obstet Gynecol 35:211, 1990.

41. **Costello C, Hillis SD, Marchbanks PA, Jamieson DJ, Peterson HB,** US Collaborative Review of Sterilization Working Group, The effect of interval tubal sterilization on sexual interest and pleasure, Obstet Gynecol 100:511, 2002.

42. **Rulin MC, Turner JH, Dunworth R, Thompson D,** Post tubal sterilization syndrome: a misnomer, Obstet Gynecol 151:13, 1985.

43. **DeStefano F, Huezo CM, Peterson HB, Rubin GL, Layde PM, Ory HW,** Menstrual changes after tubal sterilization, Obstet Gynecol 62:673, 1983.

44. **Rulin MC, Davidson AR, Philliber SG, Graves WL, Cushman LF,** Changes in menstrual symptoms among sterilized and comparison women: a prospective study, Obstet Gynecol 79:749, 1989.

45. **DeStefano F, Perlman J, Peterson HB, Diamond E,** Long-term risk of menstrual disturbances after tubal sterilization, Am J Obstet Gynecol 152:835, 1985.

46. **Kjer J, Knudsen L,** Hysterectomy subsequent to laparoscopic sterilization, Eur J Obstet Gynecol 35:63, 1990.

47. **Stergachis A, Shy KK, Gouthaus LC, Wagner EH, Hecht JA, Anderson G, Normand EH, Raboud J,** Tubal sterilization and the long-term risk of hysterectomy, JAMA 264:2893, 1990.

48. **Shy KK, Stergachis A, Grothaus LG, Wagner EH, Hecht J, Anderson G,** Tubal sterilization and risk of subsequent hospital admission for menstrual disorders, Am J Obstet Gynecol 166:1698, 1992.

49. **Thranov I, Hertz JB, Kjer JJ, Andresen A, Micic S, Nielsen J, Hancke S,** Hormonal and menstrual changes after laparoscopic sterilization by Falope-rings or Filshie-clips, Fertil Steril 57:751, 1992.

50. **Wilcox LS, Martinez-Schnell B, Peterson HB, Ware JH, Hughes JM,** Menstrual function after tubal sterilization, Am J Epidemiol 135:1368, 1992.

51. **Rulin MC, Davidson AR, Philliber SG, Graves WL, Cushman LF,** Long-term effect of tubal sterilization on menstrual indices and pelvic pain, Obstet Gynecol 82:118, 1993.

52. **Carmona F, Cristóbal P, Casamitjana R, Balasch J,** Effect of tubal sterilization on ovarian follicular reserve and function, Am J Obstet Gynecol 189:447, 2003.

53. **Peterson HB, Jeng G, Folger SG, Hillis SA, Marchbanks PA, Wilcox LS, for the U.S. Collaborative Review of Sterilization Working Group,** The risk of menstrual abnormalities after tubal sterilization. U.S. Collaborative Review of Sterilization Working Group, New Engl J Med 343:1724, 2000.

54. **Miller WB, Shain RN, Pasta DJ,** Tubal sterilization or vasectomy: how do married couples make the decision? Fertil Steril 56:278, 1991.

55. **Grubb G, Refoser H, Layde PM, Rubin GL,** Regret after decision to have a tubal sterilization, Fertil Steril 44:248, 1985.

56. **Hillis SD, Marchbanks PA, Tylor LR, Peterson HB,** Poststerilization regret: findings from the United States Collaborative Review of Sterilization, Obstet Gynecol 93:889, 1999.

57. **Chandra A,** Surgical Sterilization in the United States: Prevalence and Characteristics, 1965–95, National Center for Health Statistics, Vital and Health Statistics, Series 23: No. 20, Hyattsville, Maryland, 1998.

58. **Schmidt JE, Hillis SD, Marchbanks PA, Jeng G, Peterson HB,** Requesting information about and obtaining reversal after tubal sterilization: findings from the U.S. Collaborative Review of Sterilization, Fertil Steril 74:892, 2000.

59. **Trussell J, Guilbert E, Hedley A,** Sterilization failure, sterilization reversal, and pregnancy after sterilization reversal in Quebec, Obstet Gynecol 101:677, 2003.

60. **Jamieson DJ, Kaufman SC, Cosstello C, Hillis SD, Marchbanks PA, Peterson HB,** US Collaborative Review of Sterilization Working Group, A comparison of women's regret after vasectomy versus tubal sterilization, Obstet Gynecol 99:1073, 2002.

61. **Vemer HM, Colla P, Schoot DC, Willensen WN, Bierkens PB, Rolland R,** Women regretting their sterilization, Fertil Steril 46:724, 1986.

62. **Wilcox LS, Chu SY, Peterson HB,** Characteristics of women who considered or obtained tubal reanastomosis: results from a prospective study of tubal sterilization, Obstet Gynecol 75:661, 1990.

63. **Vessey M, Huggins G, Lawless M, McPherson K, Yeates D,** Tubal sterilization: findings in a large prospective study, Br J Obstet Gynaecol 90:203, 1983.

64. **WHO,** Mental health and female sterilization: report of a WHO collaborative study, J Biosoc Sci 16:1, 1984.

65. **Siegler AM, Hulka J, Peretz A,** Reversibility of female sterilization, Fertil Steril 43:499, 1985.

66. **Dubuisson JB, Chapron C, Nos Z, Morice P, Aubriot FX, Garnier P,** Sterilisation reversal: fertility results, Hum Reprod 10:1145, 1995.

67. **Smith GL, Taylor GP, Smith KF,** Comparative risks and costs of male and female sterilization, Am J Public Health 75:370, 1985.

68. **Jamieson DJ, Costello C, Trussell J, Hillis SD, Marchbanks PA, Peterson HB, for the U.S. Collaborative Review of Sterilization Working Group,** The risk of pregnancy after vasectomy, Obstet Gynecol 103:848, 2004.

69. **Marquette CM, Koonin LM, Antarsh L, Gargiullo PM, Smith JC,** Vasectomy in the United States, 1991, Am J Public Health 85:644, 1995.

70. **Kendrick JS, Gonzales B, Huber DH, Grubb GS, Rubin G,** Complications of vasectomies in the United States, J Fam Pract 25:245, 1987.

71. **Schuman LM, Coulson AH, Mandel JS, Massey Jr FJ, O'Fallon WM,** Health status of American men — a study of post-vasectomy sequelae, J Clin Endocrinol 46:697, 1993.

72. **Manson JE, Ridker PM, Spelsberg A, Ajani U, Lotufo PA, Hennekens CH,** Vasectomy and subsequent cardiovascular disease in US physicians, Contraception 59:181, 1999.

73. **Giovanucci E, Ascherio A, Rimm EB, Colditz GA, Stampfer MJ, Willett WC,** A prospective cohort study of vasectomy and prostate cancer in US men, JAMA 269:873, 1993.

74. **Giovanucci E, Tosteson TD, Speizer FE, Ascherio A, Vessey MP, Colditz GA,** A retrospective cohort study of vasectomy and prostate cancer in US men, JAMA 269:878, 1993.

75. **Hayes RB, Pottern LM, Greenberg R, Schoenberg J, Swanson GM, Liff J, Schwartz AG, Brown LM, Hoover RN,** Vasectomy and prostate cancer in US blacks and whites, Am J Epidemiol 137:263, 1993.

76. **Hsing AW, Wang RT, Gu FL, Lee M, Wang T, Leng TJ, Spitz M, Blot WJ,** Vasectomy and prostate cancer risk in China, Cancer Epidemiol Biomark Prev 3:285, 1994.

77. **Sidney S, Quesenberry Jr CP, Sadler MC, Guess HA, Lydick EG, Cattolica EV,** Vasectomy and the risk of prostate cancer in a cohort of multiphasic health-checkup examinees: second report, Cancer Causes Control 2:113, 1991.

78. **Moller H, Knudsen LB, Lynge E,** Risk of testicular cancer after vasectomy: cohort study of over 73,000 men, Br Med J 309:295, 1994.

79. **Rosenberg L, Palmer JR, Zauber AG, Warshauer E, Strom BL, Harlap S, Shapiro S,** The relation of vasectomy to risk of cancer, Am J Epidemiol 140:431, 1994.

80. **Zhu K, Stanford JL, Daling JR, McKnight B, Stergachis A, Brawer MK, Weiss NS,** Vasectomy and prostate cancer: a case-control study in a health maintenance organization, Am J Epidemiol 144:717, 1996.

81. **John EM, Whittemore AS, Wu AH, Kolonel LN, Hislop TG, Howe GR, West DW, Hankin J, Dreon DM, The C-Z, Burch JD, Paffenbarger Jr RS,** Vasectomy and prostate cancer: results from a multiethnic case-control study, J Natl Cancer Inst 87:662, 1995.

82. **Lynge E, Knudsen LB, Müller H,** Vasectomy and testis and prostate cancer, Fertil Control Rev 3:8, 1994.

83. **Healey B,** Does vasectomy cause prostate cancer? JAMA 269:2620, 1993.

84. **Bernal-Delgado E, Latour-Pérez J, Pradas-Arnal F, Gómez-López LI,** The association between vasectomy and prostate cancer: a systematic review of the literature, Fertil Steril 70:191, 1998.

85. **Cox B, Sneyd MJ, Paul C, Delahunt B, Skegg DC,** Vasectomy and risk of prostate cancer, JAMA 287:3110, 2002.

86. **Krieger JN, Nirapathpongporn A, Chaiyaporn M, Peterson G, Nikolaeva I, Akridge R, Ross SO, Coombs RW,** Vasectomy and human immunodeficiency virus type 1 in semen, J Urol 159:820, 1998.

87. **Hendry WF,** Vasectomy and vasectomy reversal, Br J Urol 73:337, 1994.

88. **Belker AM, Thomas AJ, Fuchs EF, Konnak JM, Sharlip ID,** Results of 1,469 microsurgical vasectomy reversals by the vasovasostomy group, J Urol 145:505, 1991.

89. **Li S-Q, Goltein M, Zhu J, Huber DH,** The no scalpel vasectomy, J Urol 145:341, 1991.

90. **Kumar V, Kaza RM, Singh I, Singhal S, Kumaran V,** An evaluation of the no-scalpel vasectomy technique, Br J Urol 83:283, 1999.

91. **Nirapathpongpom A, Huber DH, Krieger JN,** No scalpel vasectomy at the King's birthday vasectomy festival, Lancet 335:894, 1990.

92. **Glazier DB, Marmar JL, Mayer E, Gibbs M, Corson SL,** The fate of cryopreserved sperm acquired during vasectomy reversals, J Urol 161:463, 1999.

93. **Winters SJ, Marshall GR,** Hormonally-based male contraceptives: will they ever be a reality? J Clin Endocrinol Metab 73:464A, 1991.

94. **Waites GMH,** Development of methods of male contraception: impact of the World Health Organization Task Force, Fertil Steril 80:1, 2003.

95. **Wang C, Swerdloff RS,** Male hormonal contraception, Am J Obstet Gynecol 190:S60, 2004.

96. **Waites GMH, Wang C, Griffin PD, Gossypol:** reasons for its failure to be accepted as a safe, reversible male antifertility drug, Int J Androl 21:8, 1998.

97. **Kessel E,** Quinacrine sterilization: an assessment of risks for ectopic pregnancy, birth defects and cancer, Adv Contracep 14:81, 1998.

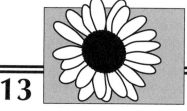

13

Induced Abortion

Contraception is more effective and convenient than ever, but our modern methods are far from perfect. Even the most conscientious couples can experience contraceptive failure. In the past, failure of contraception meant another, sometimes unwanted, birth or recourse to dangerous, secret abortion. The most ancient medical texts indicate that abortion has been practiced for thousands of years. Induced abortion did not become illegal until the 19th century, as a result of changes in the teachings of the Catholic Church (life begins at fertilization) and, in the United States, the efforts of the American Medical Association to have greater regulation of the practice of medicine.

In the 1950s, uterine aspiration led to much safer abortion, and beginning in Asia, induced abortion was gradually legalized in the developed countries of the world. This trend reached the United States from Western Europe in the late 1960s when California, New York, and other states rewrote their abortion laws. The U.S. Supreme Court followed the lead of these states in 1973 in the "Roe versus Wade" decision that limited the circumstances under which "the right of privacy" could be restricted by local abortion laws. By 1980, legal abortion became the most common surgical procedure performed in the United States.

The number of abortions performed in the United States has been decreasing since a peak was reached in 1990, totaling 1.33 million in 1993 and 1.18 million in 1997, with the greatest decline among teenagers.[1-3] This is partly because the number of pregnancies in the United States has been decreasing and the proportion of reproductive-aged women younger than age 30 is also decreasing.[4] Accounting for underreporting, a more accurate

387

estimate indicated about 1.36 million induced abortions in 1996 and 1.31 million in 2000, the lowest number since 1976.[5, 6] The proportion of abortions performed in hospitals has steadily declined, reaching 5% in 2000. The proportion handled by specialized abortion clinics has increased, while the percentage of abortions performed by physicians in their own offices has remained low, about 2% of all abortions.[6, 7] More than 50% of abortions are obtained by women younger than 25 (about 20% under the age of 20), with the rate peaking at ages 18–19, and about 80% are unmarried.[1, 3, 8]

In the United States, the decline in the annual number of induced abortions has been greater than the decline in the annual number of births.[2] Possible explanations include a reduction in unintended pregnancies (better contraception) and a greater willingness to experience a pregnancy; however, another important factor is reduced access to abortion providers (a major problem for women not living in a metropolitan area) and regulatory restrictions in recent years that have created difficulties and obstacles for women seeking services.[6, 7]

American teenagers are especially dependent on abortion compared with their European counterparts who are better educated about sex and use contraception more often and more effectively. In 1996, 20% of women who obtained legal abortions were adolescents.[2] In addition, from ages 20–34, American women have the highest proportion of pregnancies aborted compared with other countries, indicating a high rate of unintended pregnancy occurring beyond the teenage years. The lack of perfect contraception and imperfect use of the available methods keeps abortion with us.

First-Trimester Abortion Procedures

Approximately 90% of the 1.3 million induced abortions performed in the United States yearly are performed during the first-trimester of pregnancy, and a growing percentage are medical abortions.[1, 9] During the first-trimester, abortion morbidity and mortality rates are less than one-tenth those of abortions performed in the later midtrimester.[10] The vast majority of these operations occur in free-standing abortion clinics, although in recent years, physicians have performed larger numbers in their offices where women are less subject to the harassment that has plagued clinics.[1, 5, 6] The safety of outpatient abortion under local anesthesia is well established.

Patient Selection

The care of a patient who has decided to terminate a pregnancy begins with the diagnosis of intrauterine pregnancy and an accurate estimate of gestational age. Failure to accomplish this is the most common source of abortion complications and subsequent litigation. Tests for pregnancy, including vaginal ultrasound, should be used when accuracy is difficult.

Nearly all women who want to terminate a pregnancy in the first-trimester are good candidates for an outpatient procedure under local anesthesia. Possible exceptions include patients with severe cardiorespiratory disease, severe anemias or coagulopathies, mental disorders severe enough to preclude cooperation, and excessive concern about operative pain that is not alleviated by reassurance.

Abortions should not be undertaken for women who have known uterine anomalies or leiomyomas or who have previously had difficult first-trimester abortion procedures, unless ultrasonography is immediately available and the surgeon is experienced in its intraoperative use. Previous cesarean section or other pelvic surgery is not a contraindication to outpatient first-trimester abortion.

Counseling and Informed Consent

Counseling has played a critical role in the development of efficient and acceptable abortion services.[11] Whether abortion is accomplished in a clinic, a physician's office, or a surgical center, the functions of a counselor must be fulfilled to ensure quality patient care. These include help with decision-making, provision of information about the procedure, obtaining informed consent, provision of emotional support for the patient and her family before, during, and after the operation, and providing information about contraception.[12] Referral opportunities should be provided for prenatal care and adoption for women who choose to carry an unplanned pregnancy to term. These responsibilities can be carried out by a physician, nurse, psychologist, social worker, or a trained lay person.

The counselor must be able to make judgments about duration of gestation using the last menstrual period and reports from other clinicians, must be aware of referral opportunities for prenatal care and adoption, must know about the abortion operation itself, must be skilled and sensitive at obtaining informed consent after presenting understandable estimates of risk, must be able to give pre- and postoperative instructions and serve as a contact person for problems that arise during these periods, and must provide realistic information about contraception. Informed consent is important both for the patient's understanding of the risks of first-trimester abortion and for the legal protection of the clinician when outcomes are unsatisfactory.

Each clinic or office should have a first-trimester abortion informed consent document that defines risks such as incomplete abortion, infection, uterine perforation, transfusion, laparotomy, ectopic pregnancy, and failed abortion in terms the patient can understand. Patients should always be asked about their intentions for future child bearing, and the response recorded. The counselor should document that all preoperative responsibilities have been discharged.

Medical Methods for First-Trimester Abortion

Surgical aspiration abortion is safe and effective, but it is not available everywhere, and some women find it difficult to undergo a surgical procedure or to go to a clinic where they may be subject to loss of privacy or harassment. Nonsurgical methods make abortion available to more women and improve the circumstances under which pregnancies are terminated. Medical abortion requires no special training and can be provided by any health care provider. Two medical methods have undergone clinical testing. The progesterone antagonist mifepristone (RU 486) and the antimetabolite methotrexate have both been demonstrated to induce abortion early in pregnancy when combined with a prostaglandin.

France and China were the first countries to approve the marketing of the medical abortifacient mifepristone, a synthetic relative of the progestational agents in oral contraceptives. Mifepristone acts primarily, but not totally, as an antiprogestational agent. Both progesterone and mifepristone form hormone-responsive element-receptor complexes that are similar, but the mifepristone complex has a slightly different conformational change (in the hormone-binding domain) that prevents full gene activation. The agonistic activity of this progestin antagonist is due to its ability to activate certain, but not all, of the transcription activation functions on the progesterone receptor. The dimethyl (dimethylaminophenyl) side chain at carbon 11 is the principal factor in its antiprogesterone action. There are three major characteristics of its action that are important: a long half-life, high affinity for the progesterone receptor, and active metabolites.

It is likely that abortion with mifepristone is the result of multiple actions. Although mifepristone does not induce labor, it does open and soften the cervix (this may be an action secondary to endogenous prostaglandins). Its major action is its blockade of progesterone receptors in the endometrium. This leads to a disruption of the embryo and the production of prostaglandins. The disruption of the embryo and perhaps a direct action on the trophoblast lead to a decrease in human chorionic gonadotropin (hCG) and a withdrawal of support from the corpus luteum. The success rate is dependent on the length of pregnancy—the more dependent the pregnancy is on progesterone from the corpus luteum, the more likely that the progesterone antagonist, mifepristone, results in abortion.

A single 600-mg oral dose of mifepristone has been followed a day later by the administration of a prostaglandin analogue. Several analogues have been used, but the most widely available and best tolerated is misoprostol, 800 μg administered vaginally.[13] The combination allows a reduction in dose of both agents. When administered in the first 8 weeks of pregnancy, this medical termination carries success and complication rates similar to that achieved with vacuum curettage.[14] However, medical abortion is associated with more discomfort and bleeding.[15] Misoprostol is a stable, orally active synthetic analogue of prostaglandin E_1, available commercially for the treatment of peptic ulcer. Combined with mifepristone, it provides an effective, simple, inexpensive, method that can be administered at home.[16–19] In the large U.S. trial of 600 mg mifepristone followed by 400 μg misoprostol orally, there was a 1% failure rate under 7 weeks of pregnancy and 9% from 8 weeks to 9 weeks.[20] Termination occurred in 50% of the women within 4 hours after misoprostol administration and 75% within 24 hours.

Based on worldwide experience, the regimen with the least side effects and cost, but equally good efficacy, is a combination of a lower dose of oral mifepristone (200 mg), followed 24–72 hours later by the vaginal administration of 800 mg misoprostol.[18, 19, 21–24] A randomized, comparison trial demonstrated that the vaginal dose of misoprostol could be self-administered at home 6–8 hours after the mifepristone without any loss of efficacy.[25] The drugs can even be administered simultaneously with only a slight decrease in efficacy.[26] Repeated doses of misoprostol have been recommended for the management of delayed expulsion.

The combined mifepristone-prostaglandin analogue method is usually restricted to pregnancies that are not beyond 9 weeks' gestation. However, a regimen using a higher dose of misoprostol (administered vaginally) achieved a 95% complete abortion rate in women at 9–13 weeks' gestation.[27] Other progesterone antagonists have been developed, but only mifepristone has undergone extensive abortion trials. It seems unlikely that mifepristone could have serious adverse effects, and there have been none reported. As of 2005, there were 3 deaths in the United States associated with mifepristone induced abortions; these deaths have been the consequence of bleeding and infection, not a direct adverse effect of the drug.

Mifepristone is most noted for its abortifacient activity and the political controversy surrounding it. However, the combination of its agonistic and antagonistic actions can be exploited for many uses, including contraception, therapy of endometriosis, induction of labor, treatment of Cushing's syndrome, and, potentially, treatment of various cancers. Doses of 2 to 5 mg per day inhibit ovulation and produce amenorrhea in over 90% of cycles, and in a pilot study of 50 women, there were no pregnancies.[28]

Lack of progesterone antagonists in the United States prompted use of methotrexate as an abortifacient in the same dose used to treat ectopic pregnancy, 50 mg intramuscularly per square meter of body surface area.[29] Later, a single 75-mg intramuscular dose was demonstrated to be as effective.[30] Methotrexate has also been administered orally in doses of 25 or 50 mg.[31] As with mifepristone, a prostaglandin is added to promote expulsion of the uterine contents, and again vaginal misoprostol is the most useful analogue. The first trials demonstrated that if the prostaglandin (800 µg misoprostol vaginally) was given a week after the injection of methotrexate, this method could be almost as effective as mifepristone.[32] Like mifepristone, efficacy diminishes with advancing gestation beyond 7 weeks since the last menstrual period.[33–35] Because methotrexate takes longer to act than mifepristone, the prostaglandin is used a week after the initial treatment and is repeated a day later if expulsion has not occurred. Methotrexate is easily available and inexpensive. It has been used in low doses to treat psoriasis and rheumatoid arthritis, as well as ectopic pregnancy, without adverse effects. It is, however, a known teratogen that can be deadly in high doses, and its use as an abortifacient results in prolonged bleeding and a prolonged time to abortion (up to a month in some cases). *Mifepristone is preferred by clinicians who have experience with both methods, and when mifepristone is available, it is better to avoid the use of methotrexate.*

Prostaglandin alone can be nearly as effective as a combination of drugs.[36] Relatively high success rates have been reported with multiple dosing,[37] but the most effective regimen and the best method of administration remain to be determined.[38] The administration of 800 µg misoprostol daily for 3 days has been reported to be very effective late in the first-trimester (10–12 weeks).[39] In very early gestation, a single vaginal dose of 800 µg misoprostol or multiple doses within 24 hours is as effective as the usual combination of mifepristone and oral misoprostol.[37, 40]

One word of caution regarding misoprostol, the synthetic prostaglandin E_1 analogue: it is now recognized that infants born to pregnant women exposed to misoprostol have an increased risk of abnormal vascular development resulting in Möbius's syndrome (congenital facial paralysis with or without limb defects) and defects such as equinovarus and arthogryposis.[41, 42] Although the risk is low, this possibility must be considered in decision-making when the various methods for first-trimester abortion are considered.

Careful prospective follow-up assessments can detect no health differences in women who have medical abortions compared with women who have abortions by vacuum aspiration.[43] Although women having medical abortions experience more bleeding and cramping, with appropriate counseling and support, women are equally satisfied with surgical and medical abortions.[44] Most importantly, medical abortion provides a method to overcome the difficulties associated with obtaining a surgical abortion.

First-Trimester Surgical Abortion Technique

The most widely used technique for first-trimester abortions is vacuum curettage.[6, 45, 46] The procedure is performed using local anesthesia (a paracervical block). Cervical dilation is accomplished with tapered Pratt dilators. Some surgeons recommend the preoperative insertion of cervical tents. These are osmotic dilators of dried seaweed or synthetic hydrophilic substances that are left in place from a few hours (synthetic) to overnight (seaweed).[47] Mifepristone (RU 486), the progesterone antagonist, produces preoperative cervical dilation equally effectively, and the ease of its single oral dose makes it a more attractive choice, but oral mifepristone requires a long pretreatment (24–36 hours).[48] Vaginal misoprostol (400 μg) dilates the cervix as effectively as *Laminaria* when given 4 hours prior to the procedure, and it is relatively inexpensive.[49] After the procedure, the patient is observed for 1–2 hours before returning home.

A standard set of simple instruments is satisfactory for termination of most first-trimester pregnancies:

> Graves medium open-sided vaginal speculum.
> Bierer atraumatic tenaculum.
> Foerster sponge forceps, curved.
> Pratt or Denniston cervical dilators, sizes 13
>   through 43 French.
> Medicine bowl (50 mL) for local anesthetic.
> Stainless steel bowl (500 mL) for antiseptic solution.
> Uterine curette, size 2 Sims.

Disposable equipment and supplies recommended for each procedure:

> Chloroprocaine (Nesacaine) 1%, 20 mL.
> Atropine, 0.4 mg (1 mL).
> Syringe, 10 cc plastic with control grip for cervical block.
> Syringe, 5 cc for intravenous administration of analgesics.
> Needle, 25-gauge (1.5 inch) for paracervical block.
> Needle, 25-gauge (0.5 inch) for intravenous medications.
> Gauze sponges, 4 x 4.
> Cotton balls.
> Clear plastic collection tubing with clear plastic handle, 11 mm
>   inside diameter (or a hand-held, 50-cc uterine
>   evacuation syringe).
> Cannulas for uterine evacuation; rigid, clear plastic, 7 mm

through 12 mm outside diameter, straight and curved.
Cannulas; whistle-tip, flexible plastic, 5 mm through 8 mm
outside diameter.
Topical antiseptic (e.g., povidone-iodine), 50 mL.

The instrument tray should be kept as simple as possible because unnecessary instruments disturb patients, increase costs, and waste time. For example, if cervical dilation is accomplished preoperatively, it may not be necessary to have cervical dilators in the tray.[50, 51]

The treatment room should be equipped with an electric vacuum pump that reaches adequate negative pressures (greater than 60 mm Hg) quietly and rapidly. The operating table should provide comfortable knee support for the patient in lithotomy position. Foot slings or stirrups are not desirable; knee crutches are much better because the patient can relax her legs, allowing the crutches to hold them apart. Ideally, the table should provide Trendelenburg position so that the surgeon can alter the angle of vision and vasovagal reactions can be treated by lowering the patient's head. A wheeled bucket should stand at the end of the table in front of the surgeon's stool, which must be height adjustable and have wheels. Two stools or tall chairs should be set at the head of the operating table for the counselor and the patient's support person, if one is with her.

The Uterine Aspiration Procedure

Patient Preparation. Correct position on the operating table helps the patient to relax and the surgeon to complete the procedure quickly; both factors are critical for pain relief. The patient should be invited to empty her bladder before she enters the treatment room (unless a full bladder is needed for intraoperative sonography). She should recline on the table and rest her legs in the padded knee crutches, achieving a comfortable dorsal lithotomy position with her buttock margins beyond the end of the table. Obese women should be positioned even further down so that the handle of the speculum can lie between the buttocks. Intravenous premedications are administered immediately before or after assuming the lithotomy position but not prior to reclining on the table because their relaxing effect is disturbed by ambulation. Oral medications are used cautiously because gastrointestinal absorption is unpredictable, and some of them (e.g., diazepam) can have long-lasting effects. Analgesic medications can be most comfortably administered by direct intravenous push with a 25-gauge, 0.5-inch needle, or through a heparin-lock cannula. A continuous infusion is necessary only in special circumstances, when patients with sickle cell disease or severe hyperemesis need hydration, for example, or when venous access might be difficult in an emergency.

Analgesia can be obtained with intravenous fentanyl (Sublimaze) 2 μg/kg given in 50 or 100 μg increments, or butorphanol (Stadol) 2 mg. Atropine, 0.4 mg (1 mL), mixed with the analgesic agent or with the local anesthetic for the cervical block provides protection against vasovagal responses to cervical manipulation. For anxiety, midazolam (Versed), 1–3 mg, is preferable to diazepam because it does not irritate veins, has a faster onset of action, and is eliminated sooner than diazepam. It can be mixed with the other agents, but when given with a narcotic like fentanyl, the mixture must be injected more slowly, over a period of 1–2 minutes, depending on the dose. Oral premedications should be given approximately 30–45 minutes before the procedure, such as a combination of 1 or 2 tablets of Vicodin, 800 mg Ibuprofen, and 5–10 mg diazepam. The use of intravenous sedation requires the availability of emergency equipment and medication (reversal agents such as nalorphan and flumazenil) to manage respiratory distress.

Cervical Assessment, Exposure, and Local Anesthesia. Before administering sedation and analgesia, a bimanual examination is performed, during which any previously placed hydrophilic dilators and sponges can be removed and the size and position of the uterus assessed. It is essential to know the direction and degree of uterine flexion. The degree of cervical dilation present can be estimated with an examining finger. After the exam, gloves are exchanged for new sterile ones, and a "no touch" technique is followed with intrauterine instruments throughout the remainder of the abortion procedure. Cleaning the vulva or labia with antiseptic does not reduce the incidence of infection and makes relaxation difficult for the patient. A Weissman-Graves open-sided speculum is slowly and gently placed in the vagina and opened as widely as possible without causing the patient discomfort to fully expose the cervix. After receiving intravenous analgesia, most patients do not find a widely opened speculum painful. The vaginal vault and cervix can then be gently cleaned with an antiseptic.

Cervical Block Technique. A well-placed cervical block relieves the pain of cervical dilation and is important even for the patient whose cervix is already dilated because it also relieves the pain of cervical manipulation. The block should be placed at least 2 minutes before uterine evacuation begins; a longer wait is preferable. A 10–20-cc control grip syringe is filled with 1% chloroprocaine (Nesacaine, preferred for its rapid metabolism) and a 25-gauge, 1.5-inch needle is attached. A deeply placed block provides better pain relief than a shallow one.[52] Inject about 2 mL, 1 cm deep into the cervical lip, the anterior lip for an anteverted uterus or posterior lip for a retroverted uterus. The injected lip is grasped with a Bierer atraumatic tenaculum so that the curve of the tenaculum does not obscure the view of the cervix (curve up for an anterior uterus, down for a posterior uterus). Apply traction to the tenaculum and observe the angle at which the cervix passes back into the lateral fornices. Bend the needle at its hub to about the same angle by pressing it on a sterile surface. Hold the syringe lightly at the end of the plunger and select a point at 3 o'clock, 1–2 cm lateral to the external os. Insert the needle tip at this point immediately beneath the cervical mucosa and slide it under the mucosa to the needle's hub so that the needle is completely buried. This places the needle tip near the paracervical plexus. Inject 7 mL in the plexus and another 1 mL as the needle is withdrawn from under the mucosa, so that the nerves that pass under the mucosa after leaving the plexus are anesthetized. The procedure is repeated on the other side at 9 o'clock, using a second syringe.

If extensive cervical dilation is anticipated, injection of the uterosacral ligaments at 5 and 7 o'clock in the posterior vaginal fornix provides a more profound cervical block, but for most minor cervical dilations, uterosacral injections cause more pain than they prevent.

Cervical Dilation Technique. If the cervix has not been dilated preoperatively,[50, 51] mechanical dilation with Pratt-type dilators (finely tapered and closely graduated) is usually required prior to uterine evacuation. Dilation should not exceed that needed for rapid (less than 5 minutes) uterine aspiration. A ten-mm diameter (a size 21 Pratt dilator) is the maximum needed for gestations under 12 weeks.

Select the smallest dilator likely to easily enter the cervical canal, holding it in the middle like a pencil to feel which end is larger. The smaller end is advanced to the internal os with the curve directed posteriorly. When the resistance of the internal os is felt, begin to rotate the dilator (if the fundus is not posteriorly positioned) 180 degrees so that the curve is directed anteriorly as it passes into the uterine cavity. If the curve of the dilator (and all other instruments passed into the uterine cavity) is always directed posteriorly as it enters the external os, perforation of posterior uteri is avoided. Failure to detect a posterior uterus is the most common cause of uterine perforation at the time of first-trimester abortion.

If firm resistance is encountered at the internal os, the procedure is repeated using a smaller dilator. If resistance is slight to moderate, the tip of the dilator is passed through the internal os into the uterine cavity completing the 180 degrees rotatory motion as it enters the cavity. It is essential to distinguish the characteristic rubbery, spring-like resistance of the internal cervical os from the softer, nonspecific resistance of cervical stroma to avoid developing a false passage with a misdirected dilator.

If a dilator is slippery with mucus or blood, a gauze sponge held around the middle prevents slippage. Progressively larger dilators are used, without skipping increments, until adequate dilation is achieved; about 1 mm diameter for every week of gestation. Pratt dilators are labeled with their circumferences in millimeters; divide by 3 to obtain their diameter, the measurement used for uterine aspiration cannulas. Avoid excessive force to obtain dilation. If dilation is difficult, consider 4-hour treatment with vaginal misoprostol (400 μg).[49] Vaginal misoprostol, 600 μg, is recommended for routine use in nulliparous women after 10 weeks' gestation.

Uterine Aspiration. All that is needed for rapid, safe uterine evacuation in early pregnancy is a cannula and a source of vacuum. Manufacturers have made both available in several varieties. Rigid, clear plastic cannulas increase in diameter by 1 mm increments from 6 through 16 mm. Flexible plastic cannulas increase from 4 mm through 12 mm in diameter. Rigid cannulas are manufactured in both straight and angulated types. Straight cannulas cause less pain when the cannula is rotated inside the uterine cavity, but curved cannulas provide easier access to the cavity and cornual areas of a retro- or anteroflexed uterus. The choice depends upon the patient's anatomy and the surgeon's preference. Flexible (soft) cannulas are useful for gestations up to 10 weeks, using minimal cervical dilation or when anatomic abnormalities, such as cervical myomas and uterine septae or duplications, distort the pathway to the gestational sac.

It is best to select a cannula of the largest size that easily passes the internal os; too small a cannula results in loss of intrauterine vacuum and prolongs the operation, while too large a cannula is painful. The cannula (and any other instrument that enters the uterine cavity) should not be touched; only the portions of those instruments that remain outside the cavity may be handled because "sterile" gloves can become contaminated.

As the cannula passes into the uterine cavity, the vacuum pump is turned on by the clinician with a foot switch or, if using a manual syringe, the syringe pinch valves are released. A negative pressure of 50–70 mm Hg assures rapid and complete evacuation and does not injure the myometrium. The cannula tip is advanced to the uterine fundus where it is rotated at approximately one revolution per second. During rotation, the cannula is gradually and gently withdrawn to the external os. Just as its tip exits the cervix, the negative pressure is released with the thumb valve on the handle, not with the pump switch. The cannula is again advanced into the uterine cavity, rotated and withdrawn to the external os. If uterine contents continue to appear in the plastic cannula and the evacuation hose, this procedure is repeated, rotating the cannula first clockwise and then counterclockwise until flow into the cannula and through the hose ceases. At this point the cannula tip is withdrawn from the external os, again taking care to release pressure with the thumb valve on the hose handle just as the tip leaves the external os. This timing of vacuum release is important to avoid leaving uterine contents behind or drawing vaginal mucosa into the tip of the suction cannula, a painful experience for the patient.

Manual uterine aspiration with a handheld syringe avoids the need for electricity and can be used in any setting. The Ipas and Milex syringes are available in the United States, and each requires the creation of a vacuum at different times. With the Ipas syringe, the valve is closed and the plunger pulled out before placement of the cannula. With the Milex syringe, the vacuum is created after the cannula is placed into the uterus. Both syringes have a lock to maintain the vacuum. The manual vacuum aspiration syringe requires emptying into a specimen container each time it is withdrawn if more than one aspiration is needed (as it usually is beyond 7 weeks). The syringe, unlike the cannula, need not be sterile; therefore, the aspirated contents should not be expelled from the syringe through the cannula, but the cannula should be detached before emptying the syringe.

Sometimes flow through the cannula stops because the placenta or its fragments are too large to pass. Flow can usually be restored simply by releasing pressure with the thumb valve (don't switch off the pump motor) and quickly restoring it by closing the valve. If this technique doesn't work, releasing and restoring vacuum while the cannula is advanced a few centimeters into the cavity and then quickly withdrawn again in a pumping motion almost always restores flow. Rotation of the cannula during the "pumping" maneuver also helps to fragment the placenta, allowing it to pass through the cannula. If the cannula remains plugged despite these attempts to clear it, simply withdraw the cannula, releasing the vacuum at the external os, but not before, and remove the plug from the cervix or the end of the cannula with ring forceps. The manual vacuum syringe must be emptied and its vacuum restored.

Comparisons of electric and manual uterine aspiration indicate no differences between the two in regard to results, complications, and acceptability by patients.[53-55] Patient and clinician choice should be the primary determinant of the source of vacuum for uterine aspiration

When all flow of uterine contents and most flow of blood has ceased and when the contraction of the uterus around the cannula makes rotation increasingly difficult, the clinician can assume that the uterus is evacuated. Completeness of the evacuation may then be evaluated using a malleable, sharp curette, 5–10 mm in breadth. Larger curettes are used in later gestations, but a no. 2 is right for most first-trimester abortions. A systematic approach to curettage helps ensure that no area of the uterine cavity is missed. First, place the tip of the curette in the right uterine cornu and withdraw it to the internal os. Repeat this motion with 2 or 3 withdrawals across the anterior uterine fundus and a final one from the left cornu. Turn the curette over and withdraw it 3 or 4 times in succession from left to right, moving across the posterior uterine wall.

During curettage, the empty uterine cavity should provoke a gritty sensation with each stroke of the curette and should feel triangular and symmetrical. Deviations from these findings can indicate retained products of conception, myomas, or uterine anomalies. If curettage reveals a slick area of uterine wall, repeated suctioning in which the cannula's open tip is applied firmly to the abnormal area of the uterus may demonstrate retained fetal, or, more likely, placental fragments. When these are suctioned out, the cavity should be reevaluated with the sharp curette. The sharp curettage is not used to remove uterine contents (the suction cannula does that) but to assess the completeness of evacuation. The whistle-tip of a flexible plastic cannula can provide the same sensation of complete uterine evacuation.

The abortion procedure is completed by again inserting the cannula through the cervical canal to the uterine fundus, switching on the vacuum pump or releasing the pinch valve on the manual syringe and rotating and withdrawing the cannula a final time to remove any fragments left behind. At the end of the abortion procedure, the uterus should be firmly contracted around the cannula. Application of vacuum to the uterine cavity should elicit only a small amount of blood and air bubbles, and when the cannula is withdrawn for the final time, only a small trickle of blood should run from the cervical os. The tenaculum is then removed, the cervical lip inspected for bleeding, the blood remaining in the vagina suctioned or sponged away, and the speculum gently withdrawn. The patient's vulva can then be cleaned and gently dried.

Postoperative Care. After a surgical abortion under local anesthesia nearly all patients can comfortably walk to a nearby recovery area. They may sit in chairs or lie down. Reclining chairs are ideal because patients recover more quickly sitting but can lie back if they prefer or if they have a syncopal episode. Vital signs should be taken on the operating table immediately after the procedure and at least one more time in the recovery room before discharge. In addition, perineal pads should be inspected for bleeding at least once before discharge. Patients should not be discharged until they ambulate independently to the bathroom, take sips of fluids, and show complete recovery from the effects of operative medications. This recovery period generally requires at least 30 minutes, and some patients need to remain longer.

At the time of discharge, patients are again informed of the 3 signs of possible complications: increasing bleeding, increasing pain, and fever. They are instructed to take their temperature for the next 3 mornings and given a thermometer if they do not have one. They are given a telephone number at which they can seek advice and answers to questions at any time during the day or night. An opportunity is given to ask final questions about contraception. Patients can begin taking oral contraceptives that night. If the preoperative hematocrit was less than 35, a daily iron supplement for 2 months is indicated. Patients who are still under the influence of preoperative medications should leave in the company of a responsible adult. A follow-up visit approximately 1 month after an abortion is strongly recommended to enhance contraceptive choices and compliance. In addition, a screening hCG level at the follow-up visit would detect cases of undiagnosed gestational trophoblastic neoplasia at an early stage.[56]

Complications of Induced Abortion

Public health authorities have demonstrated that the legalization of abortion reduced maternal morbidity and mortality more than any single development since the advent of antibiotics to treat puerperal infections and blood banking to treat hemorrhage. The number of American women reported as dying from abortion declined from nearly 300 deaths in 1961, to only 6 in 1985, 10 in 1992, and 4 in 1999, or about *0.6 deaths for every 100,000 legal abortions.*[45, 57] For comparison, in 1990, the maternal death rate for childbirth in the United States was 10 per 100,000 births, and for ectopic pregnancy, approximately 50 per 100,000 cases,[10, 58, 59] and, in 1992, 17 deaths were associated with spontaneous miscarriage.[45]

The most important determinants of abortion mortality are duration of gestation and type of anesthesia: later abortions and general anesthesia are more hazardous.[60–62] As with mortality, morbidity rates vary primarily with duration of pregnancy, but other factors are important as well, including type of operation, age of patient, type of anesthesia, operator's skill, and method of cervical dilatation. More experienced clinicians and younger, healthier women are less likely to have complications.

Major and minor complications in a series of 170,000 first-trimester abortion patients were as follows:[63]

Major Complications (Hospitalization Required)

Retained tissue	27.7 per 100,000 induced abortions
Sepsis	21.2
Uterine perforation	9.4
Hemorrhage	7.1
Inability to complete	3.5
Intrauterine plus tubal pregnancy	2.4

Minor Complications (Managed in Clinic or Office)

Mild infection	462.0 per 100,000 induced abortions
Reaspiration same day	180.8
Reaspiration later	167.8
Cervical stenosis	16.5
Cervical tear	10.6
Underestimated gestation	6.5
Convulsive seizure	4.0

The possibility that abortion can result in longer term complications has been examined in more than 150 studies.[64] There is no evidence for any adverse consequences of vacuum aspiration abortion for subsequent fertility,[65, 66] pregnancies,[67, 68] or increased risk for ectopic pregnancy.[69, 70] Second-trimester abortions do not increase the rate of preterm delivery or midtrimester fetal losses.[71] Multiple induced abortions do not increase the risk of a subsequent ectopic pregnancy but may increase the rate of preterm delivery in subsequent pregnancies.[72, 73] The long-term effects of second-trimester abortion may depend on the method used.[74] A French study disagrees with these conclusions, finding a slightly increased risk of ectopic pregnancy in women with a prior induced abortion and no previous ectopic pregnancy, and Chinese and Danish studies found a small increase in the risk of spontaneous miscarriage following surgically induced abortions.[75-77]

The psychological sequelae of elective abortion have been studied and debated. The evidence largely indicates that depression is less frequent among women postabortion compared with postpartum; that women denied abortion experience resentment for years; and that the children born after abortion is denied have social, occupational, and interpersonal difficulties lasting into early adulthood.[78] However, some have found that depression is observed at a higher rate among women with a history of induced abortions.[79, 80]

Conflicting results have been reported in over 20 studies examining the risk of breast cancer associated with the number of abortions (especially induced abortions) experienced by individual patients.[81, 82] Concern for an adverse effect has been based on the theoretical suggestion that a full-term pregnancy protects against breast cancer by invoking complete differentiation of breast cells, but abortion increases the risk by allowing breast cell proliferation in the first-trimester of pregnancy but not allowing the full differentiation that occurs in later pregnancy. In these studies there has been a major problem of recall bias; women who develop breast cancer are more likely to reveal truthfully their history of induced abortion than healthy women. In studies that avoided recall bias (e.g., by deriving data from national registries instead of personal interviews), the risk of breast cancer was identical in women with and without induced abortions.[83, 84] More careful case-control studies have also failed to link a risk of breast cancer with induced or spontaneous abortions.[85, 86]

Because the risk of breast cancer following abortion (based on poorly controlled studies) was misrepresented in public information provided by the U.S. National Cancer Institute and some state governments, a collaborative reanalysis of the data from 53 studies including 83,000 women with breast cancer in 16 countries was conducted by leading British epidemiologists.[87] In studies that collected data prospectively, no relationship was detected between the risk of breast cancer and spontaneous or induced abortion history. A link was present only in some studies that collected data retrospectively. The misleading findings in the retrospective studies almost assuredly resulted from the inclination of women who developed breast cancer to disclose previous induced abortion more frequently than other women.

Safe abortion is still unavailable to many women in parts of Asia, Africa, and Latin America.[88] Therefore, many women resort to clandestine, unsafe abortions, accounting for about 20% of the world's maternal mortality. These deaths are preventable.[89] It has been estimated that in 2000 there were 19 million unsafe abortions in the world, about 1 in 10 pregnancies.[90] Family planning services that provide effective contraceptive choices as well as access to safe abortion early in pregnancy are essential for societies to achieve desired fertility rates and a healthy female population.

Immediate Postoperative Complications of First-Trimester Abortion

Postoperative complications of elective abortions are classified as either immediate or delayed. Uterine perforation and uterine atony are examples of immediate complications. Delayed complications can occur several hours to several weeks after the operation. These usually present as complaints of bleeding, pain, or continuing symptoms of pregnancy. Complication rates are similar for both the manual and electric methods of vacuum aspiration.[54]

Excessive Bleeding Immediately after Aspiration

By far the most common cause of unusually heavy postabortal bleeding is retained products of conception. Rates in large series vary from 0.2 to 0.6%.[63] Patients with retained products of conception occasionally present several weeks after an abortion, but most report excessive bleeding within 1 week. Severe pain or pelvic tenderness suggests that infection is also present. Treatment is prompt aspiration of the uterus with the largest cannula that passes the cervix.

Excessive blood loss occurring promptly after uterine evacuation can result from uterine atony, retained products of conception, uterine perforation, or cervical laceration. A pelvic bimanual examination and visualization of the cervix distinguishes among these. Uterine atony, marked by a soft, nontender uterine fundus and a steady trickle of dark blood from the cervix, is initially treated by uterine massage, the intramuscular injection of 0.2 mg ergonovine (Methergine), and repeated uterine assessment before discharge. If bleeding persists it may be necessary to repeat this injection and continue oral treatment (ergonovine, 0.2 mg tid for 3 days). If blood loss is great enough to cause tachycardia or hypotension, an intravenous infusion of lactated Ringer's solution should be started. If the response to ergonovine is inadequate, prompt transvaginal, intrauterine injection of 250 μg 15-methyl $PGF_{2\alpha}$ usually restores uterine tone. Misoprostol (five 200 μg tablets) as a rectal suppository or held under the tongue also causes uterine contraction.[91]

If bleeding is excessive and pelvic examination reveals a slightly tender uterus somewhat larger than expected, the possibility of retained fetal or placental tissue must be considered. Bleeding unresponsive to uterotonic agents also suggests retained tissue. The uterine cavity should then be re-evaluated with the largest sharp curette that passes through the cervix. If more than 30 minutes have lapsed since the procedure, a second paracervical block and additional parenteral analgesia may be required. If the uterine cavity is asymmetrical or lacks a gritty surface, it should be reaspirated with the largest cannula that passes the cervix. If nothing can be aspirated, an ultrasonographic evaluation of the uterus should be conducted with the cannula in the uterine cavity. Sonography may reveal unsuspected uterine anomalies, such as an additional uterine horn or a septum, may demonstrate that the cannula is not actually within the uterine cavity, or may localize the retained products. Evacuation can then be carried out under direct ultrasonographic monitoring.

If there are no other explanations for excessive bleeding, a clotting disorder is possible. The diagnosis is made by assessing the clotting capacity of blood in a tube, measuring platelet and fibrinogen levels, as well as prothrombin and partial thromboplastin times. The values of fibrinogen degradation products may also be helpful in following this problem. Patients suspected of having disseminated intravascular coagulation (DIC) should have lost fluid volume rapidly replaced with whole blood, or, lacking that, lactated Ringer's solution, and be transferred to a facility with a blood bank that can provide specific replacement products such as fresh frozen plasma and cryoprecipitate. DIC can occur as an isolated condition or can accompany other complications such as hemorrhage, amniotic fluid embolus, or anesthetic toxicity.

Uterine Perforation

Perforation of the uterus during first-trimester abortion occurs from 1 to 2 times per 1,000 operations.[92] Most commonly, perforations occur in the midfundal area because the clinician failed to identify a retroverted or retroflexed uterus prior to uterine sounding or cervical dilation. Preventive measures are preoperative cervical dilation, a bimanual examination immediately before every abortion procedure to determine uterine position, and elimination of uterine sounding.[93] If the uterus is not palpable, its location should be determined sonographically, or the direction of the cervical canal should be cautiously determined using a small caliber cervical dilator with its curve directed posteriorly as it traverses the cervical canal. If these measures are taken, many first-trimester perforations can be avoided.[63] Uterine perforation rarely results in significant blood loss. The patient's vital signs, hematocrit, and abdominal pain and tenderness indicate the rare event of intraabdominal hemorrhage. Patients who do not have significant blood loss, and for whom uterine evacuation is already completed, should be observed for 2 or 3 hours postoperatively. If their vital signs and hematocrit remain stable and they are without pain, patients can be discharged with cautions to telephone or return should pain or bleeding occur later.

If perforation has occurred and the uterus has not been completely evacuated, evacuation can usually be completed under ultrasonographic guidance by passing a flexible or rigid plastic cannula into the uterine cavity, taking care to avoid the perforation. To improve the image, fill the bladder when using an abdominal sector transducer, or use a small vaginal transducer. When ultrasonography is immediately available, laparoscopy is rarely needed to guide uterine evacuation.

Cervical Laceration

Cervical trauma is a relatively uncommon and rarely serious complication of first-trimester abortion, occurring about once per 100 abortions. It is more common when general anesthesia and forceful cervical dilation are employed.[94, 95] Bleeding from the tenaculum site is unusual if an atraumatic (Bierer) tenaculum is used. Tenaculum site bleeding can usually be controlled by direct application of a sponge (ring) forceps to the bleeding site; the metal should be applied directly to the bleeding site, and the ring completely closed and left in place for 1–2 minutes. Cervical lacerations that continue to bleed can be sutured with 00 chromic catgut or polyglycolic braided suture; a single figure of eight usually suffices.

Acute Hematometra

Postabortal hematometra or the "post abortion syndrome" occurs in about one in every 200 abortions and is most common in late first-trimester and early second-trimester abortions (11–14 weeks).[96] It is easily diagnosed and should be promptly treated. Symptoms include the rapid onset of post abortion pelvic pain, within an hour or two of surgery, without increased vaginal bleeding or changes in vital signs. Pelvic examination reveals a very tender and distended uterus. Treatment is prompt suction evacuation of the accumulated clot and blood, providing immediate relief, followed by intramuscular ergonovine, 0.2 mg, and 2 days of oral treatment, 0.2 mg tid.

Syncopal Episodes During or After Abortion

Syncopal episodes can be caused by vasovagal reaction, hyperventilation, toxic or allergic reactions to local anesthetics, or shock. Vasovagal reactions are by far the most common cause. The reaction ranges from uneasiness and diaphoresis to severe bradycardia and hypotension. Vasovagal reaction is usually diagnosed by noting bradycardia in response to cervical manipulation or dilation. Lowering the patient's head provides relief. Severe reactions can be treated with subcutaneous or intravenous atropine, 0.6 mg. Since mild vasovagal reactions are a common response to cervical manipulation, the routine use of a prophylactic dose of atropine, 0.4 mg, intravenously with the analgesic agent or cervically with the anesthetic is highly recommended.

Hyperventilation can be a cause of syncope in abortion patients. It is a response to anxiety and sometimes occurs when patients "over breathe" as

405

a relaxation technique for local anesthesia. It is often accompanied by an inability to breathe comfortably and circumoral paresthesia. Lightheadedness may progress to actual syncope as a result of cerebral vasoconstriction and peripheral vasodilation. It is prevented by helping the anxious patient to breathe deeply but slowly. Recovery is accelerated by re-breathing expired air from a paper bag to increase pCO_2.

Reactions to local anesthetics used in the paracervical block have a wide range of manifestations, including syncope. A majority of reactions are toxic and occur because the block is injected into a highly vascular area. Direct intravenous injection causes immediate ringing in the patient's ears, occasionally accompanied by paresthesias and lightheadedness. A more profound reaction leads to dizziness and, finally, syncope. Severe reactions are marked by seizures. Duration of the toxic reaction depends on the rapidity with which the anesthetic agent is cleared from the bloodstream. The amino esters (procaine and chloroprocaine) are rapidly hydrolyzed by plasma cholinesterase. Chloroprocaine is hydrolyzed 3–4 times faster than procaine and has a half-life of only 21 seconds. Amino amide local anesthetics (lidocaine, mepivacaine, bupivacaine) are metabolized at a much slower rate, and some of their metabolites can themselves cause toxic reactions. The elimination half-life of lidocaine, for example, is 1.6 hours. Metabolism occurs primarily in the liver rather than in the blood as for the ester anesthetics. A severe toxic reaction can result in sinus bradycardia, atrioventricular (AV) block, or even asystole. Severe hypotension, unconsciousness, generalized convulsions, and respiratory arrest can follow.[97] With ester anesthetics, these reactions are self-limited and rarely require treatment. With amide anesthetics, treatment consists of cardiopulmonary resuscitation support. Seizures can be controlled with intravenous midazolam, 2–4 mg.

Inadequate Products of Conception and Ectopic Pregnancy

Failure to identify fetal or placental tissue after first-trimester pregnancy termination results from failure to aspirate the uterus, failure to detect products of conception in the aspirated specimen, or ectopic pregnancy. Since ectopic pregnancy is a life-threatening condition, each office or clinic should have a system for managing patients who have inadequate products of conception following uterine aspiration.

Counselors, nurses, and physicians should be alert to the possibility of an ectopic pregnancy in patients who report bleeding episodes since their last menstrual period, pelvic pain prior to requesting abortion, or who have risk factors such as a previous ectopic pregnancy, salpingitis, or tubal surgery. The possibility of an ectopic pregnancy should be considered when the physical examination reveals a uterus that seems small for the reported duration of gestation, presence of an adnexal mass, or the presence of unilateral pelvic tenderness. Offices or clinics that perform a high proportion of abortions early in gestation (prior to 8 weeks) have a special responsibility to diagnose ectopic pregnancy because patients with this condition may seek abortion prior to the onset of symptoms that would suggest the diagnosis.

For patients at high risk of ectopic pregnancy, a pelvic examination should be carried out immediately prior to uterine aspiration to assess uterine size and position and to detect adnexal tenderness or masses. If history and physical examination suggest that ectopic pregnancy is a possibility, the uterus should, if possible, be aspirated under sonographic guidance. If the cannula can be identified in the uterine cavity but no gestational sac is seen, ectopic pregnancy should be suspected. Occasionally an adnexal pregnancy is actually seen, but this cannot be counted on to diagnose ectopic pregnancy.

Following aspiration, all collected tissue should be flushed from the hose and cannula with an isotonic solution for examination. If the aspirate is flushed with water, the villi collapse, making them difficult to identify, and the opportunity to confirm an intrauterine pregnancy can be lost. In earlier gestations, villi are easiest to detect when the washed tissue is placed in a white, translucent plastic container (the kind typically used for pathological specimens) and spread over the bottom making the clear, tubular villi obvious in the light transmitted through the container. Another widely used method is to empty the washed material into a clear flat dish of isotonic solution that can then be set on a horizontally placed light source such as a slide viewer or an x-ray box. Light shining up through the bottom of the container makes easier the distinction between decidual tissue and the products of conception such as the gestational sac, the decidua capsularis, chorionic villi, and the embryo. A magnifying hand lens is also helpful, especially in early gestations.

If the clinician cannot positively identify evidence of intrauterine gestation in the specimen, it should be sent to a pathologist with the diagnosis of "possible ectopic pregnancy" and a request for multiple sections to identify villi. Villi remaining in the uterus after a spontaneous miscarriage can be difficult to identify without staining because with time they lose their fluid content. Since the pain and bleeding of spontaneous miscarriage can be hard to distinguish from ectopic pregnancy, the pathologist should be informed of both possibilities.

If visual examination of the uterine aspirate does not confirm an intrauterine pregnancy, the clinician must make certain that the uterus is really empty. The best approach is to repeat a pelvic examination to detect uterine anomalies, such as a uterus didelphys, and adnexal masses or tenderness that might have been missed at the preoperative evaluation. Uterine aspiration should be repeated using intraoperative sonographic guidance, if available, to ensure that the cannula is correctly placed in the uterine cavity. If the cavity is, in fact, found to be empty, pregnancy should be confirmed with a test for the beta subunit of human chorionic gonadotropin (hCG). A highly sensitive urine test is sufficient. If such a test is positive, and if the patient is at high risk for an ectopic pregnancy from history, signs, or symptoms, treatment is indicated. If the test is positive but there are no risk factors for ectopic pregnancy, spontaneous abortion must be considered, and the hCG levels must be assessed over the following days. If hCG has not decreased or if signs or symptoms of an ectopic pregnancy develop, the patient should be treated surgically or medically with methotrexate, depending on the size of the pregnancy and the clinical situation.

Delayed Complications

Delayed complications of abortion are those occurring several hours to several weeks after the operation. The vast majority of these occur within the first week following the operation, which is why postabortion follow-up should occur within a week of the procedure.

These complications can be classified by the symptoms they produce: bleeding, pain, or continuing symptoms of pregnancy. All three kinds of symptoms can be present in some patients (e.g., those with an ectopic pregnancy) while others can present with only a single symptom.

Delayed Bleeding

By far the most common cause of unusually heavy postabortal bleeding is retained products of conception, which follows one of every 200 abortions.[63] Patients with retained products of conception occasionally present several weeks after an abortion, but the great majority report excessive bleeding within 1 week. Patients may also report uterine contractions, but severe pain or pelvic tenderness suggests that infection is also present. If bleeding has been significant, the cervical os usually is dilated and clots may be present in the vagina and cervical canal. Treatment is aspiration of the uterus with the largest cannula that passes the cervix. Cervical dilation to 10 mm is occasionally required. Local anesthesia as described for the abortion procedure usually suffices.

Infection

Infection is sometimes marked by uterine bleeding; although without retained products of conception, the volume of blood loss is usually modest. Fever and uterine tenderness are the most common signs of postabortal endometritis, occurring in about 0.5% of cases.[63] Some studies indicate that prophylactic antibiotics reduce the risk of postabortal infection.[98, 99] Most clinicians agree that women at risk of pelvic infection benefit from the use of prophylactic antibiotics prior to induced abortion; others state that women who have not had a previous delivery should receive prophylaxis, and still others believe that all abortion patients would benefit from prophylactic antibiotics.[100, 101] A meta-analysis of antibiotics at the time of induced abortion unequivocally concluded that prophylactic antibiotics should be routinely used without exceptions.[102] Because both gonorrhea and chlamydia, as well as other organisms, can cause postabortion infections, a tetracycline is the best drug for prophylaxis. Doxycycline, 100 mg an hour before the abortion and 200 mg 30 minutes afterward, is the most convenient and comprehensive regimen.[103] Tetracycline, 500 mg once before and once after the operation, is also acceptable. Metronidazole, 400 mg an hour before and 4–8 hours afterward, has been tested and is effective treatment for patients with bacterial vaginosis detected at the time of abortion.[104, 105]

Patients who present with uterine tenderness, fever, and bleeding require antibiotic treatment as well as uterine reaspiration. The treatment regimen depends on the severity of the infection. Patients who have fevers above 37° (101° F) and signs of peritoneal as well as uterine tenderness require hospitalization and intravenous antibiotics. Outpatient treatment should be reserved for patients whose signs and symptoms are confined to the uterus; doxycycline, 100 mg bid for 10 days, metronidazole, 500 mg bid for 7 days, amoxicillin and clavulanic acid (Augmentin), 250 mg tid for 7 days, or azithromycin, 1 g as a single dose, depending on the suspected cause, are all appropriate treatments.

Cervical Stenosis

Patients who experience amenorrhea or hypomenorrhea and cyclic uterine pain after first-trimester abortion may have stenosis of the internal os.[106] This condition is more common among women whose abortions are done in the early first-trimester with a minimum of cervical dilation and a small diameter, flexible plastic cannula. A possible explanation is that the whistle tip of this type of cannula abrades the internal os and the minimal dilation allows the abraded areas to heal in contact. The result is an inability to pass menstrual effluent and accompanying pain. The condition is easily treated with cervical dilation under paracervical block using Pratt dilators.

Rh Sensitization

Approximately 4% of Rh-negative women become sensitized following an induced abortion (a lower proportion in first-trimester and a higher proportion in second-trimester abortions).[107] Subsequent hemolytic disease of the newborn can be prevented by administering 50 mg of Rh immune globulin to all Rh-negative, Du-negative women undergoing abortion. A standard 300 mg dose has been administered for second-trimester abortion, but 150 mg is adequate according to a British controlled trial.[108]

Abortion in the Second-Trimester

Second-trimester abortions can be accomplished surgically or medically. The surgical procedure is termed *dilation and evacuation* or *extraction* (D & E). Several approaches have been used for the medical termination of pregnancy. These include the vaginal, intramuscular, or intraamniotic administration of prostaglandins and the intraamniotic injection of hypertonic saline or urea. The D & E procedure has been considered safer and less expensive than the medical methods and better tolerated (and thus preferred) by patients.[109-111] However, increasing experience in the United Kingdom with an inexpensive combination of mifepristone and misoprostol is demonstrating a high level of safety and efficacy.[112] Misoprostol alone (400 μg vaginally every 3 hours) is also effective.[113]

In 1996, only 4% of induced abortions occurred at 16–20 weeks of gestation and 91% of these were by D&E; 1.5% occurred at 21 weeks or later, and 79% of these were by D&E.[45] By 2000, only 0.17% of all abortions were late abortions.[6]

The training, experience, and skills of the clinician are the primary factors that limit the gestational age at which abortion can be safely performed. Advanced gestational age by itself incurs increased risks for all types of complications. These are multiplied when the duration of pregnancy is discovered, after beginning uterine evacuation, to be beyond the experience and skill of the clinician or capacity of the equipment. Uterine perforation, infection, bleeding, amniotic fluid embolism, and anesthetic reactions are increased as gestational age increases.[109, 114]

When errors in estimating gestational age require the clinician to use unfamiliar instruments or techniques that are not frequently practiced, the increased duration of the procedure can cause problems. Efforts to sedate or relieve pain by administering additional drugs increase the risk of toxic reactions or overdosage. If a change from local to general anesthesia is undertaken, the patient is at much greater risk of anesthetic complications. Finally, if complications caused by advanced gestational age necessitate transfer of the patient to clinicians who are not familiar with uterine evacuation techniques, the patient may undergo unnecessarily extensive surgery, such as hysterectomy, with all the risks inherent in emergency procedures.

Although menstrual history and physical examination are adequate estimators of gestational duration for the great majority of patients in early pregnancy, uterine ultrasonography offers a reliable alternative when these are in doubt. For patients whose pregnancies may exceed 16 weeks or be near the limit of a particular clinician, or when complicating conditions are suspected such as ectopic pregnancy, uterine malformations, myomas, multiple or other abnormal gestations, fetal demise, or when uterine size and menstrual dates disagree, ultrasonographic measurements should be obtained. Published, generally accepted scales for converting crown-rump length, femur length, and biparietal diameter to menstrual weeks should be consistently applied to images provided by experienced sonographers. These measurements should be photographically documented for the patient's medical record. During D&E operations, real-time sonography helps the clinician to accurately direct intrauterine forceps and can reduce the risk of uterine perforation, one of the primary hazards of D&E abortion.[115]

Preoperative cervical dilation with hydrophilic dilators (*Laminaria* or Dilapan) is essential for surgical second-trimester abortion.[47] Local rather than general anesthesia also makes second-trimester abortion safer.[116, 117] Some patients are not good candidates for surgical procedures of any kind under local anesthesia, but others may have special reasons to prefer that an abortion be performed under general anesthesia. Patient requests should be seriously considered, but the clinician also has a responsibility to inform the patient of the risks and benefits of local versus general anesthesia.

Oral, vaginal, intramuscular, or intraamniotic administration of prostaglandins, and the intraamniotic injection of hypertonic saline or urea are the medical methods of second-trimester abortion. The combination of mifepristone and misoprostol has been effectively used.[118] They all require the patient to go through labor in a hospital. The D&E procedure is less expensive than medical methods, and it is better tolerated by patients.[110, 114]

In the United Kingdom, prostaglandin analogues are favored for a noninvasive method of second-trimester abortion. A combination of the progesterone antagonist, mifepristone, (a single, oral 200-mg dose of mifepristone administered 36 hours before prostaglandin treatment) and an E prostaglandin analogue (misoprostol) administered orally or vaginally is highly effective, and the combination allows a lesser dose of both agents, which results in fewer side effects.[112] In addition, this combination does not require the use of cervical *Laminaria* for dilatation.

References

1. **Henshaw SK, Van Vort J,** Abortion services in the United States, 1991 and 1992, Fam Plann Perspect 26:100, 1994.

2. **Centers for Disease Control and Prevention,** Abortion Surveillance—United States, 1999, MMWR 52:1, 2002.

3. **Jones RK, Darroch JE, Henshaw SK,** Patterns in the socioeconomic characteristics of women obtaining abortions in 2000–2001, Persp Sexual Reprod Health 34:226, 2002.

4. **Deardorff KE, Montgomery P, Hollmann FW,** U.S. population estimates by age, sex, race, and Hispanic origin: 1990 to 1995, U.S. Department of Commerce, Economics and Statistics Administration, Bureau of the Census, Washington, D.C., 1996.

5. **Henshaw SK,** Abortion incidence and services in the United States, 1995–1996, Fam Plann Perspect 30:263, 1998.

6. **Finer LB, Henshaw SK,** Abortion incidence and services in the United States in 2000, Persp Sexual Reprod Health 35:6, 2003.

7. **Henshaw SK, Finer LB,** The accessibility of abortion services in the United States, 2001, Persp Sexual Reprod Health 35:16, 2003.

8. **Henshaw SK,** Induced abortions: a world review, 1990, Fam Plann Perspect 22:76, 1990.

9. **Koonin L, Smith J, Ramick M,** Abortion surveillance—United States, 1993 and 1994, MMWR 46:23, 1997.

10. **Lawson H, Frye A, Atrash H, Smith J, Schulman H, Ramick M,** Abortion mortality, United States, 1972 through 1987, Am J Obstet Gynecol 171:1365, 1994.

11. **Landy U, Lewit S,** Administrative, counseling, and medical practices in National Abortion Federation facilities, Fam Plann Perspect 14:257, 1982.

12. **Landy U,** Abortion counseling—a new component of medical care, Clinics Obstet Gynecol 13:33, 1986.

13. **El-Rafaey HJ, Rajasekar D, Abdalla M, Calder L, Templeton A,** Induction of abortion with mifepristone (RU 486) and oral or vaginal misoprostol, New Engl J Med 332:983, 1995.

14. **Silvestre L, Dubois C, Renault M, Rezvani Y, Baulieu EE, Ulmann A,** Voluntary interruption of pregnancy with Mifepristone (RU 486) and a prostaglandin analogue, New Engl J Med 322:645, 1990.

15. **Jensen JT, Astley SJ, Morgan E, Nichols M,** Outcomes of suction curettage and mifepristone abortion in the United States. A prospective comparison study, Contraception 59:153, 1999.

16. **Thong KJ, Baird DT,** Induction of abortion with mifepristone and misoprostol in early pregnancy, Br J Obstet Gynaecol 99:1004, 1992.

17. **Peyron R, Aubeny E, Targosz V, Silvestre L, Renault M, Elkik F, Leclerc P, Ulmann A, Baulieu EE,** Early termination of pregnancy with mifepristone (RU 486) and the orally active prostaglandin misoprostol, New Engl J Med 328:1509, 1993.

18. **Schaff EA, Eisinger SH, Stadalius LS, Franks P, Gore BZ, Poppema S,** Low-dose mifepristone 200 mg and vaginal misoprostol for abortion, Contraception 59:1, 1999.

19. **Schaff EA, Fielding SL, Westhoff C, Ellertson C, Eisinger SH, Stadalius LS, Fuller L,** Vaginal misoprostol administered 1, 2, or 3 days after mifepristone for early medical abortion: A randomized trial, JAMA 284:1948, 2000.

20. **Spitz IM, Bardin CW, Benton L, Robbins A,** Early pregnancy termination with mifepristone and misoprostol in the United States, New Engl J Med 338:1241, 1998.

21. **Ashok PW, Penney GC, Flett GMM, Templeton A,** An effective regimen for early medical abortion: a report of 2000 consecutive cases, Hum Reprod 13:2962, 1998.

22. **Schaff EA, Fielding SL, Westhoff C,** Randomized trial of oral versus vaginal misoprostol 2 days after mifepristone 200 mg for abortion up to 63 days of pregnancy, Contraception 66:247, 2002.

23. **Hamoda H, Ashok PW, Flett GMM, Templeton A,** Medical abortion at 64 to 91 days of gestation: a review of 483 consecutive cases, Am J Obstet Gynecol 188:1315, 2003.

24. **von Hertzen H, Honkanen H, Piaggio G, Bartfai G, Erdenetungalag R, Gemzell-Danielsson K, Gopalan S, Horga M, Jerve F, Mittal S, Ngoc NT, Peregoudov A, Prasad RN, Pretnar-Darovec A, Shah RS, Song S, Tang OS, Wu SC, WHO Research Group on Post-ovulatory Methods of Fertility Regulation,** WHO multinational study of three misoprostol regimens after mifepristone for early medical abortion. I: Efficacy, Br J Obstet Gynaecol 110:808, 2003.

25. **Creinin MD, Fox MC, Teal S, Chen A, Schaff EA, Meyn LA, for the MOD Study Trial Group,** A randomized comparison of misoprostol 6 to 8 hours versus 24 hours after mifepristone for abortion, Obstet Gynecol 103:850, 2004.

26. **Creinin MD,** in press.

27. **Ashok PW, Flett GM, Templeton A,** Termination of pregnancy at 9–13 weeks' amenorrhoea with mifepristone and misoprostol, Lancet 352:542, 1998.

28. **Baird DT, Brown A, Cheng L, Critchley HO, Lin S, Narvekar N, Williams AR,** Mifepristone: a novel estrogen-free daily contraceptive pill, Steroids 68:1099, 2003.

29. **Creinin MD, Vittinghoff E, Keder L, Darney PD, Tiller G,** Methotrexate and misoprostol for early abortion: a multicenter trial. I. Safety and efficacy, Contraception 53:321, 1996.

30. **Creinin MD,** Medical abortion with methotrexate 75 mg intramuscularly and vaginal misoprostol, Contraception 56:367, 1997.

31. **Creinin MD,** Oral methotrexate and vaginal misoprostol for early abortion, Contraception 54:15, 1996.

32. **Creinin M, Darney P,** Methotrexate and misoprostol for early abortion, Contraception 48:339, 1993.

33. **Creinin MD, Vittinghoff E,** Methotrexate and misoprostol vs misoprostol alone for early abortion. A randomized controlled trial, JAMA 272:1190, 1994.

34. **Creinin MD, Park M,** Acceptablility of medical abortion with methotrexate and misoprostol, Contraception 52:41, 1995.

35. **Hauskenecht RU,** Methotrexate and misoprostol to terminate early pregnancy, New Engl J Med 333:538, 1995.

36. **Koopersmith TB, Mishell Jr DR,** The use of misoprostol for termination of early pregnancy, Contraception 53:237, 1996.

37. **Carbonell JLL, Rodríguez J, Velazco A, Tanda R, Sánchez C, Barambio S, Chami S, Valero F, Marí J, de Vargas F, Salvador I,** Oral and vaginal misoprostol 800 μg every 8 h for early abortion, Contraception 67:457, 2003.

38. **Blanchard K, Winikoff B, Ellertson C,** Misoprostol used alone for the termination of early pregnancy. A review of the evidence, Contraception 59:209, 1999.

39. **Carbonell Esteve JL, Varela L, Velazco A, Cabezas E, Tanda R, Cabezas E, Sánchez C,** Early abortion with 800 μg of misoprostol by the vaginal route, Contraception 59:219, 1999.

40. **Jain JK, Meckstroth KR, Mishell Jr DR,** Early pregnancy termination with intravaginally administered sodium chloride solution-moistened misoprostol tablets: historical comparison with mifepristone and oral misoprostol, Am J Obstet Gynecol 181:1386, 1999.

41. **Pastuszak AL, Schüler L, Speck-Martins CE, Coelho K-EFA, Cordello SM, Vargas F, Brunoni D, Schwarz IVD, Larrandaburu M, Safattle H, Meloni VFA, Koren G,** Use of misoprostol during pregnancy and Möbius' syndrome in infants, New Engl J Med 338:1881, 1998. ⋅

42. **Gonzalez CH, Marques-Dias MJ, Kim CA, Sugayama SMM, Da Paz JA, Huson SM, Holmes LB,** Congenital abnormalities in Brazilian children associated with misoprostol misuse in first trimester of pregnancy, Lancet 351:1624, 1998.

43. **Howie FL, Henshaw RC, Naji SA, Russell IT, Templeton AA,** Medical abortion or vacuum aspiration? Two year follow-up of a patient preference trial, Br J Obstet Gynaecol 104:829, 1997.

44. **Elul B, Ellertson C, Winikoff B, Coyaji K,** Side effects of mifepristone-misoprostol abortion versus surgical abortion. Data from a trial in China, Cuba, and India, Contraception 59:107, 1999.

45. **Koonin LM, Stauss LT, Chrisman CE, Montalbano MA, Bartlett LA, Smith JC,** Centers for Disease Control Abortion Surveillance: United States, 1996, MMWR 48:1, 1999.

46. **Centers for Disease Control and Prevention,** http://www.cdc.gov, 2004.

47. **Darney PD, Atkinson E, Hirabayashi K,** Uterine perforation during second trimester abortion by cervical dilation and instrumental extraction: a review of 15 cases, Obstet Gynecol 75:441, 1990.

48. **World Health Organization Task Force on Postovulatory Methods of Fertility Regulation,** Cervical ripening with mifepristone (RU-486) in late first trimester abortion, Contraception 50:461, 1994.

49. **MacIsaac L, Grossman D, Balistreri E, Darney P,** A randomized controlled trial of laminaria, oral misoprostol, and vaginal misoprostol before abortion, Obstet Gynecol 93:766, 1999.

50. **Darney P, Dorward K,** Cervical dilation before first-trimester elective abortion: a controlled comparison of meteneprost, laminaria and hypan, Obstet Gynecol 70:397, 1987.

51. **Kline S, Meng H, Munsick R,** Cervical dilation from laminaria tents and synthetic osmotic dilators used for 6 hours before abortion, Obstet Gynecol 86:931, 1995.

52. **Wiebe ER,** Comparison of the efficacy of different local anesthetics and techniques of local anesthesia in therapeutic abortions, Am J Obstet Gynecol 167:131, 1992.

53. **Edelman A, Nichols MD, Jensen J,** Comparison of pain and time of procedures with two first-trimester abortion techniques performed by residents and faculty, Am J Obstet Gynecol 184:1564, 2001.

54. **Goldberg AB, Dean G, Kang MS, Youssof S, Darney PD,** Manual versus electric vacuum aspiration for early first-trimester abortion: a controlled study of complication rates, Obstet Gynecol 103:101, 2004.

55. **Dean G, Cardenas L, Darney P, Goldberg A,** Acceptability of manual versus electric aspiration for first trimester abortion: a randomized trial, Contraception 67:201, 2003.

56. **Seckl MJ, Gillmore R, Foskett M, Sebire NJ, Rees H, Newlands ES,** Routine terminations of pregnancy—should we screen for gestational trophoblastic neoplasia? Lancet 364:705, 2004.

57. **Elam-Evans LD, Strauss LT, Herndon J, Parker WY, Bowens SV, Zane S, Berg CJ,** Centers for Disease Control and Prevention, Abortion surveillance—United States, 2000, MMWR 52:1, 2003.

58. **Lawson H, Atrash H, Saftlas A,** Ectopic pregnancy surveillance, United States, 1970–1986, MMWR 38:11, 1989.

59. **Berg CJ, Atrash HK, Koonin LM, Tucker M,** Pregnancy-related mortality in the United States, 1987–1990, Obstet Gynecol 88:161, 1996.

60. **Grimes DA, Schulz KF, Cates Jr W, Tyler Jr CW,** Local versus general anesthesia: which is safer for performing suction curettage abortions, Am J Obstet Gynecol 135:1030, 1979.

61. **Peterson HB, Grimes DA, Cates Jr W, Rubin GL,** Comparative risk of death from induced abortion at 12 weeks' gestation performed with local versus general anesthesia, Am J Obstet Gynecol 141:763, 1981.

62. **Buehler J, Schulz K, Grimes D, Mogue C,** The risk of serious complications from induced abortion: do personal characteristics make a difference? Am J Obstet Gynecol 153:14, 1985.

63. **Hakim-Elahi E, Tovell H, Burnhill M,** Complications of first trimester abortions: a report of 170,000 cases, Obstet Gynecol 76:129, 1990.

64. **Hogue C,** Impact of abortion on subsequent fertility, Clin Obstet Gynecol 13:96, 1986.

65. **Stubblefield PG, Monson RR, Schoenbaum SC, Wolfson CE, Cookson DJ, Ryan KJ,** Fertility after induced abortion: a prospective follow-up study, Obstet Gynecol 63:186, 1984.

66. **Daling J, Weiss N, Voigt I, Spadoni LR, Soderstrom R, Moore DE, Stadel BV,** Tubal infertility in relation to prior induced abortion, Fertil Steril 43:389, 1985.

67. **Schoenbaum S, Monson R, Stubblefield P, Darney PD, Ryan KJ,** Outcome of the delivery following an induced or spontaneous abortion, Am J Obstet Gynecol 136:19, 1980.

68. **Frank PI, McNamee R, Hannaford PC, Kay CR, Hirsch S,** The effect of induced abortion on subsequent pregnancy outcome, Br J Obstet Gynaecol 98:1015, 1991.

69. **Daling J, Chow W, Weiss N, Metch BT, Soderstrom R,** Ectopic pregnancy in relation to previous induced abortion, JAMA 253:1005, 1985.

70. **Atrash HK, Strauss LT, Kendrick JS, Skjeldestad FE, Ahn YW,** The relation between induced abortion and ectopic pregnancy, Obstet Gynecol 89:512, 1997.

71. **Kalish RB, Chasen ST, Rosenzweig LB, Rashbaum WK, Chervenak FA,** Impact of midtrimester dilation and evacuation on subsequent pregnancy outcome, Am J Obstet Gynecol 187:882, 2002.

72. **Skjeldestad FE, Gargiullo PM, Kendrick JS,** Multiple induced abortions as risk factor for ectopic pregnancy. A prospective study, Acta Obstet Gynecol Scand 76:691, 1997.

73. **Henriet L, Kaminski M,** Impact of induced abortions on subsequent pregnancy outcome: the 1995 French national perinatal survey, Br J Obstet Gynecol 108:1036, 2001.

74. **MacKenzie I, Fox A,** A prospective self-controlled study of fertility after second trimester prostaglandin-induced abortion, Am J Obstet Gynecol 158:1137, 1988.

75. **Tharaux-Deneux C, Bouyer J, Job-Spira N, Coste J, Spira A,** Risk of ectopic pregnancy and previous induced abortion, Am J Public Health 88:401, 1998.

76. **Sun Y, Che Y, Gao E, Olsen J, Zhou W,** Induced abortion and risk of subsequent miscarriage, Int J Epidemiol 32:449, 2003.

77. **Zhou W, Olsen J,** Are complications after an induced abortion associated with reproductive failures in a subsequent pregnancy? Acta Obstet Gynecol Scand 82:177, 2003.

78. **Dagg PKB,** The psychological sequelae of therapeutic abortion—denied and completed, Am J Psychiatr 148:578, 1991.

79. **Thorp JM, Jr., Hartmann KE, Shadigian E,** Long-term physical and psychological health consequences of induced abortion: review of the evidence, Obstet Gynecol Survey 58:67, 2003.

80. **Cougle JR, Reardon DC, Coleman PK,** Depression associated with abortion and childbirth: a long-term analysis of the NLSY cohort, Med Sci Monit 9:CR105, 2003.

81. **Andrieu N, Clavel F, Gairard B, Piana L, Bremond A, Lansac JH, Flamant R, Renaud R,** Familial risk of breast cancer and abortion, Cancer Detect Prev 18:51, 1994.

82. **Daling JR, Malone KE, Voigt LF, White E, Weiss NS,** Risk of breast cancer among young women: relationship to induced abortion, J Natl Cancer Inst 86:1584, 1994.

83. **Rookus MA, van Leeuwen FE,** Induced abortion and risk for breast cancer: reporting (recall) bias in a Dutch case-control study, J Natl Cancer Inst 88:1759, 1996.

84. **Melbye M, Wohlfahrt J, Olsen JH, Frisch M, Westergaard T, Helweg-Larsen K, Andersen PK,** Induced abortion and the risk of breast cancer, New Engl J Med 336:81, 1997.

85. **Ye Z, Gao DL, Qin Q, Ray RM, Thomas DB,** Breast cancer in relation to induced abortion in a cohort of Chinese women, Br J Cancer 87:977, 2002.

86. **Mahue-Giangreco M, Ursin G, Sullivan-Halley J, Berstein L,** Induced abortion, miscarriage, and breast cancer of young women, Cancer Epidemiol Biomarkers Prev 12:209, 2003.

87. **Collaborative Group on Hormonal Factors in Breast Cancer, Breast Cancer and Abortion:** collaborative reanalysis of data from 53 epidemiological studies, including 83,000 women with breast cancer from 16 countries, Lancet 363:1007, 2004.

88. **Kulczycki A, Potts M, Rosenfield A,** Abortion and fertility regulation, Lancet 347:1663, 1996.

89. **Darney P,** Maternal deaths in the less developed world, Int J Gynecol Obstet 26:177, 1988.

90. **Ahman E, Shah I,** Unsafe abortion: worldwide estimates for 2000, Reprod Health Matters 10:13, 2002.

91. **Goldberg A, Greenberg M, Darney P,** Misoprostol and pregnancy, New Engl J Med 344:38, 2001.

92. **Lindell G, Flam F,** Management of uterine perforations in connection with legal abortions, Acta Obstet Gynecol Scand 74:373, 1995.

93. **Grimes D, Schulz K, Cates Jr W,** Prevention of uterine perforation during curettage abortion, JAMA 257:2108, 1983.

94. **Cates Jr W, Schulz K, Grimes D,** The risks associated with teenage abortion, New Engl J Med 379:621, 1983.

95. **Schulz KF, Grimes DA, Cates Jr W,** Measures to prevent cervical injury during suction curettage abortion, Lancet i:1182, 1983.

96. **Sands RX, Burnhill MS, Hakim-Elahi E,** Post-abortal uterine atony, Obstet Gynecol 43:595, 1974.

97. **Grimes DA, Cates Jr W,** Deaths from paracervical anesthesia used for first trimester abortion, New Engl J Med 295:1397, 1976.

98. **Brewer C,** Prevention of infection after abortion with a supervised single dose of doxycycline, Br Med J 281:780, 1980.

99. **Hodgson JE, Major B, Portmann K, Quattlebaum FW,** Prophylactic use of tetracycline for first trimester abortions, Obstet Gynecol 45:574, 1975.

100. **Park T-X, Flock M, Schulz KF, Grimes DA,** Preventing febrile complications of suction curettage abortion, Am J Obstet Gynecol 152:252, 1985.

101. **Darj E, Stralin E, Nilsson S,** The prophylactic effect of doxycycline on postoperative infection rate after first trimester abortion, Obstet Gynecol 70:755, 1987.

102. **Sawaya GF, Grady D, Kerlikowske K, Grimes DA,** Antibiotics at the time of induced abortion: the case for universal prophylaxis based on a meta-analysis, Obstet Gynecol 87:884, 1996.

103. **Levallois P, Rioux J,** Prophylactic antibiotics for suction curettage abortion: results of a clinical controlled trial, Am J Obstet Gynecol 158:100, 1988.

104. **Heisterberg L, Petersen K,** Metronidazole prophylaxis in elective first trimester abortion, Obstet Gynecol 65:371, 1985.

105. **Larsson PG, Platz-Christensen JJ, Thejls H, Forsum U, Pahlson C,** Incidence of pelvic inflammatory disease after first trimester legal abortion in women with bacterial vaginosis after treatment with metronidazole: a double-blind, randomized study, Am J Obstet Gynecol 166:100, 1992.

106. **Hakim-Elahi E,** Postabortal amenorrhea due to cervical stenosis, Obstet Gynecol 48:723, 1976.

107. **Grimes D, Ross W, Hutchen R,** Rh immunoglobulin utilization after spontaneous and induced abortion, Obstet Gynecol 57:261, 1977.

108. **Medical Research Group,** Report by the working party on the use of anti-D immune globulin for the prevention of isoimmunization of Rh-negative women during pregnancy: controlled trial of various anti-D dosages in suppression of Rh following pregnancy, Br Med J ii:75, 1974.

109. **Peterson WF, Berry FN, Grace MR, Gulbranson CL,** Second trimester abortion by dilatation and evacuation: an analysis of 11,747 cases, Obstet Gynecol 62:185, 1983.

110. **Kafrissen M, Schulz K, Grimes D, Cates Jr W,** Midtrimester abortion: intra amniotic instillation of hyperosmolar urea and prostaglandin F2α v dilatation and evacuation, JAMA 251:916, 1984.

111. **Ferris LE, McMain-Klein M, Colodny N, Fellows GF, Lamont J,** Factors associated with immediate abortion complications, Can Med Assoc J 154:1677, 1996.

112. **Ashok PW, Templeton A, Wagaarachi PT, Flett GMM,** Midtrimester medical termination of pregnancy: a review of 1002 consecutive cases, Contraception 69:51, 2004.

113. **Jain J, Kuo J, Mishell Jr DR,** A coomparison of two dosing regimens of intravaginal misoprostol for second-trimester pregnancy termination, Obstet Gynecol 93:571, 1999.

114. **Grimes DA, Schulz KF, Cates Jr W, Tyler CW,** Midtrimester abortion by dilation and evacuation, New Engl J Med 296:1141, 1977.

115. **Darney PD, Sweet RL,** Routine intraoperative ultrasonography for second trimester abortion reduces the incidence of uterine perforation, J Ultrasound Med 8:71, 1989.

116. **Mackay T, Schulz K, Grimes D,** Safety of local versus general anesthesia for second trimester dilatation and evacuation abortion, Obstet Gynecol 66:661, 1985.

117. **Atrash H, Chelk T, Hogue C,** Legal abortion and general anesthesia, Am J Obstet Gynecol 158:420, 1988.

118. **El-Rafaey H, Templeton A,** Induction of abortion in the second trimester by a combination of misoprostol and mifepristone: a randomized comparison between two misoprostol regimens, Hum Reprod 10:475, 1995.

14

Interpreting Epidemiologic Reports

Clinical practice is the ultimate distillate of evidence, judgment, and experience. The safety, side effects, and benefits of contraception are established by epidemiologic studies. The clinician must determine whether the data derived from epidemiologic studies are clinically relevant and useful. The incorporation of the data into clinical practice depends upon that determination. In this chapter, we provide a guide for interpreting epidemiologic reports, a guide intended to help clinicians make appropriate determinations regarding epidemiologic data and, ultimately, to apply this information properly in clinical practice.

The Hierarchy (in descending order) of Epidemiologic Studies

I. Randomized Controlled Trials

A randomized trial is a true clinical experiment in which an intervention is compared with a standard treatment, no treatment, or a placebo, with allocation to treatment by chance. More than one comparison can be made within a study.

Advantages: Provides scientific, epidemiologic proof.

Disadvantages: Very expensive and time-consuming. Only a limited number of hypotheses can be evaluated in any one study.

Example: The Women's Health Initiative

II. Observational Studies
(Nonexperimental Studies: Observation Without Intervention)

Cohort studies: A prospective follow-up over a long period of time of a large group of individuals. Also referred to as longitudinal or follow-up studies. Exposure information is collected from all subjects who are disease-free, and subjects are followed over time to determine who develops disease.

Advantages:	A relatively accurate estimation because of large numbers, can evaluate changes over time, avoids recall bias.
Disadvantages:	Expensive, lengthy in time, and subject to biases (particularly selection bias and surveillance bias) making the two groups being compared unequal.
Example:	The Nurses' Health Study

Case-control studies: A retrospective comparison of a group of individuals with a condition or problem compared with a carefully selected control group. Subjects are selected according to specific inclusion and exclusion criteria. The exposure history of those with disease and those with no disease is collected and compared.

Advantages:	Relatively quick and inexpensive because of small sample sizes.
Disadvantages:	Subject to biases and errors.
Example:	WHO Collaborative Study of Cardiovascular Disease and Steroid Hormone Contraception

Cross-sectional studies: A description of a group of individuals at one point in time.

Advantages:	A reliable method to estimate prevalence, quick and inexpensive.
Disadvantages:	Cannot assess changes over time and very susceptible to sampling error (the group is not representative of the actual population of interest).
Example:	The Health and Nutritional Examination Survey

III. Clinical Reports

A case series: A collection of similar cases that suggests more than a chance or coincidental occurrence.

A case report: An anecdotal report that serves to bring attention to a possible problem or condition.

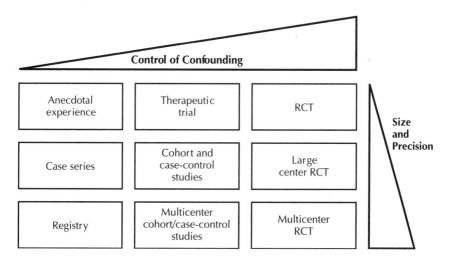

Possible Confounders and Biases of Importance

Confounders: Factors associated with the disease and the exposure, such as age, body weight, smoking, family history, duration of oral contraceptive use, preferential prescribing, healthy user effect.

Biases: Errors due to study design.

Detection or Surveillance Bias: Systematic errors in methods of ascertainment, diagnosis, or verification of cases. Not everyone in the study population has equal access to or utilization of medical interventions and diagnostic tests.

Publication Bias: Negative (null) studies and studies that confirm old results tend not to be published. An important source of bias in meta-analysis.

Reporting or Recall Bias: Inaccurate memory and dishonesty introduce errors.

Selection Bias: Differences in characteristics between those selected for study (cases) and those in the control group, such as preferential prescribing, family history, preferential referral of patients, healthy user effect. For case-control studies, the source of the controls is important. Hospital-based controls are less likely to be representative of the general population than population-based controls. It is best to choose controls by random selection, but this is not always possible. Selection bias in a cohort study can result in differences between exposed and unexposed groups.

Information or observer bias: A flaw in measuring exposure or outcome that produces different results between comparison groups. Nonresponse by subjects or patients lost to follow-up can produce differences in cohort studies.

A Guide To Epidemiologic Terms Commonly Used
Relative Risk:

The ratio of the risk among those exposed to the risk among the unexposed or the ratio of the cumulative incidence rate in the exposed and the unexposed. Also called risk ratio. In its simplest definition, relative risk compares the rate of disease in two groups, one of which has been exposed to something that is believed to either increase or decrease the risk of that disease.

Odds Ratio:

The odds ratio is the measure of association calculated in case-control studies when the prevalence of disease events is low; the estimate and interpretation are similar to relative risk.

Confidence Interval (CI):

The range of relative risk that would include 95% of the subjects being studied; the range of relative risk within which the true magnitude of effect lies, given the study data, with a certain degree of assurance. To be statistically significant, a reduced relative risk (a beneficial effect) requires the larger number (the right hand number) to be less than 1.0 (thus, both numbers are less than 1.0). An increased relative risk (an adverse effect), to be statistically significant, requires the smaller number (the left hand number) to be greater than 1.0 (thus, both numbers are greater than 1.0).

The tighter (more narrow) the range, the more precise the conclusion. The wider the CI, the more imprecise the conclusion, usually because of small numbers of study subjects.

Attributable risk:

The difference in actual incidence between exposed and unexposed groups, providing a realistic estimate of the change in incidence in a given population. A modest increase in relative risk produces only a small number of cases when clinical events are rare, such as venous thromboembolism and arterial thrombosis in young women.

Important Points

Epidemiology is a tool to detect disease patterns in large populations. Epidemiologic studies do not prove causation; they identify associations between diseases and certain factors.

A relative risk in the range of 1.0–2.0 represents an increased risk but a weak association.

The clinical significance of an increase in risk is influenced by the rate of the disease in the general (unexposed) population (attributable risk). If the rate of the disease in the unexposed population is 10% and the relative risk is 1.4, an exposed person has a disease risk of 14%. If the rate of disease in the unexposed population is only 1%, then the same relative risk of 1.4 increases the actual disease risk by only 1.4%.

Criteria that strengthen the conclusion that an epidemiologic finding is clinically real include the following:

1. The strength of the association (the larger the relative risk, the more likely it is real).
2. Consistency, uniformity, and agreement among many studies.
3. A dose-response relationship (either with dose of a drug or an increasing effect with increasing time of exposure).
4. Biological plausibility of the finding (known mechanisms by which exposure could cause or influence disease).
5. An appropriate temporal relationship (the amount of time between exposure and development of disease is appropriate according to the pathogenesis of the disease).

U.S. Preventive Task Force Evidence Grading Scheme

Quality of Evidence

Level I	Evidence from at least 1 properly designed randomized controlled trial.
Level II-1	Evidence from well-designed, nonrandomized, controlled trial.
Level II-2	Evidence from well-designed cohort or case-control studies.
Level II-3	Evidence from cross-sectional studies or uncontrolled studies.
Level III	Evidence from descriptive case reports, case series, or expert/committee opinions.

Strength of Recommendation

A	Good and consistent scientific evidence to support recommendation.
B	Limited or inconsistent (fair) evidence to support recommendation.
C	Insufficient evidence to recommend for or against conclusion.
D	Fair evidence against the recommendation.
E	Good evidence against the recommendation.

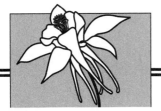

Epilogue

And so we reach our final paragraph. We do so with optimism. This book documents, within a tick of planet Earth's time, tremendous accomplishments in contraception. These accomplishments reflect initiative, creativity, and dedication. There is reason to believe, as we do, that these human traits will persevere, and we will meet the contraceptive challenges of the future.

Index